Books ar.

The Cranio-cervical Syndrome

Acquisitions editor: Heidi Allen
Development editor: Myriam Brearley
Production controller: Anthony Read
Desk editor: Jane Campbell
Cover designer: Helen Brockway

The Cranio-cervical Syndrome
Mechanisms, assessment and treatment

Editor

Howard Vernon, DC, FCCS, FCCRS, FICC

Associate Dean of Research
Canadian Memorial Chiropractic College, Toronto, Ontario, Canada

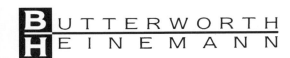

BUTTERWORTH
HEINEMANN

OXFORD   AUCKLAND   BOSTON   JOHANNESBURG   MELBOURNE   NEW DELHI

Butterworth-Heinemann
Linacre House, Jordan Hill, Oxford OX2 8DP
225 Wildwood Avenue, Woburn, MA 01801-2041
A division of Reed Educational and Professional Publishing Ltd

℞ A member of the Reed Elsevier plc group

First published 2001

British Library Cataloguing in Publication Data
The cranio-cervical syndrome: mechanisms, assessment and
  treatment
  1. Cervical syndrome
  616.7'3

Library of Congress Cataloguing in Publication Data
The cranio-cervical syndrome: mechanisms, assessment, and treatment/editor, Howard Vernon.
  p.cm.
  Includes bibliographical references and index.
  ISBN 0 7506 4495 8
  1. Neck pain. 2. Headache. 3. Cervical vertebrae – Diseases. I. Vernon, Howard, D.C.
  [DNLM: 1. Headache – diagnosis. 2. Cervical Vertebrae – physiopathology.
  3. Headache – therapy. 4. Neck Pain – therapy. WL 342 C891 2001]
  RD763.C66
  616.8'491–dc21   2001018465

ISBN 0 7506 4495 8

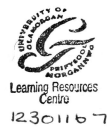
Composition by Scribe Design, Gillingham, Kent
Printed and bound by MPG Ltd, Bodmin, Cornwall

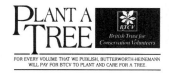

Table of Contents

Foreword

This text on 'The Cranio-Cervical Syndrome' deals with a constellation of conditions that may present a variety of features and problems for the patient with cervical and cranial pain and dysfunction and difficulties for the clinician trying to treat them. Indeed, the conditions have often evoked considerable controversy since there are varying views on their occurrence, aetiology, pathogenesis, diagnosis and management. A major factor underlying the controversial nature of this topic has been the limited understanding of the pathophysiology, biomechanics and neural mechanisms that contribute to pain and associated neuromuscular dysfunction of the head and neck. Another factor is the complex anatomical arrangement and inter-related functions, and dysfunctions, of the structures in this region of the body. As Dr Vernon points out in the introduction to this text, the cranio-cervical junction is a complicated amalgam of bony structures, articulations, supporting tissues and nerves.

Fortunately, there are emerging new insights into the processes underlying cranial and cervical pain and associated neuromuscular disorders. There have been some remarkable insights into these processes in the past few years as a consequence of an enhanced focus of basic science research, largely using experimental animal models, into cranial and cervical pain and motor mechanisms and an increased research interest in behavioural and psychosocial factors influencing pain. This has resulted in a more solid scientific foundation upon which to base diagnosis and management. It therefore follows that extensively reviewed and well-reasoned texts, correlating and reconciling the latest research advances in this field with prudent clinical practice, are essential. These are features of this text. Dr Vernon is to be commended for garnering the contributions of acknowledged experts, who collectively cover the many disciplines that bear on this topic. The book is essential reading for those interested in mechanisms of cranial and cervical pain and dysfunction, and the clinical approaches to diagnose and manage disorders in the region. This book should prove invaluable to clinical practitioners dealing with these problems, as well as to basic and clinical scientists with an interest in the latest knowledge of the mechanisms underlying many aspects of pain and dysfunction in the head and neck.

Barry J. Sessle
Professor and Dean
Faculty of Dentistry, University of Toronto

Preface

INTRODUCTION

What is the cranio-cervical syndrome? Simply put, it is a constellation of symptoms and conditions that have their origin in mechanical dysfunction of the cranio-cervical junction. Let's work backwards with that definition. What is the cranio-cervical junction? The occipital bone (known as C0) of the skull or cranium forms the first joint of the spine via its occipital condyles and the superior surfaces of the articulating facets of the atlas or C1 lateral masses. The atlas, or first cervical vertebra, acts as a link between the skull and the cervical spine, bringing the C2 vertebra, or axis, into a complex of articulations known as the upper cervical spine. This three-joint complex is arguably the most unique and complex joint in the entire spine.

Structurally, it is composed of three bony elements that share virtually no similarities between each other or any of the other vertebrae. The occipital condyles are formed around the outer margin of the foramen magnum; they are convex joint surfaces whose angle in the transverse plane is among the most obtuse in the spine, virtually locking the skull in rotation on the atlas. They are shaped so as to have a higher slope anteriorly, fitting into the concave surfaces of the atlas superior articulating surfaces, and thereby permitting one of the largest ranges of flexion/extension at any spinal joint.

The atlas is a ring-shaped vertebra with two lateral masses and four prominences, two tubercles front and back and two of the largest transverse processes of any vertebra. The axis is certainly the most irregularly shaped of the vertebrae, with a large central superior protuberance, the odontoid process or dens, two large downward-sloping superior articulating joint surfaces and a bifid spinous process. The primary joints between these bones do not contain an intervertebral disc. That is reserved for the C2–C3 articulation as the first of the 'regular' cervical intervertebral joints. There are important secondary articulations between the dens and the atlas ring, which, together with a complex array of ligaments, stabilize the atlas and maintain the patency of the uppermost spinal canal.

It should be no surprise that, when all of the joint surface configurations with their complex ligaments are taken into account, the instantaneous axis of rotation within this joint complex lies in the middle of the atlas ring, placing the least rotational strain on its vital contents.

The entire junctional region is supported by a complex of unique ligaments as well as a wide variety of long, medium-sized and short muscles, these latter being so unique as to merit their own label as the 'suboccipital' muscles. The arrangements and anatomical courses of the first three spinal nerves arising from these three segments are also among the most unique in the whole spine.

So the cranio-cervical junction is the most complex triad of bony structures, articulations, supporting tissues and nerves in the mobile human spine. It has adapted to perform numerous vital functions including (1) support of the skull and its vital contents, the brain, the specialized sense organs of sight, smell, hearing and balance and the oro-facial region, (2) configuring the orientation of the cranium in space so as to subserve the vital sensory functions of balance and sight, (3) providing the maximum mobility of the cranium while still providing the maximum protection to its vital contents and the optimal dynamic capacity of the cranial sensorium, (4) acting as a self-contained receptor organ of the balance system, consisting of specialized receptors in the ligaments and muscles of the upper cervical joints, and (5) housing the structures that form the centre of neural processing of pain for the entire cranio-facial region.

What is 'mechanical dysfunction' of the cranio-cervical junction? Each manipulative school has its own nomenclature for this condition. The term traditionally used by chiropractors, 'subluxation', is somewhat historical, and the modern term 'fixation' is more in line with those of osteopathy, manual medicine and physiotherapy, who use the terms 'somatic dysfunction', 'blockage' and 'lesion', respectively. The characteristic, which underlies all of these terms, is a non-pathological reduction of spinal joint mobility, or hypomobility. This state is associated with (causally or as an effect) local and referred pain, as well as muscle spasm, or hypertonicity, and tenderness. These muscular manifestations often take the form of myofascial dysfunction, which has become known as tender or trigger points in musculoskeletal medicine.

The 'Taxonomy of Chronic Pain' from the International Association for the Study of Pain [1] has recognized the generic term 'segmental dysfunction', and defined it as follows:

(Cervical) spinal pain ostensibly due to excessive strains sustained by the restraining elements of a single spinal motion segment.

Clinical features: (Cervical) spinal pain, with or without referred pain, which can be aggravated by selectively stressing a particular spinal segment.

Diagnostic criteria: All of the following should be satisfied:

1. The affected segment must be identified.
2. The patient's pain is aggravated by clinical tests that selectively stress the affected segment.

3. Stressing adjacent segments does not reproduce the patient's pain.

Pathology: Unknown. Presumably involves excessive strain incurred during activities of daily living by structures such as the ligaments, joints or intervertebral disc of the affected segment.

This is the definition we will use in this text for the mechanical spinal dysfunction associated with the cranio-cervical syndrome.

What are the types of conditions that form the constellation of disorders that make up the 'cranio-cervical syndrome'? According to Edmeads, [2], the first mention of the upper neck as a cause of head pain is attributed to Liveing, in 1864. Since then, numerous authors have expanded on this concept. In the 1920s, Barre and Lieou [3] proposed that a variety of cranial disorders including migraine, dizziness and other autonomic dysfunctions could have their origin in disturbances of vertebral arterial circulation arising from either injury or degenerative changes in the upper cervical spine. In the late 1940s Bartschi-Rochaix [4] coined the term 'migraine cervicale' for headache arising from this region. In the 1950s, De Jong and colleagues [5,6] showed that anaesthetization of the upper cervical joints in monkeys produced nystagmus and ataxic gait.

At nearly the same time, Skillern [7] coined the term 'greater occipital-trigeminal neuralgia' and recognized the intimate connection between these two neural watersheds, while Kerr and his colleagues [8] reported on the convergence of upper cervical nociceptive input with that of the spinal tract of the trigeminal nerve, by observing referred cranial pain from C1 nerve rootlets irritated during posterior cranial surgery. While some have gone on to call this unique neural connectivity the 'Kerr phenomenon', it has been more properly called the 'medullary dorsal horn' by Gobel *et al.* [9], and the 'trigemino-cervical nucleus' by Bogduk [10], arguably the greatest anatomist of the region.

While these various terms (and others, such as 'headache of cervical origin', 'vertebragenous headache', 'neck-tongue syndrome', 'greater occipital neuralgia') all reflected the special interests of numerous clinicians in this region, it is probably the works of Bogduk from the early 1980s onwards [11–14] and the work of Sjasstad *et al.* [15–17] in coining the term 'cervicogenic headache' (1983) which have contributed most to our current understanding of the clinical implications of upper cervical mechanical dysfunction. This work firmly cemented the idea that headache and cranial pain could arise from the upper cervical region.

When one adds the work of European authors on cervicogenic vertigo to this [18–20], the picture becomes complete. Whether through trauma such as whiplash injury or through repetitive strain from work-related or postural strain, or even, as a minority of authors claim, through the trauma of the birth process, dysfunction of the cranio-cervical tissues may manifest as headache, cranial pain, dizziness, mandibular and ocular dysfunction. These clinical conditions may have profound implications for the psychosocial wellbeing of the sufferer, as chronic pain in this region produces profound effects on concentration, mood state, and vocational and avocational capabilities.

Once said, it is clear that these very same symptoms may arise from a great many other pathological conditions, and so one of the greatest challenges in defining and managing the cranio-cervical syndrome is the differential diagnosis of mechanical versus organic origins of such conditions. The former may be managed by a wide variety of conservative approaches, while the latter must be referred to the appropriate medical specialist for diagnosis and treatment.

This introduction has laid out the framework for this text. In 1986, I was privileged to work with an outstanding team of experts in the production of a text entitled *The Upper Cervical Syndrome: Chiropractic Diagnosis and Treatment* (Williams and Wilkins, 1998). I was grateful for the success which that text garnered; but, as the years passed, I realized that a reprise was necessary. The current volume is not really a second edition of the first, but an entirely new enterprise, developed with arguably an even more talented cast of authors. The breadth of expertise in this collective of authors is truly remarkable. Their most important feature, as a group, is that they are truly representative of the full spectrum of disciplines involved in the area. They are experts in anatomy, neurosciences, clinical diagnostics, chiropractic and medical practice. This text is, then, a very deliberate attempt to engage in a multidisciplinary exploration of a unique and important clinical condition.

The text begins with contributions from the basic sciences. Dr Gregory Cramer, whose text on spinal anatomy is now a classic, outlines the anatomical landscape of the cranio-cervical region. His chapter is a welcome departure from the typical treatment of anatomy because of his special emphasis on the clinically important elements, a style that he has developed with mastery.

The following two chapters are written by world-renowned experts in their fields; Dr Frances Richmond together with Dr Corneil summarizes a career's worth of work in her exposition on the sensory mechanisms of the upper cervical region, particularly as they apply to posture and balance. Dr James Hu applies his two decades of research into cranio-facial pain mechanisms to a superb chapter which broadens that topic to include upper cervical nociceptive mechanisms, providing a 'unified field theory' of cervico-cranial-facial pain. These three chapters provide an outstanding basis for the rest of the text.

The next section involves basic clinical mechanisms, and starts with a review of the radiological investigation of this area by Dr Marshall Deltoff. Radiological anomalies are highly common in the cranio-cervical region, and Dr Deltoff's chapter provides the reader with ample illustrations of this phenomenon. The next chapter is provided by the world's leading authority on the clinical anatomy of the upper cervical spine, Dr Nik Bogduk. No one has been better able to combine sophisticated and detailed anatomical investigations with innovative clinical research into the blend of scholarship that Dr Bogduk brings to all of his work. In this chapter, he describes the clinical basis of upper cervical pain and its referral to the cranial region. His work provides a broader basis for 'cervicogenic headache', making Bogduk its leading proponent. Dr Ray Brodeur completes this section with a superb review of the unique biomechanics of the upper cervical region. This topic has both basic and clinical applications, as an understanding of normal function is the foundation for any of the therapeutic approaches whose aim is to improve or even restore mechanical function as part of the healing process.

The final section is on clinical matters. Here, the emphasis is on conservative treatment approaches, particularly those of manual medicine. Dr Vernon writes two chapters on tension-type (TTH) and cervicogenic headaches (CH). The first of these is a review of the clinical features of each of these common forms of headaches. The criteria for clinical classification as well as epidemiology and treatment utilization are detailed. This is followed by a section on the clinical assessment of cranio-cervical dysfunction in these headache categories. One of the sub-themes of this section is that while the criteria for classification of the headache characteristics of TTH and CH as presented by the International Headache Society [21] appear to distinguish these two types of headaches, there is still a belief among many that dysfunction of the cranio-cervical spine has an important role in both.

This theme is reinforced by the second of Vernon's chapters which consists of a systematic review of all randomized clinical trials of complementary and alternative therapies for TTH and CH. This chapter is an update of an original investigation with colleagues McDermaid and Hagino, which was first published in *Complementary Therapies in Medicine* [22].

Drs Rothbart and Gale follow with a description of the current medical approach to the management of headaches associated with cranio-cervical dysfunction. Again, the apparent distinctiveness of the definitions of TTH and CH is blurred by this comprehensive medical approach targeted to cranio-cervical dysfunction. The authors present their outcomes of this form of treatment in chronic headache.

Drs Reitav and Hamovitch continue with an important contribution on the psychosocial aspects of head and neck pain. Their admonition to approach patients with these complaints from a biopsychosocial perspective is crucial to successful management in this often difficult area of practice. They go further by providing a review of the instruments available to the office-based practitioner to systematically assess the affective, cognitive and experiential dimensions of head and neck pain.

Whiplash-associated disorder (WAD) is probably the most common clinical entity involving traumatic injury to the upper cranio-cervical region. Drs Teasell and Shapiro provide an excellent update on whiplash-associated disorders, their assessment and treatment. He sifts through the current debates

on the role of zygapophyseal joint injury and its treatment by anaesthetic blockades and presents a rational approach to cranio-cervical symptoms resulting from WAD.

Dr Beidermann gives us a true gem in his dissertation on manual therapy in children with special emphasis on what he calls 'Kinetic Imbalance of the Suboccipital Spine' (KISS). Dr Biedermann is, first and foremost, a clinician, but one with well-recognized expertise in this important but controversial area of practice. Perhaps not all will agree with his premises and practices; but, hopefully, all will agree that he presents them in a thoughtful, precise and dispassionate manner. The data he presents from his large case volume should make a compelling argument that our interest in the health of the cranio-vertebral region should begin early in the lives of our patients, as it will have a profound influence on subsequent developmental patterns.

Dr Tjell then provides an excellent review of the integration of the cranio-cervical region with balance function. The clinical application of this premise lies in appreciating the role of cranio-vertebral dysfunction in disequlibrium and the all-too-common experience of cervical vertigo, particularly after whiplash-type injury to the cervical spine. Tjell first provides the neuro-anatomical and neurophysiological background to cervical vertigo. Then he provides his recommendations for clinical practice in assessing and managing this disorder. Postural and balance retraining are central to this management, while manual therapy offers an important adjunct.

Finally, Dr McDermaid provides a comprehensive review of the major adverse effect of manual therapy in the cranio-vertebral spine – cerebrovascular accidents, particularly involving the vertebral artery. While much has been written on this topic, and certain comprehensive case reviews are mandatory for a thorough review of the clinical manifestation of this problem, McDermaid provides a fresh insight into the theories and mechanisms underlying this rare but unfortunate problem.

Finally, a brief word about the format of this text, or, more specifically, the lack of it. The efforts of each of these esteemed authors deserve careful and thorough reading. This is becoming a forgotten art in our times of cyber-communication with graphical, user-friendly interfaces between writers and consumers. In this text, the chapters stand on their own, demanding your full attention. There are no 'learning objectives' or 'take home messages' or 'key concept' dialogue boxes to pop up like pedagogic dandelions. The only concession I have made in this direction is to provide the e-mail addresses of each author, and the reader is encouraged to 'speak' directly to any authors this way.

As editor, I have been blessed with outstanding contributors whose leading-edge work and high scholarly standards have made putting together this text a true labour of love.

On their behalf, I would like to thank all the people who supported their work during its development. I also thank the editorial staff at Butterworth-Heinemann, particularly Mary Seager, who accepted my proposal and shepherded it through the editorial approval process, and Judy Elias who assisted me in the production of the text. I would also like to express my appreciation to the Canadian Memorial Chiropractic College, which has supported me through all my endeavours.

I dedicate this text to my father and to his four grandchildren. He would love to have read this one, too, and I know they will.

Howard Vernon DC FCCS
Canadian Memorial Chiropractic College

REFERENCES

1. Merskey H , Bogduk N (eds.). Classification of chronic pain. Descriptions of Chronic Pain Syndromes and Definitions of Pain Terms. 2nd edn. Seattle, WA: IASP Press, pp. 94–95, 1994.
2. Edmeads J. Headaches and head pains associated with diseases of the cervical spine. *Med Clin N Am* 1979;**62**:533–541.
3. Barre J. Sur un syndrome sympathetique cervicale posterieure et sa cause frequente: l'arthrite cervicale. *Rev Neurol* 1926;**45**:1246.
4. Bartschi-Rochaix W. *Migraine Cervicale: Des Encephale Syndrome Nach Halswerbeltrauma.* Bern: Huber, 1949.
5. De Jong PTVM, de Jong JMBV, Cohen B, Jongkees LBW. Ataxia and nystagmus induced by injection of local anesthetics in the neck. *Ann Neurol* 1977;**1**:240–246.
6. De Jong JMBV, Bles W, Bovenker G. Nystagmus, gaze shift and self-motion perception during sinusoidal head and neck rotation. *Ann NY Acad Sci* 1981;**374**:590–599.
7. Skillern PG. Great occipital trigeminus syndrome as revealed by induction block. *Arch Neurol Psychiatr* 1954;**72**:335–340.
8. Kerr FW. Structural relation of the trigeminal spinal tract to the upper cervical roots and the solitary nucleus in the cat. *Exp Neurol* 1961;**4**:131–148.
9. Gobel S. An EM analysis of the transsynaptic effects of peripheral nerve injury subsequent to tooth pulp extirpations on neurons in laminae I and II of the medullary dorsal horn. *J Neurosci* 1984;**4**:2281–2290.
10. Bogduk N, Corrigan B, Kelly P, Schneider G, *et al.* Cervical headache. *Med J Aust* 1985;**143**:202–207.
11. Bogduk N, Marsland A. On the concept of third occipital nerve headache. *J Neurol Neurosurg Psychiatr* 1986;**49**:775–780.
12. Bogduk N. Cervical causes of headache and dizziness. In *Modern Manual Therapy of the Vertebral Column* (ed. GP Grieve), Edinburgh: Churchill Livingstone, pp. 289–302, 1986.
13. Bogduk N, Marsland A. The cervical zygapophyseal joints as a source of neck pain. *Spine* 1988;**13**:610–617.
14. Lord S, Barnsley L, Wallis BJ, Bogduk N. Third occipital nerve headache: a prevalence study. *J Neurol Neurosurg Psychiatr* 1994;**57**:1187–1190.
15. Sjaastad O, Saunte C, Hovdahl H, Breivik H, *et al.* Cervicogenic headache: a hypothesis. *Cephalalgia* 1983;**3**:249–256.
16. Sjaastad O, Fredricson TA, Stolt-Neilsen A. Cervicogenic headache, C2 rhizopathy and occipital neuralgia: a connection. *Cephalalgia* 1986;**6**:189–195.
17. Fredrickson TA, Hovdahl H, Sjaastad O. Cervicogenic headache: clinical manifestations. *Cephalalgia* 1987;**7**:147–160.
18. Hulse M. Disequilibrium caused by functional disturbance of the upper cervical spine: clinical aspects and differential diagnosis. *J Man Med* 1983;**1**:18–23.
19. Simon H, Moser M. Der zervicalnystagmus aus manual-medizinishcer sicht. *Man Med* 1977;**15**:47–51.
20. Mahlstedt K, Westohen M, Konig K. Therapy of functional disorders of the craniovertebral joints in vestibular disease. *Laryngorhinootologie* 1992;**71**:246–250.
21. International Headache Society Classification and Diagnostic Criteria for Headache Disorders, Cranial Neuralgias and Facial Pain. *Cephalalgia* 1988, Suppl. 7.
22. Vernon H, McDermaid C, Hagino C. Systematic review of randomized clinical trials of complementary/alternative therapies in the treatment of tension-type and cervicogenic headache. *J Comp Therap Med* 1999;**7**:142–155.

List of contributors

Heiner Bierdermann, MD
Private practice,
18, Victor Jacobslei, Antwerp, Belgium
hb@manmed.org

Nikolai Bogduk, MD PhD DSc Dip Anat
Professor of Anatomy and Musculoskeletal
Medicine, University of Newcastle, Bone and
Joint Institute, Royal Newcastle Hospital,
Australia
tlambert@newcastle.edu.au

Ray Brodeur, DC, PhD
Ergonomics Research Laboratory, Michigan
State University, USA
brodeur@ergo.msu.edu

B. Corneil, PhD
CIHR Group in Sensory-Motor Systems,
Department of Physiology, Queen's University
Kingston, Ontario, Canada

Gregory Cramer, DC, PhD
Professor of Anatomy,
National College of Chiropractic, Department
of Anatomy, Illinois, USA
gcramer@national.chiropractic. edu

Marshall N. Deltoff, BSc, DC, DACBR, FCCR(C)
Director, Images Radiology Consultants,
Toronto, Ontario
arnied@sprint.ca

George Gale MBBS, FRCPC, DAAPM
Private practice
Toronto, Ontario, Canada
reception@rothbart.com

Carol Hagino BSc, MBA, MSC(Cand)
Research Department, Canadian Memorial
Chiropractic College, Toronto, Ontario,
Canada
chagino@cmcc.ca

Gregory Hamovitch, PhD
Canadian Memorial Chiropractic College,
Toronto, Ontario, Canada
ghamovitch@cmcc.ca

James Hu, PhD
Associate Professor, Faculty of Dentistry, Oral
Physiology Laboratory, University of Toronto,
Toronto, Ontario, Canada
James.hu@utoronto.ca

Cameron McDermaid, DC
Clinical Researcher, Division of Graduate
Studies and Research, Canadian Memorial
Chiropractic College, Toronto, Ontario, Canada
cmcdermaid@cmcc.ca

Jan Reitav, PhD
Canadian Memorial Chiropractic College,
Toronto, Ontario, Canada
jreitav@cmcc.ca

Frances Richmond, BNSc PhD
Professor of Physiology, Director MRC Group
in Sensory-Motor Neuroscience, Department
of Physiology, Queens University, Kingston,
Ontario, Canada
fjr@biomed.queensu.ca

Peter Rothbart, MD
Private practice, Toronto, Ontario, Canada
reception@rothbart.com

Allan P. Shapiro, PhD
Adjunct Professor, Department of Psychology and Physical Medicine and Rehabilitation, The University of Western Ontario, London, Ontario, Canada

Robert Teasell, MD, FRCPC
Professor of Medicine, University of Western Ontario, London, Ontario, Canada
robert.teasell@lhsc.on.ca

Carsten Tjell, MD PhD
Senior Consultant, Department of Otorhino-laryngology, Central Hospital, Sweden
carsten.tjell@vgregion.se

Howard Vernon, DC FCCS PhD (cand)
Associate Dean of Research, Canadian Memorial Chiropractic College, Toronto, Ontario, Canada
hvernon@cmcc.ca

Chapter 1

Clinical anatomy of the cranio-cervical syndrome*

Gregory D. Cramer

INTRODUCTION

This entire book is devoted to discussing a phenomenon confronted by a typical clinician every hour of the working day – that is, pain. More specifically, this text is devoted to headache and head pain and how that pain can, in some instances, be related to the cervical region. To help serve this function, this chapter will attempt to answer the questions, 'what are some of the potential causes of an individual patient's neck and head pain?' and 'what are some of the potential mechanisms involved in neck and head pain?' Let us, for the sake of discussion, take the case of a patient, and let's call him Mr B. Mr B. is a 45-year-old college professor who has had neck pain and headaches during the past 6 months and is still seeking relief. A person like Mr B. is not that rare. This chapter will discuss the possible causes of neck and headache pain with a patient like Mr B. in mind.

The topic of head pain is similar to a complex puzzle with many different pieces. If we again consider our patient, Mr B., factors such as his general health, his age, the harmony of his family life and his working environment can all be pieces of Mr B.'s pain puzzle [1]. In this chapter we will be focusing on only a few pieces of this puzzle.

* Adapted from: Anatomy of the Cervical Spine with Respect to Head Pain. *Topics in Clinical Chiropractic* 1998;**5**:1–10, with permission.

One of the most important purposes of this chapter is to provide the anatomical framework for the other chapters in this book. Therefore, with Mr B. and this other related purpose in mind we will be discussing the following topics:

I.   Definitions related to nociception and pain
II.   Pain generators of the neck and their innervation
III. Nociceptive (pain) pathways from the neck
IV.   Somatic referred pain
V.   Pain generators of the head and their innervation
VI.   Nociceptive (pain) pathways from the head
VII. Referral of pain related to neck and head pain

DEFINITIONS RELATED TO NOCICEPTION AND PAIN

Before being able to properly discuss the topic of neck and head pain we need to define a few terms related to pain. Firstly, we need to differentiate between the terms *nociception* and *pain*.

Nociception

Nociception can be defined as 'the neural mechanisms involved in signalling and modulating noxious stimuli' [2]. Therefore, nociception is the stimulation of receptors, often as a result of tissue damage, and the subsequent transmission by the nervous system of impulses related to these stimuli. Put in a very crude sense, nociception can be thought of as impulses travelling along a highway of nerves that extends from the peripheral regions of the body to the spinal cord and higher neural centres of the brain.

Pain

Pain has been defined by the International Association for the Study of Pain as 'An unpleasant sensory and emotional experience associated with actual or potential tissue damage, or described in terms of such damage'. The Committee on Taxonomy of the above mentioned society goes on to state, ... 'If they [people experiencing pain] regard their experience as pain and if they report it in the same ways as pain caused by tissue damage, it should be accepted as pain' [3]. Therefore, not all pain is the result of a nociceptive stimulus received and transmitted by a sensory receptor of a peripheral nerve [4]. More specifically, pain is the patient's interpretation (perception) of nociceptive information. Pain is significantly influenced by a person's early experiences with nociception and higher centres of the central nervous system are used in this interpretive process. For example, Mr B. is most probably receiving nociceptive input from something in his neck or head. He is interpreting this as pain. The degree of Mr B.'s discomfort may be related to his early experiences with noxious stimuli.

Another term that is currently being used is *pain generator*. For purposes of our discussion let us use the following definition.

Pain generator

A pain generator is any structure containing nociceptive nerve endings. Pain generators of the spine include the muscles, ligaments (including joint capsules), vertebrae, intervertebral discs and the neural elements themselves. Therefore, Mr B. is probably experiencing pain as a result of nociceptive input arising from a pain generator in his neck or head.

Lastly, we need to define the term *pain referral*. More specifically we need to define the term *somatic referred pain*. In this paper the following definition will be used.

Somatic referred pain

Somatic referred pain is nociception generated by a musculoskeletal structure [muscle, ligament (including capsule), bone, etc.] that is felt in a region larger than or distant to the area immediately surrounding the damaged tissue itself. An example of somatic referred pain is illustrated by the work of Bogduk and Marsland [5]. These investigators studied 24 consecutive patients with neck pain. Fourteen of the patients had headaches along with neck pain. These investigators injected the posterior primary divisions innervating the zygapophysial joints (Z joints) of the 24 individuals with a local anaesthetic (bupivacaine), and they confirmed their methods on several individuals by directly injecting the Z joints with a local anaesthetic mixed with a corticosteroid (methylprednisolone). Seventeen of the patients had complete, temporary relief of all symptoms. The pain patterns relieved by injecting into the C2–C3 Z joints included the regions of the orbits, forehead, vertex of the skull, suboccipital region and superior aspect of the back of the neck; injection of the C3–C4 Z joints relieved pain in the posterior aspect of the entire neck; and injecting the C5–C6 Z joints relieved pain extending onto the 'cape' region of the base of the neck, insertion of the trapezius muscle and superior aspect of the shoulder region (Figure 1.1). These pain patterns relieved by Z joint anaesthetic injections are examples of somatic

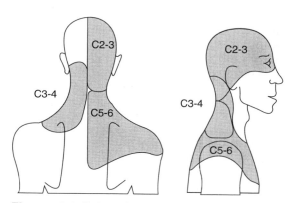

Figure 1.1 *Pain referral patterns relieved by anaesthetizing the zygapophysial joints indicated in the shaded regions. (From: Bogduk N, Marsland A. The cervical zygapophysial joints as a source of neck pain. Spine 1988;**13**:610–617, with permission.)*

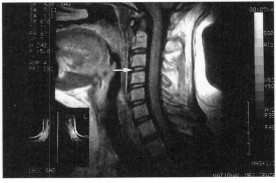
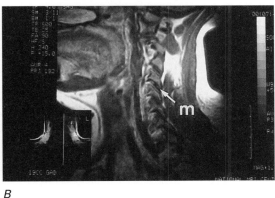

A *B*

Figure 1.2 *Mid-sagittal (A) and parasagittal (B) MRI scans showing several of the possible pain generators of the neck. In (A) the anterior aspect of the C3–C4 annulus fibrosus is identified by the arrow. The outer third of the annulus fibrosus is a potential pain generator. Vertebral bodies can be seen superior and inferior to the annulus fibrosus. The periosteum of the vertebrae themselves can also be a source of nociception arising from the neck. In (B), m = paraspinal muscles. In addition, the arrow indicates a zygapophysial (Z) joint. Both the paraspinal muscles and the capsular ligaments of the Z joints are potential sources of neck pain that can refer to the head.*

referred pain. The pain patterns represent referral from the nociceptors associated with the Z joint capsule or conceivably from the subchondral bone of the articular processes that make up the Z joint. These are somatic structures and therefore the pain that is experienced distant to these structures can best be termed *somatic referred pain.*

The preceding definitions begin to paint a picture of neck pain, head pain and pain referral. The work of Campbell and Parsons [6] helps to complete the picture. These investigators found that pain arising from almost any structure innervated by the upper four cervical nerves may refer to the head, resulting in head pains and headaches. The sentiments of this statement have also been reiterated by more recent authors [7–9], although these more recent authors are convinced the upper three cervical nerves, rather than the upper four cervical nerves, can be involved in the production of headaches. Therefore, head pain can arise from a variety of sources in the neck. More specifically, Mr B.'s head pain could be arising from pain generators innervated by the posterior primary divisions (dorsal rami) or anterior primary divisions (ventral rami) of the upper three cervical nerves. Recall that the anterior primary divisions of the upper three cervical nerves make up the cervical plexus. Structures innervated by the upper three cervi-

cal anterior and posterior primary divisions include the following: muscles, ligaments (including Z joint capsules), annulus fibrosus, anterior spinal dura mater and any part of the vertebrae (Figure 1.2).

PAIN GENERATORS OF THE NECK AND THEIR INNERVATION

The neural elements listed below conduct nociceptive impulses from pain generators of the neck. These nerves include the following:

- Branches of the posterior primary division (dorsal ramus)
- Branches of the anterior primary division (ventral ramus)
- Recurrent meningeal nerve
- Vertebral artery sympathetic nerve plexus

Nociception conducted by the above listed nerves then passes centrally by means of the mixed spinal nerves to the dorsal root and dorsal root ganglion to reach the spinal cord and higher centres.

Figure 1.3 shows several of the neural structures listed above.

Therefore, pain generators capable of producing neck and head pain similar to that described in the case of Mr B. can be organized

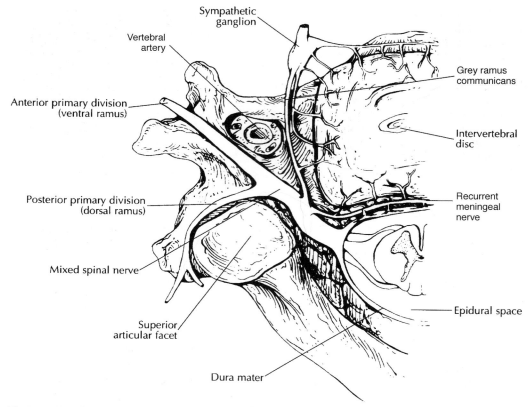

Figure 1.3 *Superior view of a cervical vertebra demonstrating the neural elements in this region. (From Figure 5–18 in Cramer G. The cervical region (Chapter 5). In: Cramer G, Darby S. (1995) Basic and Clinical Anatomy of the Spine, Spinal Cord and ANS. Mosby Year Book, St Louis, pp. 109–155.)*

by pain generators supplied by one or more of the following: (1) posterior primary divisions, (2) anterior primary divisions, (3) recurrent meningeal nerves and (4) branches of the vertebral artery sympathetic nerve plexus. Since neck and head pain can theoretically arise from any structure innervated by these nerves, each of these three nerves and the pain generators supplied by each will be briefly discussed.

This discussion should help to provide a better understanding of the types of structures that could be involved in neck and head pain.

The majority of potential pain generators of the posterior neck receive innervation from the posterior primary divisions of the mixed spinal nerves. Each posterior primary division divides into a medial branch and a lateral branch. Table 1.1 lists those structures supplied by the medial branch of the posterior primary division.

Table 1.1 Structures (pain generators) innervated by the medial branch of the posterior primary division (dorsal ramus)

- Deep back muscles (spinalis, transversospinalis group, interspinales and a portion of the intertransversarii)
- Zygapophysial joints (subchondral bone and Z joint capsule)
- Periosteum of posterior vertebral arch
- Interspinous, supraspinous, and intertransverse ligaments (possibly ligamentum flavum)
- Skin (supplied by upper cervical dorsal rami)

Some of the most important structures from a clinical perspective listed in Table 1.1 include the Z joints and the transversospinalis group of muscles. The upper cervical Z joints are very strong candidates for neck pain that refers to the head and tightness of the transversospinalis muscles (including the semispinalis cervicis and the multifidus cervicis) could be a source of neck and even head pain. Notice that the medial branch of the posterior primary division also supplies several ligaments. These include the interspinous and supraspinous ligaments (in the cervical region this is considered to be the ligamentum nuchae), the intertransverse ligament, and the ligamentum flavum. Reports of the amount of nociceptive innervation to these ligaments varies and more thorough investigation is required before the innervation to these structures will be completely understood.

The posterior primary division also gives a lateral branch. Table 1.2 lists the structures supplied by the lateral branch of the posterior primary division.

Tightness of the muscles listed above could result in neck and head pain.

Pain generators supplied by the recurrent meningeal nerve can be another source of neck pain that can refer to the head. Figure 1.4 shows the recurrent meningeal nerve re-entering the intervertebral foramen to supply the structures listed in Table 1.3.

The recurrent meningeal nerve is a unique structure. Groen *et al.* [10] stated that two to six of these structures enter the intervertebral foramen (IVF) at each vertebral level. They

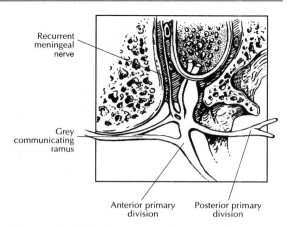

Figure 1.4 *Horizontal section through an intervertebral foramen demonstrating the recurrent meningeal nerve. (From Figure 1–16C in Cramer G. General characteristics of the spine (Chapter 2). In: Cramer G, Darby S. (1995) Basic and Clinical Anatomy of the Spine, Spinal Cord and ANS. Mosby Year Book, St Louis, pp. 17–51.)*

demonstrated a dense plexus of nerves derived from the recurrent meningeal nerve supplying the posterior longitudinal ligament. Therefore, the posterior longitudinal ligament may be a source of pain in a patient with a history of a flexion-extension type of injury. Tear or damage to the outer third of the posterior anulus fibrosus could also be a source of discomfort in a case like that of our sample patient, Mr B.

Another unique feature of the recurrent meningeal nerves is that they are irregular in their distribution. Groen *et al.* [11] found recurrent meningeal nerves taking any combination of the following courses: (1) ascending as many as four vertebral segments, (2) descending as many as four segments, and/or (3) crossing to the opposite side of the vertebral column. Such irregularity makes identifying pain patterns generated from structures innervated by the recurrent meningeal nerves extremely difficult.

In addition, the anterior longitudinal ligament and the anterior aspect of the intervertebral disc are also potential pain generators. These structures are supplied by branches of the sympathetic trunk. Other structures supplied by branches of the sympathetic trunk are listed in Table 1.4.

Table 1.2 Structures innervated by the lateral branch of the posterior primary division (dorsal ramus)

- Erector spinae muscles
- Splenius capitis
- Skin of the neck

Table 1.3 Structures innervated by the recurrent meningeal nerve

- Posterior aspect of the intervertebral disc
- Posterior longitudinal ligament
- Periosteum of posterior vertebral bodies
- Internal vertebral (epidural) veins and basivertebral veins
- Epidural adipose tissue
- Anterior aspect of the spinal dura mater

Table 1.4 Structures innervated by nerves associated with the sympathetic trunk and the grey rami communicans

- Anterior and lateral aspects of the intervertebral disc
- Anterior longitudinal ligament
- Periosteum of the anterior and lateral aspects of the vertebral bodies
- Vertebral artery (supplied by the vertebral nerve)

Also, pain can refer to the neck and head from structures innervated by the anterior primary divisions. Structures innervated by the anterior primary divisions are listed in Table 1.5.

Table 1.5 Structures innervated by the anterior primary divisions (ventral ramus)

- Referred pain from structures innervated by nerves of the cervical plexus (possible head pain) and brachial plexus (possible neck pain)
- Longus colli and capitis, rectus capitis anterior and lateralis, and part of the intertransversarii muscles

In addition, portions of the intracranial dura mater, vertebral arteries and the basilar artery are supplied by the upper four cervical nerves [12]. Disorders affecting these structures can easily refer to the neck and head. Structures within the cranial vault innervated by the upper four cervical nerves are listed in Table 1.6.

Table 1.6 Structures of the head innervated by the upper four cervical nerves

- Vessels of the posterior cranial fossa (vertebrobasilar system)
- Meninges and dural vessels of the posterior cranial fossa

Depending upon the irritated structure any one of the nerves listed in this section may be part of the pathway travelled by the nociceptive impulses that are resulting in Mr B.'s sensation of pain.

NOCICEPTIVE PATHWAYS AND SOMATIC REFERRED PAIN

Many potential pain generators have been listed in the section above. The majority of the structures listed are found in the neck. Yet, pain arising from them can be felt in the head. Earlier we defined somatic referred pain as pain generated by a skeletal or related (bone, joint, ligament, muscle) structure which is felt in an area distant to the structure(s) generating the pain. We then gave the example of somatic referred pain provided by the work of Bogduk and Marsland [5] in which they injected the upper cervical Z joints with a local anaesthetic and relieved pain felt in the head, neck, and cape region covering the upper thorax and shoulder. Another example of somatic referred pain can be found in the work of Campbell and Parsons [6]. These investigators injected hypertonic saline (salt water) into trigger points detected in the suboccipital region. The patients reported feeling pain in a wide variety of locations including the following: mandible, nose, orbital region, frontal region (forehead), auriculomastoid region, superior occipital region, inferior occipital region, suboccipital region and the shoulder. With the exception of pain in the suboccipital region, the areas of pain reported by the patients in Campbell and Parsons' [6] study represent somatic referred pain.

The quality of somatic referred pain is a constant, nagging ache that is difficult to pinpoint in location. To discuss the mechanism of somatic referred pain we first need to briefly review the primary pathway for conducting nociceptive input. This pathway is found in the anterior and lateral aspect of the spinal cord and is sometimes referred to as the lateral spinothalamic tract. This pathway is reviewed in outline form below and is illustrated in Figure 1.5.

Anterior lateral quadrant (lateral spinothalamic tract)

I. Incoming nociceptive afferents (first order neurons) have many options upon entering the cord (participation in withdrawal reflex, modulation of nociception and/or transmission of nociception by stimulation of tract cells). These incoming afferents can

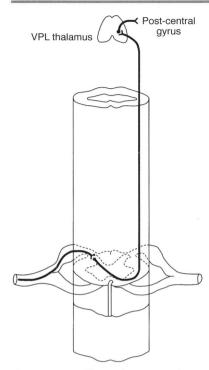

VPL thalamus

Post-central gyrus

Figure 1.5 *The primary pathway for conducting nociceptive input, the lateral spinothalamic tract or neospinothalamic tract. (From Figure 2–6 in Cramer G and Darby S. (1995) Anatomy related to spinal subluxation (Chapter 2). In: Gatterman M, ed.* **Foundations of chiropractic: Subluxation.** *Mosby Year Book, St Louis, pp. 18–34.)*

be dispersed superiorly or inferiorly as many as four spinal cord segments in the dorsolateral tract of Lissauer.

II. Tract cells of the anterior lateral quadrant (second order neurons):

A. Have their origin in laminae I, IV–VII of the spinal grey mater [2]. They receive excitatory input from primary nociceptive afferents or from interneurons stimulated by primary afferents.

B. Cross (axons of the tract cells cross) the midline within the spinal cord (ventral white commissure).

C. Tract cell axons ascend in the anterior lateral quadrant of the spinal cord.

D. Tract cell axons continue to ascend the medulla, pons, and midbrain as the spinal lemniscus – collateral fibres are given off to the medullary and pontine reticular formations and the periaqueductal grey

matter of the midbrain (paleospinothalamic tract).

E. Tract cell neurons continue to the thalamus – synapse in the ventral posterolateral (VPL) thalamic nucleus.

F. The third order neurons originating in the VPL of the thalamus project to the postcentral gyrus of the cerebral cortex via the internal capsule and the corona radiata. These fibres terminate in a somatotopic arrangement (homunculus). The VPL of the thalamus and the primary sensory cortex (postcentral gyrus) are necessary for the accurate localization of painful stimuli.

The referral of pain can occur in several locations along this pathway. The following represents a model for the mechanisms of such somatic referred pain.

Mechanism of somatic referred pain

1. Incoming afferents conducting nociception can disperse superiorly or inferiorly as many as four spinal cord segments before synapsing on a tract cell. This dispersal of incoming afferents transmitting nociception to the spinal cord may cause decreased accuracy in the ability to localize the region of tissue damage (Figure 1.6).

2. In addition, afferents from different regions of the body converge onto the same pool of spinal cord tract cells. For example, input from the C2–C3 Z joint, semispinalis and multifidus cervicis muscles, ligamentum nucha, C3–C4 intervertebral disc and several other structures could conceivably converge onto the same pool of tract cell neurons. This convergence of incoming afferents onto tract neurons may also decrease the ability of an individual to accurately localize the region of tissue damage (Figure 1.7).

3. These same phenomena (1 and 2, above) can also occur in the VPL of the thalamus. This may further decrease accuracy of localizing tissue damage.

4. The back region (particularly the neck region) of the sensory homunculus of the primary sensory cortex is very small and is

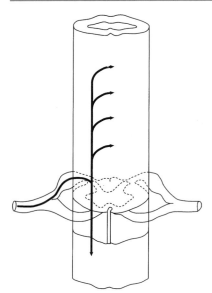

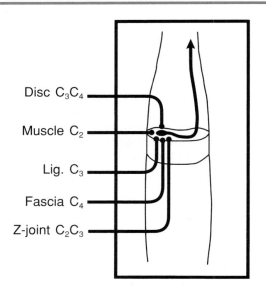

Figure 1.6 *Dispersion of incoming afferents in the spinal cord. Incoming afferents conducting nociception can disperse superiorly or inferiorly in the tract of Lissauer up to four spinal cord segments before synapsing on a tract cell. This dispersion may be one reason for decreased accuracy in the ability of humans to localize a region of tissue damage.*

Disc C_3C_4
Muscle C_2
Lig. C_3
Fascia C_4
Z-joint C_2C_3

Figure 1.7 *Convergence of afferents from several sources onto the same spinal cord tract cell. This convergence of incoming afferents onto tract neurons may also decrease a patient's ability to accurately localize a region of tissue damage.*

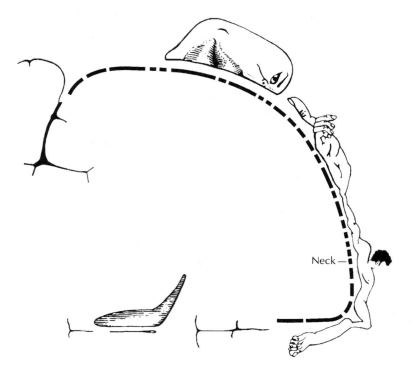

Neck

Figure 1.8 *Sensory homunculus. Notice how small the neck region is on the homunculus and how closely related it is to the suboccipital and occipital regions. These features of the homunculus also help explain the broad referral of neck pain to the posterior head.*

very closely related to the posterior region of the head (Figure 1.8). Therefore, a great deal of overlap can occur. This also helps to explain the broad referral of neck pain to the posterior head. Referral to the anterior aspect of the head is explained below.

The phenomena listed in items 1–4 above combine to allow a patient (such as Mr B.) to perceive pain in an area quite distant from the structure causing the discomfort.

Spinoreticular tracts (medullary and pontine)

The spinoreticular tracts (medullary and pontine) are also related to the perception of pain by an individual. These tracts are very similar to lateral spinothalamic tract except they conduct all somaesthetic impulses (both nociceptive impulses and touch impulses). Fibres ascend to the medullary and pontine reticular formations and these regions then project to a variety of neurological centres including the intralaminar and posterior (dorsal) nuclei of the thalamus. Third order neurons from these thalamic nuclei project diffusely to all regions of the cerebral cortex (including the hippocampal formation). This pathway seems to be involved in assigning an emotional value and a level of discomfort to a patient's pain. We mentioned previously that a person's discomfort can be related to her or his early experiences with noxious stimuli. The spinoreticular and then the reticulo-thalamo-cortical pathway may provide the mechanism that allows an individual, such as Mr B., to describe his level of pain, and allows him to compare the current discomfort level with the level of discomfort of previous experiences with pain.

PAIN GENERATORS OF THE HEAD AND THEIR INNERVATION

We have discussed a mechanism for neck pain referring to the posterior aspect of the head. To better understand the relationship between neck pain referring to the anterior aspect of the head the trigeminal nerve needs to be briefly discussed.

The three divisions of the trigeminal nerve, V1 – ophthalmic, V2 – maxillary and V3 – mandibular, supply sensory innervation (including nociception) to the majority of the pain generators of the head. These pain generators include those associated with the orbit, cornea, conjunctiva, paranasal sinuses and nasal mucosa, oral cavity, anterior two-thirds of the tongue, tooth pulp, gingiva, periodontal membrane, temporomandibular joint, dura mater of the anterior and middle cranial fossae and skin of the face (Figure 1.9) [12]. In addition, the cavernous sinus nerve plexus surrounding the internal carotid artery consists of sympathetic fibres, parasympathetic fibres and fibres from the ophthalmic and maxillary divisions of the trigeminal nerve. A lesion in this region of the cavernous sinus could produce headache accompanied by autonomic symptoms [13].

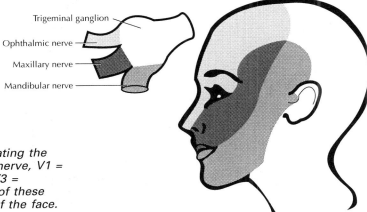

Figure 1.9 *Illustration demonstrating the three divisions of the trigeminal nerve, V1 = ophthalmic, V2 = maxillary and V3 = mandibular, and the distribution of these nerves onto the anterior aspect of the face.*

NOCICEPTIVE (PAIN) PATHWAYS FROM THE HEAD

The next step in understanding the interaction between head pain and neck pain is to discuss the pathway associated with nociception transmitted from the pain generators innervated by branches of the trigeminal nerve. Nociceptive input arising from these pain generators follows branches of the trigeminal nerve proximally and then courses into the brainstem. These fibres then descend through the pons, medulla and approximately the upper three cervical spinal cord segments (Figure 1.10). These descending fibres make up what is known as the spinal tract of the trigeminal nerve. Synapses with second order neurons occur in the adjacent spinal nucleus of the trigeminal nerve. These synapses occur throughout the length of the spinal nucleus of the trigeminal, including the region within the upper three cervical spinal cord segments. The second order fibres then ascend to the thalamus (ventral posterior medial nucleus). Here the second order neurons synapse with third order neurons and the third order neurons project to the cerebral cortex. Table 1.7 summarizes the key features of this pathway.

REFERRAL OF PAIN RELATED TO NECK AND HEAD PAIN

The most important feature of this pathway for our present discussion is the fact that the spinal tract and adjacent spinal nucleus of the trigeminal nerve descend to the upper three

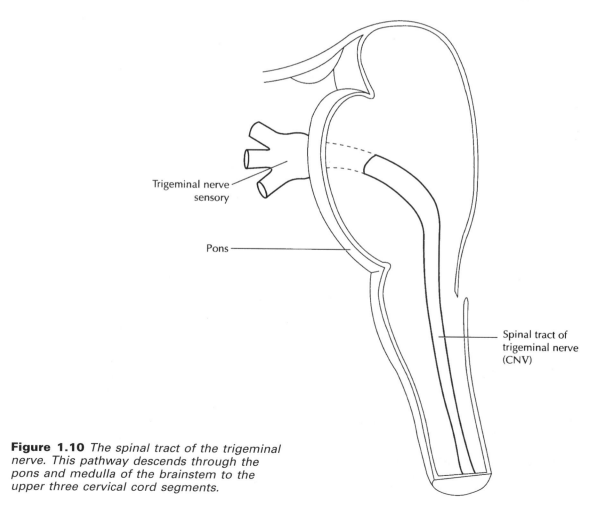

Figure 1.10 *The spinal tract of the trigeminal nerve. This pathway descends through the pons and medulla of the brainstem to the upper three cervical cord segments.*

Trigeminal nerve sensory

Pons

Spinal tract of trigeminal nerve (CNV)

Table 1.7 Pathway for nociception arising from pain generators supplied by the trigeminal nerve

- Trigeminal nerve
- Spinal tract of the trigeminal nerve
- Spinal nucleus of the trigeminal nerve (most synapse in pars caudalis – C1–C3 spinal cord segments)
- Ventral trigeminothalamic tract (crosses to opposite side)
- Thalamus [synapse in ventral posteromedial thalamic nucleus (VPM)]
- Primary sensory cortex (postcentral gyrus) – somatotopic representation (face region of homunculus)

nal nerve is intermixed with the dorsal horn of the upper two to three cervical spinal cord segments (nucleus posteromarginalis and substantia gelatinosa) (Figure 1.12). This is also the region that receives nociceptive information from the upper three cervical cord segments. Because of the intermixing of trigeminal fibres with those of the cervical spinal cord, this area of the posterior dorsal horn of the upper two to three cervical spinal cord segments is frequently described as the trigeminospinal nucleus [2,14] or the trigeminocervical nucleus [15]. Many upper cervical dorsal horn neurons in this region receive afferents from both nerves of upper cervical spinal cord segments and the trigeminal nerve [15]. Of additional interest is the fact that many afferent fibres coursing through the upper cervical dorsal roots ascend to the medulla and synapse on cells of the spinal nucleus of the trigeminal nerve after entering the spinal cord. These facts serve as the

cervical spinal cord segments (Figure 1.11). The spinal tract of the trigeminal nerve intermingles with the posterolateral region of the spinal cord occupied by the tract of Lissauer. In addition, the spinal nucleus of the trigemi-

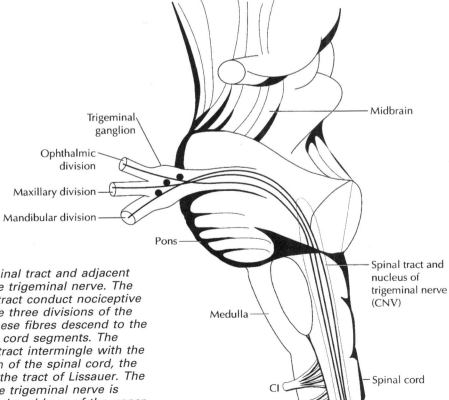

Figure 1.11 *The spinal tract and adjacent spinal nucleus of the trigeminal nerve. The fibres of the spinal tract conduct nociceptive information from the three divisions of the trigeminal nerve. These fibres descend to the upper three cervical cord segments. The fibres of the spinal tract intermingle with the posterolateral region of the spinal cord, the region occupied by the tract of Lissauer. The spinal nucleus of the trigeminal nerve is intermixed with the dorsal horn of the upper two to three cervical spinal cord segments.*

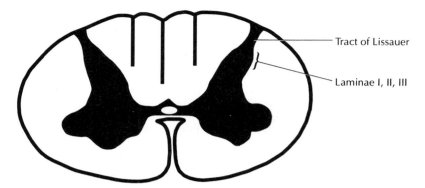

Tract of Lissauer

Laminae I, II, III

Figure 1.12 *Illustration of a horizontal section through an upper cervical spinal cord segment. The spinal nucleus of the trigeminal nerve is intermixed with the dorsal horn of the upper two to three cervical spinal cord segments (shown as laminae I, II, and III). This is also the region of the dorsal horn of the spinal cord that receives nociceptive information from the upper three cervical cord segments. Because of the intermixing of trigeminal fibres with those of the cervical spinal cord, this area of the dorsal horn of the upper two to three cervical cord segments is frequently described as the trigeminospinal nucleus (see text). The intermixing of fibres in this location serves as the neuroanatomical basis for head pain referring to the neck and for neck pain referring to the anterior head.*

neuroanatomical basis for head pain referring to the neck and for neck pain referring to the anterior head in a patient like Mr B. [15,16]. This serves as an additional neuroanatomical basis for neck pain referring to the anterior head.

Because of the complex nature of pain referral related to nociception arising from the neck and head, one can see that a thorough examination of cranial nerves, neck and head, is required in a case such as that presenting as Mr B.

SUMMARY

This chapter began by discussing the case of a sample patient, Mr B., who presented with neck and head pain. To begin consideration of the potential causes of this type of pain and the mechanisms of action that might be involved, several definitions related to neck and head pain (nociception, pain, pain generator, somatic referred pain) were presented. Pain generators of the neck and the nociceptive pathways associated with these pain generators were then explored. This led to a discussion of somatic referred pain. Because neck and head pain can also originate in the

head and because pain originating in the neck can refer to the anterior head, pain generators of the head and nociceptive pathways associated with these pain generators were discussed next. The chapter concluded with a discussion of how pain referral from pain generators of the head could be perceived by a patient like Mr B. to be arising from the neck and, also, how pain arising from a pain generator in the neck could be perceived by Mr B. to be arising from the head, as headache pain.

Several structures that can cause neck and head pain and the neuroanatomical basis of neck pain as a cause of headache have been discussed in this chapter. The remaining chapters in this book are extremely important because they further explain the mechanisms behind this type of pain referral, the differential diagnosis of headache and the treatment of headaches.

ACKNOWLEDGMENTS

The author would like to gratefully acknowledge Drs Carolyn Scott, Adam Wilding and Nathaniel R. Tuck, Jr, for help with the manuscript and preparation of figures.

REFERENCES

1. Haldeman S. The neurophysiology of spinal pain. In *Principles and Practice of Chiropractic.* (ed. S Haldeman) 2nd edn, Norwalk, Connecticut: Appleton and Lange, 1992.
2. Parent A. *Carpenter's Human Neuroanatomy*, 9th edn, Baltimore, Maryland: Williams and Wilkins, 1996.
3. Merskey H, Bogduk N (eds). *Classification of Chronic Pain: Descriptions of Chronic Pain Syndromes and Definitions of Pain Terms*, 2nd edn, Seattle, Washington: IASP Press; 1994.
4. Weinstein WH. The perception of pain. In *Managing Low Back Pain*, 2nd edn, (ed. W Kirkaldy-Willis), New York: Churchill Livingstone, 1988.
5. Bogduk N, Marsland A. The cervical zygapophysial joints as a source of neck pain. *Spine* 1988;**13**:610–617.
6. Campbell DG, Parsons CM. Referred head pain and its concomitants. *J Nerv Mental Diseases* 1944;**99**:544–551.
7. Bogduk N. The rationale for patterns of neck and back pain. *Patient Management* 1984;**13**:17–28.
8. Aprill C, Dwyer A, Bogduk N. Cervical zygapophyseal joint pain patterns II: A clinical evaluation. *Spine* 1990;**15**:453–457.
9. Dwyer A, Aprill C, Bogduk N. Cervical zygapophyseal joint pain patterns I: A clinical evaluation. *Spine* 1990;**15**:458–461.
10. Groen GJ, Baljet B, Drukker J. Nerves and nerve plexuses of the human vertebral column. *Am J Anat* 1990;**188**:282–296.
11. Groen GJ, Baljet B, Drukker J. The innervation of the spinal dura mater: anatomy and clinical implications. *Acta Neurochirurgica* 1988;**92**:39–46.
12. Williams PL, Bannister LH, Berry MM, Collins P, *et al. Gray's Anatomy*, 38th edn, Edinburgh: Churchill Livingstone, 1995.
13. Darby S, Cramer G. Pain generators and pain pathways of the head and neck. In *Chiropractic Approach to Head Pain*, (ed. D Curl), Baltimore: Williams and Wilkins, 1994.
14. Brodal A. *Neurological Anatomy*. New York: Oxford University Press, 1981.
15. Bogduk N. The anatomical basis for cervicogenic headache. *J Manip Physiol Ther* 1992;**15**:67–70.
16. Sessle BJ. Neurophysiological mechanisms related to craniofacial and cervical pain. *Topics in Clinical Chiropractic* 1998;**5**:36–38.

Further reading

Darby S, Cramer G. Pain generators and pain pathways of the head and neck. In *Chiropractic Approach to Head Pain*, (ed. D Curl), Baltimore: Williams and Wilkins, 1994.

Cramer G, Darby S. Pain of spinal origin. In *Basic and Clinical Anatomy of the Spine*, (eds. G Cramer and S Darby), *Spinal Cord, and ANS*. St. Louis: Mosby Yearbook, 1995.

Cramer G, Darby S. Clinical anatomy of spinal subluxation. In *Foundations of Chiropractic Subluxation* (ed. M Gatterman), St Louis: Mosby Yearbook, 1995.

Chapter 2

Afferent mechanisms in the upper cervical spine

Frances J. R. Richmond and Brian D. Corneil

INTRODUCTION

The tissues that surround the vertebral column contain a rich and varied collection of sensory receptors. The cutaneous mechanoreceptive system is primarily *exteroceptive*; it supplies information about deformation of the skin and hair and is supplied by relatively large nerve fibres. A second system sensitive to temperature, chemical changes and tissue damage is distributed throughout all cervical tissues and is served by fine nerve axons and endings. These fine afferent fibres are part of an important *nociceptive* system that warns the nervous system about damage or deterioration of nuchal structures. The muscle and joint receptors together form a *proprioceptive* system that continually updates the nervous system about body posture and movement by monitoring muscle activity and joint angle change. A particularly high density of proprioceptors is present in the muscles of the neck. Despite the wealth of sensory input from neck-muscle proprioceptors, this system is less potent than the similar system in limb muscles, which can produce short segmental reflexes, such as stretch reflexes in homonymous muscles. However, neck muscle afferents have strong projections to higher brain centres and it is these centres that appear to have key roles in the monitoring and integration of the proprioceptive input that controls body posture and movement. Distortions of nuchal sensory signals induced by damage,

anaesthesia or vibratory stimulation cause changes in perceptions of head and body position, disruption of postural reflexes and problems with balance and locomotion.

THE EXTEROCEPTIVE SYSTEM

The cervical spinal cord has eight sets of segmental nerves that together supply the skin from the face to the arm (Figure 2.1). The first cervical segment supplies the smallest dermatome (cutaneous receptive field), one that is confined to the dorsal scalp. The second cervical segment supplies a much broader territory including a substantial region around the ear. Caudal spinal segments (C3, C4 and C5) supply ring-like regions of skin that encircle the neck. Cervical segments below C5 have territories that are confined to the arm and hand. Individuals seldom realize that the nerves to the skin supply individual dermatomes because the nervous system integrates the input from different segments into a single seamless map. However, the fact that dermatomes do exist can become painfully obvious in patients who suffer damage or inflammation restricted to the nerve supply of one segment. Herpes zoster is an infectious condition that commonly confines itself to the nerves of a single spinal segment. In consequence, on the rare occasion when a patient develops a herpes infection in the neck, skin lesions and changes in sensation are confined to a single cervical dermatome.

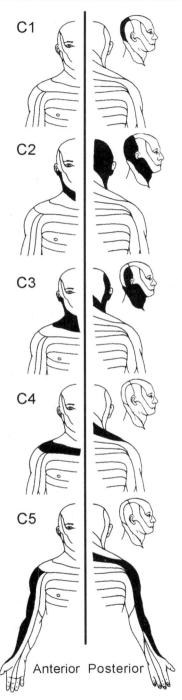

Figure 2.1 *Dermatomal organization of upper and middle cervical segments shown as shaded areas. (From* Neck Pain: Medical Diagnosis and Comprehensive Management, *Chapter 3, (eds. Borenstein, Wiesel and Boden), 1996, with permission).*

The sensory receptors responsible for recognizing mechanical events on the skin of the head and neck tend to have structures like those in other body parts, and these are described elsewhere in detail [1,2]. They include rapidly adapting mechanoreceptors such as Meissner's corpuscles and the exquisitely sensitive Pacinian corpuscles that fire very briefly when the skin is touched; hair follicle receptors that respond to transients when hairs are moved; and slowly adapting mechanoreceptors such as Merkel's discs and Ruffini endings that fire tonically for the entire period through which a stimulus is applied to the skin. The skin is also supplied by thinner Group III and IV afferent fibres that end in free endings. Many of these less differentiated receptors respond to prodding, stretching or squeezing, as well as more damaging intense stimuli (see below).

THE NOCICEPTIVE SYSTEM

The compelling sensation of pain, often associated with nuchal damage, is a complex percept that arises from centrally mediated interpretations of signals arising from high-threshold mechanoreceptors and nociceptors. The receptor system that is involved most intimately in nociception includes two main groupings of fibres, small A-delta (also called Group III) myelinated fibres supplied by axons with conduction velocities of about 10–25 m/s and unmyelinated C (also called Group IV) fibres whose conduction velocities are below 2.5 m/s. Because these fibres terminate in 'free' endings without an elaborate morphological form, it has been tempting to consider them as a homogeneous grouping. However, the responses of these receptors vary according to their locations, their history of activation and their inherent properties.

Information about damaging stimuli comes from receptors in both the skin and deep structures. Painful sensations from the skin are often considered to have two components, an 'epicritic' component that is experienced first, as a sharp, localized sensation thought to be associated with firing in A-delta fibres and a slightly delayed 'protopathic' component that is often described as 'dull' or 'burning' and is thought to be due to C fibre activation [3]. These two types of painful percepts may be mediated, at least in part, by different neuro-transmitters, substance P and somatostatin, respectively [4]. Relatively little research has been directed at understanding pain from the skin of the neck because it is presumed to be processed in much the same way as cutaneous pain in other body parts where it has been studied in great depth [5].

Pain in deeper structures has received less experimental study, although clinically it may be a more important aspect of neck pain, particularly chronic neck pain. Deep neck pain is a common and often intractable consequence of many types of neck pathology. Sensory signals responsible for such painful sensations are thought to originate from Group III and IV fibres that are distributed widely in deeper structures, such as muscle, ligaments and joints. Our understanding of sensory function arising from muscle and joint nociceptors comes largely from studies in which single fibres have been dissected from nerves that supply limb muscles or joints in experimental animals (see Mense [6] for review). In muscles, free nerve endings supplied by Group III and IV fibres are numerous. For example, Group IV fibres account for two thirds of the fibres in nerves supplying neck muscles [7] as they do in muscles of the limb [8,9]. Of these unmyelinated fibres, about half are estimated to serve a sensory role [6]. Their endings are found not only in the muscle belly but also in associated aponeuroses and fascial coverings [10,11]. The responses of these endings suggest that they could potentially have a role in both mechanoreception and nociception. Many receptors supplying Group III axons fire modestly to stretch or squeeze, and more vigorously to the intramuscular injection or intra-arterial injection of algesic chemicals, such as KCl, bradykinin or acetylcholine [10,12]. For example, Mense [13] found that about two-thirds of Group III axons and half of Group IV axons from the gastrocnemius-soleus were sensitive to algesic chemicals, a property presumed to indicate a nociceptive chemosensitivity. Group III and, more rarely, Group IV fibres are reported to fire when the muscle contracts, and some Group IV fibres respond to changes in temperature. The sensitivity of individual receptors to mechanical and chemical stimuli varies widely, leading some to suggest that receptors may be divided into

subgroups with particular response specificities (see Mense [6] for arguments). Nevertheless, many single receptors show 'polymodal' responses to mechanical, chemical and/or thermal stimulation.

Only a few studies have specifically examined nociceptors in the neck, but the work that has been done suggests that the nociceptive system is equally important. Nerves supplying rat and cat neck muscles, for example, contain at least as many unmyelinated as myelinated fibres; about 60% of the unmyelinated fibres are sensory [7,14]. Electrophysiological analyses of the Group III axons has shown that most behave as high threshold mechanoreceptors that adapt slowly to mechanical stimuli such as pinch, but are excited only rarely by the intra-arterial injection of algesic chemicals [15]. This evidence suggests that nociceptive chemosensitivity may be subserved primarily by Group IV afferent fibres, at least in normal muscle.

There is, however, a problem associated with attempts to characterize receptors in normal, undamaged tissue and then extrapolate those results to conditions in which tissues are damaged or inflamed. Unlike larger mechanoreceptors whose responses remain quite stable even when the chemical environment is changed [16], free nerve endings exhibit a property called 'sensitization' in which thresholds to stimulation diminish and firing patterns intensify after they have been stimulated intensely or exposed to noxious chemical substances (reviewed in Mense [6]). The sensitization appears to be due in part to the accumulation of humoral mediators and peptides around the receptor, as a result of tissue inflammation and damage. An important part of this process is initiated by the release of arachidonic acid from damaged cells; this triggers a biochemical cascade that stimulates the production of prostaglandins and leucotrienes (Figure 2.2). The well-known anti-inflammatory action of acetylsalicylic acid and other non-steroidal anti-inflammatory agents is related to their ability to block the production of prostaglandins in this cascade [17]. Administration of acetylsalicylic acid into muscle has been shown to decrease the firing of Group III and IV afferents to bradykinin [18].

The nerves themselves may contribute to their own sensitization by releasing endogenous compounds that affect not only the nerve

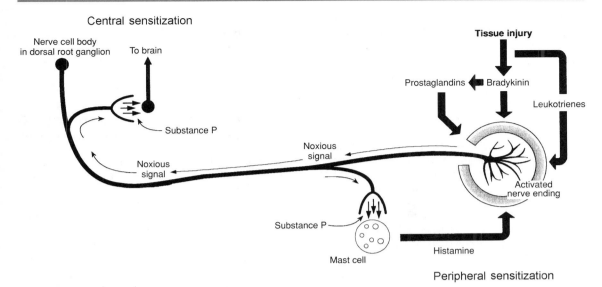

Figure 2.2 *Multiple mechanisms involved in the sensitization of receptors. Tissue inflammation results in the release of chemical mediators that increase the firing rate and sensitivity of nociceptive endings. The axons contribute to this sensitization both centrally and peripherally by releasing compounds such as substance P. (Modified from* Contemporary Conservative Care for Painful Spinal Disorders, *Chapter 6, (eds. Mayer, Mooney, Gatchel), 1991, with permission).*

ending under assault but also, through 'axon reflexes', the other branches of the same nerve axon (e.g., Levine *et al.* [5]) (Figure 2.2). Some of the compounds released from axon endings by intense C-fibre stimulation include neuropeptides such as substance P, calcitonin gene-related peptide and neurokinin A. The release of neurally derived compounds stimulates most cells to release histamine and contributes to the development of 'neurogenic' inflammation, characterized by increased blood flow, vascular permeability and leucocyte accumulation.

Free nerve endings supplied by small-calibre axons are found in soft tissues that are an integral part of joints, including cervical vertebral joints. The nerve endings are reported to be distributed in joint capsules and ligaments, but not cartilage or synovial tissues [19,20]. They are also found in cervical dura mater near the dorsal root ganglia and nerve roots [21]. However, because of the difficulties of recording from such small fibres while the joints are manipulated, most tests to characterize such endings have been conducted in knee joints of experimental animals. Here Group III and IV axons exhibit similar proper-

ties to Group III and IV fibres in muscle. Many fire in response to strong or potentially damaging mechanical stimuli [22–26]. As in other tissues, their responses to such stimuli can be sensitized by joint inflammation (e.g., Grigg *et al.* [25], Coggeshall *et al.* [27], Schaible *et al.* [28] and Guilbaud *et al.* [29]) or the application of algesic substances [30–32]. Sensitized endings then may fire vigorously even to stimuli that in normal joints would be considered innocuous and would not excite the endings. The sensitization of nociceptive endings may be an important contributing factor to the chronic pain encountered clinically in degenerative diseases or traumatic injury to the vertebral column in the neck [33].

THE PROPRIOCEPTIVE SYSTEM

The vertebral column, from the head to tail, is generally viewed to form the long axis of the body. Thus, structures close to or investing the vertebral column are described as 'axial' to distinguish them from 'appendicular' structures in the limbs. However, the neck in many mammals is an exceptionally mobile and specialized type of 'appendage'. The control of its movements is essential for many tasks that ensure survival such as finding and following objects by sight, sound and smell, killing and carrying food, eating, grooming and even mating. The necks of different animals are therefore specialized to permit a greater range and flexibility than vertebrae of the trunk.

In humans, some of the tasks carried out by lower vertebrates have been transferred as hands replaced jaws as the primary prehensile organ. Nevertheless, the unique position of the neck between head and body gives it at least three specialized roles for which sensory input will be needed. First, it must move the head in a highly controlled way throughout space to extend the movement range of the eyes, ears and mouth. Second, it must generate forces so that it can interact with external loads and respond to perturbations. In some cultures, for example, individuals commonly carry vessels or palettes weighing many kilograms by placing them on the crown of the head. Finally, it must serve a unique sensory role to relate the position of the head in space (sensed by the vestibular system) to the position of the trunk and limbs (sensed by proprioceptors elsewhere in the body).

ORGANIZATION OF SENSORY RECEPTORS

How is the neck equipped to provide sensory information about neck position and movement? Such a picture is usually thought to be constructed by integrating sensory signals from muscles and joints. In muscles, muscle spindles and Golgi tendon organs provide sensitive information about muscle length, length change and force development. In joints, Ruffini endings and Paciniform corpuscles are thought to provide signals about joint-angle change. Most is known about receptor organization in muscles because the receptors are easy to recognize using conventional microscopy and can be studied physiologically by recording from their nerve axons. Vertebral joint receptors, in contrast, are difficult to study because they are located in tissues that move with the bones. This makes it difficult to obtain the stable electrophysiological signals from their sensory axons that are

necessary in order to study their functional properties.

MUSCLE SPINDLES

The 'generic' muscle spindle

The muscle spindle is the most studied proprioceptor in the neck. As discussed below, it is also the most distinctive. Muscle spindles in neck muscles are particularly varied in structural form. The implications of those specializations can only be considered against a background understanding of 'generic' muscle spindles.

Muscle spindles are found between extrafusal fibre fascicles, where they are subject to the same shortening and lengthening perturbations experienced by the muscle in which they are located. Muscle spindles provide the nervous system with information about muscle length and rate of change of muscle length. Their sensitivity to stretch is highly developed – they can signal changes in muscle length as small as a few micrometres.

Most of what we know about muscle spindles come from experiments on cat limb muscles (see Matthews [34], Barker and Banks [35], Boyd and Smith [36] and Prochazka [37] for detailed review). Muscle spindles are typically described as single isolated receptors. In each spindle, a fusiform connective-tissue capsule encloses a number of muscle fibres, called intrafusal fibres, that are shorter and thinner than the normal (extrafusal) muscle fibres. Intrafusal fibres in a single spindle are not all the same. In mammalian species, most muscle spindles contain at least three differentiable types of muscle fibres called nuclear bag$_1$, nuclear bag$_2$ and nuclear chain fibres [38]. The nuclear bag fibres derive their unusual name from observations that muscle fibre nuclei are accumulated like marbles in a bag under the primary sensory ending in the central region of the intrafusal fibre (Figure 2.3). Nuclear chain fibres, which are thinner than nuclear bag fibres, have nuclei that are aligned in single file down their central cores. The three to seven nuclear chain fibres that are generally found in a spindle are often considered to be a homogeneous group.

However, many studies have reported that one nuclear chain fibre is longer than the others and has a different pattern of motor innervation, suggesting a specialized role in signal generation.

Nuclear bag$_1$, bag$_2$ and chain fibres can also be differentiated on the basis of their protein composition. Each type of intrafusal fibre has its own characteristic staining profile for myosin antibodies and myosin ATPase activity (e.g. Ovalle and Smith [38], Banks *et al.* [39], Rowlerson *et al.* [40], Maier *et al.* [41], Pedrosa *et al.* [42] and Kucera *et al.* [43]). These differences appear to confer specialized physiological properties on each intrafusal fibre type. The nuclear bag$_1$ fibre contracts most slowly and appears to be the fibre whose sensory ending encodes the velocity-related component of the spindle signal, whereas the other fibres contract more quickly and are thought to support sensory nerve endings important for the part of the spindle signal that is related more closely to muscle length.

Muscle spindles are innervated by two kinds of sensory endings (Figure 2.3). The ending that has been studied in greatest detail is the larger primary ending that arises from an afferent axon with a diameter in the Group I range (designated as a Ia afferent). This affer-

ent ending is located in the central region of the spindle, where it branches to form a series of coil-like endings on the central nucleated portion of each intrafusal fibre in the capsule. The sensory signal that ultimately arises from the primary ending is a blended signal from multiple 'encoders' in different terminal coils, so that its firing reflects both length of the muscle and velocity of muscle-length change. Spindles are also supplied by one or more sensory axons with thinner diameters in the Group II range. These so-called 'secondary' endings are distributed primarily to nuclear chain fibres, and innervate the intrafusal fibres at sites adjacent to the centrally placed primary ending. The signal generated by the secondary ending reflects muscle length, but is less sensitive to velocity-related events.

The ends of the intrafusal fibres are composed primarily of contractile proteins. They are contacted by a variety of motor endings whose firing causes one or more of the intrafusal fibres to shorten and stiffen (Figure 2.3). This contraction increases the sensitivity of sensory endings on the contracting fibre. The motor innervation to muscle spindles is complex (see Matthews [34], Prochazka [37], Boyd and Gladden [44] and Banks [45] for detailed review). Motor axons arise from

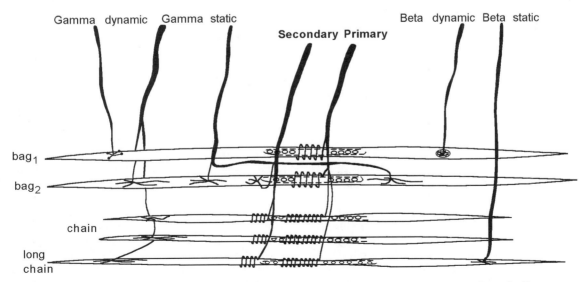

Figure 2.3 *Sensory and motor innervation of intrafusal fibres in a typical muscle spindle. Sensory endings (primary, secondary) are confined to the central portion of the intrafusal fibre. Four types of motor axons (gamma static, gamma dynamic, beta static, beta dynamic) are distributed differentially to different intrafusal fibre types (see text for further detail).*

branches of motoneurons supplying extrafusal fibres (named β-motoneurons if they innervate both extrafusal and intrafusal fibres) and also from smaller motoneurons, called δ-motoneurons, that only innervate intrafusal fibres. Each type of intrafusal fibre appears to have its own characteristic complement of motor axons. Nuclear bag$_1$ fibres are innervated by β-motoneurons that also innervate slow extrafusal fibres and a specific subset of δ-motoneurons, called 'dynamic' δ-motoneurons. By causing contractions of the nuclear bag$_1$ fibre, δ-motoneurons increase the sensitivity of the spindle to the velocity component of stretch. The nuclear bag$_2$ and chain fibres are supplied by a different group of δ-motoneurons called 'static' δ-motoneurons because they innervate fibres primarily responsible for the part of the signal that encodes muscle length. When static δ-motoneurons are active they increase the rate of spindle firing and often the spindle's sensitivity to changes in length. Within the population of static gamma axons may be further subgroupings whose relative roles are still quite poorly understood. For example, there is evidence that the nuclear bag$_2$ fibre and the nuclear chain fibres may have different patterns of motor innervation. Further, at least one of the nuclear chain fibres (generally a chain fibre extending beyond the ends of the spindle capsule) is often innervated in a specialized way, by a branch of a β-motoneuron supplying fast extrafusal fibres (a so-called 'static' β-motoneuron). The high degree of specialization in this motor system suggests that the nervous system has enormous potential to control different parts of the muscle-spindle signal by enhancing or diminishing the dynamic or static features of its response. These changes may occur as a way by which the nervous system can enhance the signal that it receives from the muscle spindle or to increase the signal to noise ratio. Changes in fusimotor activity are seen commonly when muscles are contracting or when movements must be controlled precisely [37,46]. Changes in fusimotor drive may also occur following neck pathology that results in pain. For example, Pederson and colleagues [47] have shown that injection of bradykinin into feline neck muscles provokes a sustained increase in the sensitivity of muscle spindle afferents. The increased activity is attributed to the activation of fusimotor reflexes initiated by nociceptive afferents.

Specializations in neck muscle spindles

For more than 50 years, physiologists and clinicians have been aware that neck muscles are particularly rich in muscle spindles. Voss [48,49] conducted extensive studies of muscle-spindle numbers in a range of human muscles throughout the body. He observed that the highest densities of spindles were present in muscles of the neck and digits. Cooper and Daniel [50] later commented on the 'bewildering' number of spindles in human neck muscles. Histological studies in rats and cats have also shown that neck muscles contain very large numbers of spindles [51,52]. The densities appear to be highest in the deepest neck muscles close to vertebral bones.

The characteristic morphology of the muscle spindle makes it easy to recognize in muscle cross-sections such as those shown in Figures 2.4 and 2.5. It is in such sections that anatomists first identified a characteristic difference in spindle populations of neck muscles. Whereas in most muscles, spindles are generally distributed as single isolated structures, in neck muscles they are often clustered together in groups. The size and complexity of the groups appear to increase with increasing spindle density. Thus, in superficial muscles such as trapezius, muscle spindle densities are relatively low and muscle spindles tend to be found as single units [53]. However, groupings or 'complexes' are more common in deeper muscles and most spindles appear to be part of spindle arrays in the deepest intervertebral muscles [51,52,54].

The apposition of two spindles in parallel is readily recognized in single muscle cross-sections such as that in Figure 2.5A and B. When the spindles are reconstructed in three dimensions from serial sections, it is clear that many spindles are also linked in a serial or 'tandem' structure (Figure 2.4). In these structures, two or more spindle units share at least one intrafusal fibre running through two or more capsules in succession [55,56].

One spindle unit generally has the structure typical of spindles described previously, but

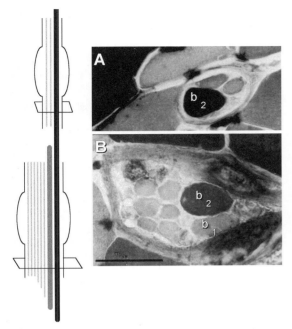

Figure 2.4 *Differences in ATPase reactivity apparent in cross-sections through intrafusal fibres of 'b₂c' (A) and 'b₁b₂c' spindles (B) intersected at levels shown in the line drawing of a tandem spindle (left). The 'b₂c' spindle contains one large profile whose intense staining is typical of a bag₂ fibre. In (B), two large profiles are present. One is stained darkly, the other more moderately, in accordance with its identity as a bag₁ fibre. The smaller, lightly stained fibres are chain fibres. Bar = 100 μm.*

the second unit is often smaller and contains fewer intrafusal fibres, usually a single nuclear bag fibre (the bag₂ fibre) from the adjoining spindle and a few intrafusal fibres that are not shared with other spindle units (Figure 2.4). This smaller, so-called 'b₂c' unit (as opposed to the more conventional 'b₁b₂c' spindle unit) generally supports only a single, centrally-placed sensory ending with a smaller axonal diameter than a typical primary ending [56].

These observations are not just interesting from an anatomical point of view. The characteristic sensory signal originating with the spindle depends on the transductive properties of nerve branches on each of the intrafusal fibres that it innervates. The loss of the bag₁ fibre deprives the 'b₂c' unit of the part of the transductive element most responsible for

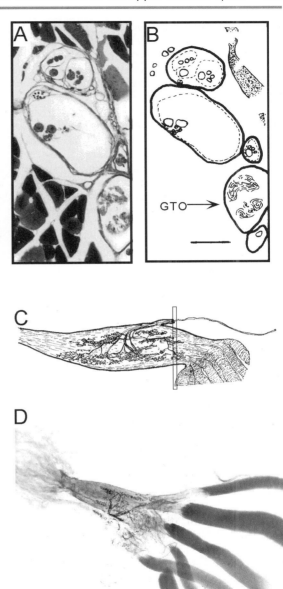

Figure 2.5 *Neck muscle-receptor anatomy. A–B: Photomicrograph (left) and line drawing (right) of a muscle-spindle complex. Numerous muscle spindle capsules are clustered side by side. A Golgi tendon organ (GTO) is also present. Its cross-sectional appearance is like that to be expected if the GTO in the line drawing (C) were to be cut crosswise at the indicated site. In (D), a GTO has been microdissected to show its attachments to several extrafusal muscle fibres. Bar = 100 μm.*

controlling the sensitivity of the velocity-related response. Signals arising from conventional and b_2c units can be differentiated experimentally by exposing spindles to the depolarizing neuromuscular blocker, succinyl-choline [57].

This differentiation suggests that the firing properties of the two spindle units also differ under conditions of dynamic gamma fusimotor drive, which should increase the firing in a b_1b_2c spindle, but not a b_2c spindle. It is not yet clear, however, if this difference is used by the nervous system to extract some special type of information that cannot be obtained from a single spindle type.

The detailed organization of muscle spindles in human neck muscles has been studied less systematically than that in homologous muscles of the cat. However, studies that have been carried out suggest a broadly similar organization. Human muscles are much larger, and densities of spindles are lower in all muscles, but the trend for deep neck muscles to have high spindle densities is found to hold true [49,50,58,59]. In addition, human neck muscles demonstrate a more heterogeneous range of spindle morphologies. Typically, some human spindles contain as many as 14 intrafusal fibres within their capsules. Nevertheless, spindles with only a single nuclear bag fibre have also been reported in deep neck muscles; these are presumably members of the tandem spindle complexes that are also found in human neck muscles ([50,60]).

GOLGI TENDON ORGANS

Golgi tendon organs (GTOs) are encapsulated receptors that are found at the musculotendinous junction rather than contractile parts of muscles (Figure 2.5) (see Proske [61] and Jami [62] for detailed reviews). The sensory axon supplying the GTO has a similar (Group Ib) diameter to that supplying the primary endings of muscle spindles. However, this axon terminates among the collagen strands at the ends of the extrafusal fibres. Here, it branches into numerous fine divisions that braid themselves amongst a group of encapsulated connective tissue bundles at the insertion points of extrafusal fibres. The muscle fibres inserting into the GTO can be fast or slow. Thus, the firing pattern of the GTO is influenced by contractions in a relatively representative

range of motor units composing the muscle around the GTO. The GTO is typically silent when the muscle is passive and unstretched. However, when the connective tissues are pulled by muscle contraction or passive muscle stretch, the straightening of the collagen strands appears to deform and depolarize the interposed receptor endings [63,64]. Firing frequency increases with the amount of stretch or contraction. Thus, the tendon organ is considered to be a 'force transducer' providing the nervous system with a force feedback signal (see Gandevia [65] for review).

Neck muscles are rich in GTOs. In cats they are found not only at the muscle ends, but also in large numbers along intramuscular tendinous inscriptions [51]. They commonly occur in association with muscle spindles, but the functional significance of this association, if any, is not known. Golgi tendon organs are highly sensitive and respond to the contraction of even a single motor unit inserting into the receptor [66–68]. Because neck-muscle motor units are often compartmentalized and confined to only a small region of the muscle (e.g., Armstrong *et al.* [69]), the large numbers of receptors may function to sample different subpopulations of motor units distributed in all muscle parts. Compartmentalization of motor units and receptors has been postulated to permit a greater degree of fine grain control over muscle function (e.g. Botterman *et al.* [70]), but it is not clear whether this opportunity is exploited by higher centres responsible for processing this sensory input.

PACINIFORM CORPUSCLES

Paciniform corpuscles are relatively small cylindrical receptors, formed by lamellations of connective tissue over the end of a sensory axon with an intermediate-sized (Group II) diameter. These receptors are widely distributed in cutaneous structures, connective tissue, muscles and joint capsules [20,52,71] (Figure 2.6). Their onion-like physical appearance resembles a smaller version of the Pacinian corpuscle. Paciniform corpuscles fire a high-frequency transient burst in response to mechanical deformation of the structure with which they are associated [22,72]. Thus they are classed as rapidly adapting mechanoreceptors thought to signal phasic events.

JOINT RECEPTORS

In 1951, McCouch and his colleagues [73] reported that section of nerves supplying the soft tissues around upper cervical joints led to the abolition of 'tonic neck reflexes', an important set of postural reflexes in which the limbs move in response to changes in head position. The receptors responsible for the effects have not yet been identified; muscle receptors are particularly numerous in intervertebral muscles, but receptors in joint capsules and ligaments may also have a role. Joints are known to contain at least two types of mechanoreceptors. Spray-like Ruffini endings (also called type I endings) are reported to be present in the fibrous joint capsules [20,74]. They are usually most sensitive to large joint excursions that stretch the joint capsules to the limits of their range although some receptors may also be active when movements occur in the joint mid-ranges [75–79]. The range and sensitivity of responses have been reported to differ from one joint to another. The differences are attributed to differences in the locations of receptors and differences in the distribution of mechanical forces in different joint capsules. Thus, it is difficult to generalize the results of experimental studies carried out on knee and hip joints, to cervical vertebral joints.

Paciniform corpuscles (also called Type II endings, [20]), are found in joint capsules and surrounding soft tissues (Figure 2.6) and are believed to fire tonically when joint capsules are stretched. Such signals may be useful in marking the beginning or end of movements, but are unlikely to give accurate information about joint position. Ligaments may also contain receptors, notably Golgi-Mazzoni endings that resemble Golgi tendon organs and adapt slowly to ligamentous stretch [80,81].

Whether these receptors are present in any significant numbers in human cervical ligaments remains to be seen.

The relative roles played by muscle, joint and cutaneous receptors in proprioception and kinaesthesia have been subject to controversy in the past (see Gandevia [65] for review). Some of the reported differences appear to depend upon the body part that is studied. For example, cutaneous input may play a larger role in proprioception in the hand than the

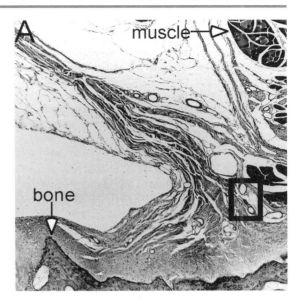

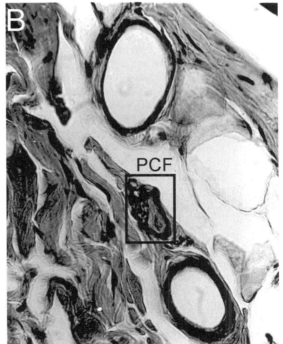

Figure 2.6 *Paciniform corpuscle in cervical joint capsule. (A) Low power photomicrograph to show the location of the receptor close to the site of connective-tissue attachment to the bone. The close proximity of intervertebral muscle is also evident. The boxed region is shown below (B) at higher magnification. The receptor (PCF) has a thickened outer capsule and modest lamellation around a central ending.*

hip. Nevertheless, it seems reasonable to expect that the nervous system uses a mix of sensory information from the periphery to construct an internal model of head position and movement; the reliance placed on different receptors in this mix may vary from joint to joint and possibly even person to person.

ROLES OF SENSORY INPUT

Deficits following sensory lesions

Sensory information from the neck enters the nervous system by way of cervical spinal roots. The importance of this sensory input for the control of movement was recognized as early as 1845, when Longet [82] reported that experimental animals staggered and seemed disoriented after neck muscles had been damaged. Magnus [83] later identified a role for these inputs in tonic neck reflexes that reorient the limbs according to changes in head posture. A number of more recent studies on experimental animals have confirmed that section of neck-muscle nerves or cervical dorsal roots is followed by postural disturbances for which animals can compensate over time (see Abrahams [84] for detailed review). In early stages of recovery, cats adopt an awkward, broad-based posture and show a reluctance to walk. Over the next few days, they exhibit consistent problems of ataxia in which the hindlimbs do not always step in time with the forelimbs. Animals tend to fall over when attempting turns and often avoid the falls by walking close to walls. Monkeys whose dorsal roots are anaesthetized have similar deficits that affect orientation and motor activity of the whole body [85]. They have difficulties in reaching and grasping an object upon which they set their gaze. The fact that they often miss the target suggests a mismatch between visual and proprioceptive cues about the position of the body in space.

The problems of gait that are seen in experimental animals probably come as no surprise to people who have suffered neck damage. Symptoms of 'cervical vertigo', including dizziness, ataxia and nystagmus, have long been recognized to follow whiplash injuries and other types of neck-muscle damage [86–88]. Such symptoms can be reproduced experimentally when neck-muscle receptors are anaesthetized [89], or stimulated by vibrating muscles on one side of the neck [90].

The use of neck-muscle vibration has been particularly useful as a tool to gain insight into some uses made of muscle-spindle input from the neck. Muscle spindles can respond to vibratory movements of only a few micrometres by synchronizing their firing with the vibratory pulses. The new level of entrained muscle-spindle firing appears to be interpreted by the nervous system as a change in muscle length and results in illusory sensations of body position in space. For example, vibration of the lateral neck in the absence of vision produces a compelling sensation described as tilting sideways or falling over [90]. This perception of falling diminishes when subjects open their eyes. Vibration of neck muscles also causes a change in the orientation of the body, usually in a direction opposite to that on which the vibration was applied [91]. Stimulation of neck extensors or flexors gives the illusion that the visual space is moving in a direction opposite to the side of stimulation [92–95]. Neck vibration also produces systematic errors in motor performance. During vibration, subjects are less accurate when asked to orient their heads in the perceived 'straight-ahead' direction or to point in a specified direction [92–94,96]. If a subject is asked to march on the spot with eyes closed, unilateral stimulation causes the subject to walk in a circle towards the side of the stimulation [90].

The importance of deep neck receptors for proprioceptive function is also suggested by tests in populations of patients with long-standing nuchal pathology. Subjects whose necks are damaged by whiplash injuries appear less able to reproduce a specified target position of the head compared with age-matched controls [97]. They also have more difficulty in reproducing a 'straight-ahead' position. These impairments are thought to reflect proprioceptive rather than motor deficits [97]. Heikkilä and Wenngren [98] also found a deterioration in the accuracy of head positioning and reported that subjects with poorer performance in the head-positioning task had more problems with oculomotor performance when following visual targets. Patients with cervico-brachial pain syndromes showed poorer postural control when balance functions were assessed during calf- or neck-muscle vibration or galvanic stimulation of vestibular nerves [99]. These results are consistent with conclusions stated by Cohen [85] from primate studies that 'neck muscle proprioception plays a very important role in maintaining proper orientation, balance and therefore motor coordination of the body'. Cohen went on to conclude: 'Indeed, it is now clear that it is as important for the organism to know the position of its head in relation to its body as it is to know the position of its head in space'.

SPINAL PROJECTIONS FROM NUCHAL AFFERENT FIBRES

The large majority of sensory axons from the neck enter the spinal cord by way of cervical dorsal roots. Even sensory fibres from trapezius and sternocleidomastoideus appear to follow this pattern although motor fibres to these muscles are routed separately through from the spinal accessory nerve (cranial nerve XI) (reviewed in Richmond *et al.* [100]). However, the possibility exists that a few axons with small calibre follow the ventral roots as they are reported to do in lumbrosacral segments [101].

Afferents from the skin have different patterns of projection than those from neck muscles. When the central processes of afferents from the skin are marked using a neuroanatomical tracer, terminations are found chiefly in the most dorsal laminae of the spinal grey matter (particularly its lateral half) and in Lissauer's tract immediately adjacent to the superficial dorsal horn [102,103]. Exposure of neck-muscle nerves to the same tracer results in a different pattern of labelling with more prominent terminations in deeper parts of the dorsal horn and intermediate laminae [103–105]. A particularly strong site of termination is the central cervical nucleus, a cell grouping in medial lamina VII that projects to the cerebellum [103,104,106]. Projections to the cerebellum are also derived from two spino-olivary pathways that take origin from cells in intermediate spinal laminae and relay through both the medial and dorsal accessory olive respectively [107]. Some connections are also made deep in the ventral horn where

motoneurons are situated [106,108–110], but monosynaptic connections are weak. Thus, it has proved very difficult to elicit monosynaptic reflexes in the neck muscles of alert or anaesthetized animals when muscle nerves or even whole dorsal roots are stimulated [111,112].

Afferents do not confine their terminations to the cervical cord. Cutaneous afferents project densely to the main cuneate and trigeminal nuclei [15]. Muscle afferents terminate in the external cuneate nucleus, the lateral part of the cuneate nucleus including cell group x, and the intermediate nucleus of Cajal (see Bakker and Abrahams [113] for detailed review and references). Information from neck afferents ultimately projects onto cells in the vestibular nuclei and the lateral reticular nucleus, where it is believed to interact with vestibular inputs [114–117]. The multiple projections provide a rich array of options by which input from the neck can reach higher centres. One centre on which much attention has been focused is the cerebellum because damage to the cerebellum results in an ataxia much like that produced by sensory damage of cervical nerves [118]. Thus, nuchal afferent projections to the cerebellum may have an important part to play in postural control. Numerous studies in which recordings were made in the cerebellum have identified projections from neck-muscle afferents to lobules IV and V of the anterior lobe [119], the flocculus [120–122], the vermal cortex and the fastigial nucleus [123–126], the paravermal cortex and interpositus nucleus [127], the cerebellar lateral zone and dentate nucleus [128]. However, neck afferents may influence the control of limb posture and gait by other pathways as well. For example, hindlimb motoneurons are facilitated by stimulation of neck afferent fibres even in animals with high spinal section, suggesting that propriospinal projections may also descend to influence motoneurons of the limbs [129].

CLINICAL IMPLICATIONS

Exteroceptive, nociceptive and proprioceptive systems provide a rich composite of information about the state of the neck. The propensity for nociceptors to become sensitized as a result of inflammatory processes may underlie many of the chronic complications following neck injury as discussed in detail later in this book. The proprioceptive system is also vulnerable to damage that leads to significant sensorimotor and postural deficits. Projections from afferent systems are diverse and complex. They appear to reflect a complex system of central processing involving several sites in the brain and spinal cord that are presumably responsible for the widespread and often unpredictable changes that follow neck damage.

REFERENCES

1. Iggo A. Cutaneous receptors. In *The Peripheral Nervous System* (ed. JI Hubbard), New York: Plenum Press, pp. 347–404, 1974.
2. Willis WD Jr, Coggeshall RE. Peripheral nerves, sensory receptors, and spinal roots. In *Sensory Mechanisms of the Spinal Cord* (eds. WD Willis Jr, RE Coggeshall), New York: Plenum Press, pp. 9–51, 1978.
3. Price DD, McHaffie JG, Stein BE. The psychophysical attributes of heat-induced pain and their relationships to neural mechanisms. *J Cog Neurosci* 1992;**4**:1–14.
4. Ohkubo T, Shibata M, Takahashi H, Inoki R. Roles of substance P and somatostatin on transmission of nociceptive information induced by formalin in spinal cord. *J Pharmacol Exper Therap* 1990;**252**:1261–1268.
5. Levine JD, Fields HL, Basbaum AI. Peptides and the primary afferent nociceptor. *J Neurosci* 1993;**13**:2273–2286.
6. Mense S. Review article. Nociception from skeletal muscle in relation to clinical muscle pain. *Pain* 1993;**54**:241–289.
7. Richmond FJR, Anstee GCB, Sherwin EA, Abrahams VC. Motor and sensory fibres of neck muscle nerves in the cat. *Can J Physiol Pharmacol* 1976;**54**:294–304.
8. Stacey MJ. Free nerve endings in skeletal muscle of the cat. *J Anat* 1969;**105**:231–254.
9. Langford LA. Unmyelinated axon ratios in cat motor, cutaneous and articular nerves. *Neurosci Let* 1983;**206**:71–78.
10. Paintal AS. Functional analysis of group III, afferent fibres of mammalian muscles. *J Physiol* 1960;**152**:250–270.
11. Bessou P, Laporte Y. Étude des récepteurs musculaires innervés par les fibres afférentes du groupe III (fibres myélinisées fines) chez le chat. *Arch Ital Biolog* 1961; **99**:293–321.
12. Mense S, Schmidt RF. Activation of group IV afferent units from muscle by algesic agents. *Brain Res* 1974;**72**:305–310.
13. Mense S. Muscular nociceptors. *J Physiol* 1977;**73**:233–240.
14. Sandoz PA, Zenker W. Unmyelinated axons in a muscle nerve. Electron microscopic morphometry of the sternomastoid nerve in normal and sympathectomized rats. *Anat Embryol* 1986;**174**:207–213.
15. Abrahams VC, Lynn B, Richmond FJR. Organization and sensory properties of small myelinated fibers in the dorsal cervical rami of the cat. *J Physiol* 1984;**347**:177–187.
16. Dorn T, Schaible H-G, Schmidt RF. Response properties of thick myelinated group II afferents in the medial articular nerve of normal and inflamed knee joints of the cat. *Somatosens Mot Res* 1991;**8**:127–136.
17. Moncada S, Ferreira SH, Vane JR. Inhibition of prostaglandin biosynthesis as the mechanism of analgesia of aspirin-like drugs in the dog knee joint. *Eur J Pharmacol* 1975;**31**:250–260.
18. Mense S. Reduction of the bradykinin-induced activity of feline group III and IV muscle receptors by acetylsalicylic acid. *J Physiol* 1982;**326**:269–283.
19. Wyke BD. Articular neurology – a review. *Physiother* 1972;**58**:94–99.
20. Wyke BD. Neurology of the cervical spinal joints. *Physiother* 1979;**65**:72–76.
21. Yamada H, Honda T, Kikuchi S, Sugiura Y. Direct innervation of sensory fibers from the dorsal root ganglion of the cervical dura mater of rats. *Spine* 1998;**23**:1524–1530.
22. Burgess PR, Clark FJ. Characteristics of knee joint receptors in the cat. *J Physiol* 1969;**203**:317–335.
23. Schaible H-G, Schmidt RF. Responses of fine medial articular nerve afferents to passive movements of knee joints. *J Neurophysiol* 1983;**49**:1118–1126.
24. Schaible H-G, Schmidt RF. Activation of groups III and IV sensory units in medial articular nerve by local mechanical stimulation of knee joint. *J Neurophysiol* 1983;**49**:35–44.
25. Grigg P, Schaible H-G, Schmidt RF. Mechanical sensitivity of group III and IV afferents from posterior articular nerve in normal and inflamed cat knee. *J Neurophysiol* 1986; **55**:635–643.
26. Cavanaugh JM, El-Bohy A, Hardy WN, Getchell TV, *et al.* Sensory innervation of soft tissues of the lumbar spine in the rat. *J Orthop Res* 1989;**7**:378–388.
27. Coggeshall RE, Hong KAP, Langford LA, Schaible H-G, *et al.* Discharge characteristics of fine medial articular afferents at rest and during passive movements of inflamed knee joints. *Brain Res* 1983;**272**:185–188.
28. Schaible H-G, Schmidt RF. Effects of an experimental arthritis on the sensory proper-

ties of fine articular afferent units. *J Neurophysiol* 1985;**54**:1109–1122.

29. Guilbaud G, Iggo A, Tegnér R. Sensory receptors in ankle joint capsules of normal and arthritic rats. *Exp Brain Res* 1985;**58**:29–40.

30. Kanaka R, Schaible H-G, Schmidt RF. Activation of fine articular afferent units by bradykinin. *Brain Res* 1985;**327**:81–90.

31. Neugebauer V, Schaible H-G, Schmidt RF. Sensitization of articular afferents to mechanical stimuli by bradykinin. *Pflugers Arch* 1989;**415**:330–335.

32. Birrell GJ, McQueen DS, Iggo A, Grubb BD. The effects of 5-HT on articular sensory receptors in normal and arthritic rats. *Br J Pharmacol* 1990;**101**:715–721.

33. Sheather-Reid RB, Cohen ML. Psychophysical evidence for a neuropathic component of chronic neck pain. *Pain* 1998;**75**:341–347.

34. Matthews PBC. *Muscle Receptors*. London: Edward Arnold, 1972.

35. Barker D, Banks RW. The Muscle Spindle. In *Myology* (eds. AG Engel, C Franzini-Armstrong), Toronto, ON: McGraw-Hill, Inc, pp 333–360, 1994.

36. Boyd IA, Smith RS. The Muscle Spindle. In *Peripheral Neuropathy* (eds. P.J. Dyck, P.K. Thomas, E.H. Lombert, R. Bunge), Saunders Co, pp. 171–202, 1984.

37. Prochazka A. Proprioceptive feedback and movement regulation. In . *Exercise: Regulation and integration of multiple system: Neural Control of Movement* (eds. L Rowell, JT Sheperd), New York: American Physiological Society, Section 12, pp. 89–126, 1996.

38. Ovalle WK, Smith RS. Histochemical identification of three types of intrafusal muscle fibers in the cat and monkey based on the myosin ATPase reaction. *Can J Physiol Pharmacol* 1972;**50**:195–202.

39. Banks RW, Harker DW, Stacey MJ. A study of mammalian intrafusal muscle fibres using a combined histochemical and ultrastructural technique. *J Anat* 1977;**123**:783–796.

40. Rowlerson A, Gorza L, Schiaffino S. Immuno-histochemical identification of spindle fibre types in mammalian muscle using type-specific antibodies to isoforms of myosin. In *The Muscle Spindle* (eds. I.A. Boyd, M.H. Gladden), London: Macmillan Press Ltd., pp. 29–34, 1985.

41. Maier A, Gambke B, Pette D. Immunohistochemical demonstration of embryonic myosin heavy chains in adult mammalian intrafusal fibers. *Histochem* 1988;**88**:267–271.

42. Pedrosa F, Butler-Browne GS, Dhoot GK, Fischman DA, *et al.* Diversity in expression of myosin heavy chain isoforms and M-band proteins in rat muscle spindles. *Histochem* 1989;**92**:185–194.

43. Kucera J, Walro JM, Gorza L. Expression of type-specific MHC insoforms in rat intrafusal muscle fibers. *J Histochem Cytochem* 1992;**40**:293–307.

44. Boyd IA, Gladden M. Review – Morphology of Mammalian Muscle Spindles. In *The Muscle Spindle* (eds. IA Boyd, MH Gladden), London: MacMillan, pp3–22, 1996.

45. Banks RW. The motor innervation of mammalian muscle spindles. *Progr Neurobiol* 1994;**43**:323–362.

46. Loeb GE, Hoffer JA. The activity of spindle afferents from cat anterior thigh muscles. II. Effects of fusimotor blockade. *J Neurophysiol* 1985;**54**:565–577.

47. Pedersen J, Sjölander P, Wenngren BI, Johansson H. Increased intramuscular concentration of bradykinin increases the static fusimotor drive to muscle spindles in neck muscles of the cat. *Pain* 1997;**70**:83–91.

48. Voss H. Untersuchungen über zahl, anordnung und länge der muskelspindeln in den lumbricalmuskeln des menschen und einiger tiere. *Anat Anz* 1937; 509–524.

49. Voss H. Zahl und Anordnung der Muskelspindeln in den unteren Zungenbeinmuskeln dem M. sternocleidomastoideus und den Bauch- und teifen Nackmuskeln. *Anatomisch Anzeiger* 1958;**105**:255–275.

50. Cooper S, Daniel PM. Muscle spindles in man; their morphology in the lumbricals and the deep muscles of the neck. *Brain* 1963; **86**:563–586.

51. Richmond FJR, Abrahams VC. Morphology and distribution of muscle spindles in dorsal muscles of the cat neck. *J Neurophysiol* 1975;**38**:1322–1339.

52. Richmond FJR, Bakker DA. Anatomical organization and sensory receptor content of soft tissues surrounding upper cervical vertebrae in the cat. *J Neurophysiol* 1982;**48**:49–61.

53. Keane J. Peripheral organization of the trapezius muscle complex in the cat. Kingston, ON: Queen's University. Thesis, pp.1–177, 1981.

54. Bakker DA, Richmond FJR. Muscle spindle complexes in muscles around upper cervical vertebrae in the cat. *J Neurophysiol* 1982; **48**:62–74.

55. Bakker GJ, Richmond FJR. Two types of muscle spindles in cat neck muscles: a histochemical study of intrafusal fiber composition. *J Neurophysiol* 1981;**45**:973–986.

56. Richmond FJR, Bakker GJ, Bakker DA, Stacey MJ. The innervation of tandem muscle spindles in the cat neck. *J Comp Neurol* 1986;**245**:483–497.

57. Price RF, Dutia MB. Properties of cat neck muscle spindles and their excitation by succinylcholine. *Exp Brain Res* 1987;**68**:619–630.

58. Amonoo-Kuofi HS. The number and distribution of muscle spindles in human intrinsic postvertebral muscles. *J Anat* 1982; **135**:585–599.

59. Amonoo-Kuofi HS. The density of muscle spindles in the medial, intermediate and lateral columns of human intrinsic postvertebral muscles. *J Anat* 1983;**136**:509–519.

60. Bakker DA, Richmond FJR. Receptor organization in human muscles: A detailed study of receptors in rectus capitis posterior major. *Soc Neurosci,* 1981;**7**:273.

61. Proske U. The Golgi tendon organ: Properties of the receptor and reflex action of impulses arising from tendon organs. In *Neurophysiology IV* (ed. R Porter), Baltimore: University Park Press, pp. 127–171, 1981.

62. Jami, L. Golgi tendon organs in mammalian skeletal muscle: Functional properties and central actions. *Physiol Rev* 1992;**72**:623–666.

63. Bridgman CF. The structure of tendon organs in the cat: A proposed mechanism for responding to muscle tension. *Anat Rec* 1968; **162**:209–220

64. Fukami Y, Wilkinson RS. Responses of isolated golgi tendon organs of the cat. *J Physiol* 1977;**265**:673–689.

65. Gandevia SC. Kinesthesia: roles for afferent signals and motor commands. In *Handbook of Physiology, Section 12* (eds. L Rowell, JT Shepherd), New York: Oxford University Press, pp. 128–172, 1996.

66. Binder MD, Kroin JS, Moore GP, Stuart DG. The response of golgi tendon organs to single motor unit contractions. *J Physiol* 1977; **271**:337–349.

67. Gregory JE, Proske U. Motor unit contractions initiating impulses in a tendon organ in the cat. *J Physiol* 1981;**313**:251–262.

68. Binder MD, Osborn CE. Interactions between motor units and golgi tendon organs in the tibialis posterior muscle of the cat. *J Physiol* 1985;**364**:199–215.

69. Armstrong JB, Rose PK, Vanner S, Bakker GJ, et al. Compartmentalization of motor units in the cat neck muscle, biventer cervicis. *J Neurophysiol* 1988;**60**:30–45.

70. Botterman BR, Binder MD, Stuart DG. Functional anatomy of the association between motor units and muscle receptors. *Am Zool* 1978;**18**:135–152.

71. Abrahams VC, Hodgins M, Downey D. Morphology, distribution and density of sensory receptors in the glabrous skin of the cat rhinarium. *J Morphol* 1987;**191**:109–114.

72. Boyd IA. The histological structure of the receptors in the knee-joint of the cat correlated with their physiological response. *J Physiol* 1954;**124**:476–488.

73. McCouch GP, Deering ID, Ling TH. Location of receptors for tonic neck reflexes. *J Neurophysiol* 1951;**14**:191–195.

74. Polacek P. Receptors of the joints: Their structure, variability and classification. Thesis, pp. 1–107, 1966.

75. Godwin-Austen RB. The mechano-receptors of costovertebral joints. *J Physiol* 1969; **202**:737–753.

76. Clark FJ, Burgess PR. Slowly adapting receptors in the cat knee joint: Can they signal joint angle? *J Neurophysiol* 1975;**38**:1448–1463.

77. Carli G, Farabollini F, Fontani G, Meucci M. Slowly adapting receptors in cat hip joint. *J Neurophysiol* 1979;**42**:767–778.

78. Baxendale RH, Ferrell WR. Discharge characteristics of the elbow joint nerve of the cat. *Brain Res* 1983;**261**:195–203.

79. Grigg P, Hoffman AH. Ruffini mechanoreceptors in isolated joint capsule: Responses correlated with strain energy density. *Somatosens Res* 1984;**2**:149–162.

80. Skoglund S. Anatomical and physiological studies of knee joint innervation in the cat. *Acta Physiol Scand* 1956;**36**:7–100.

81. Zimny ML. Mechanoreceptors in articular tissues. *Am J Anat* 1988;**182**,:16–32.

82. Longet FA. Sur les troubles qui surviennent dans l'équilibration, la station et la locomotion des animaux, après la section des parties molles de la nuque. *Gaz Med* Paris, 1845. (Cited in Biemond and De Jong (1969)) 13, 565–567).

83. Magnus R. Some results of studies in the physiology of posture (Cameron Prize lectures). *Lancet* 1926;**211**:531–536, 585–588 (2 parts).

84. Abrahams VC. Neck muscle proprioception and motor control. In *Proprioception, Posture and Emotion* (ed. D Garlick), New South Wales, Australia: The Committee in Postgraduate Medical Education, pp 103–120, 1982.

85. Cohen LA. Role of eye and neck proprioceptive mechanisms in body orientation and motor coordination. *J Neurophysiol* 1961;**24**:1–11.

86. Weeks VD, Travell J. Postural vertigo due to trigger areas in the sternocleidomastoid muscle. *J Pediatr* 1955;**47**:315–322.

87. Cope S, Ryan GMS. Cervical and otolith vertigo. *J Laryngol Otol* 1959;**73**:113–120.

88. Biemond A, De Jong J. On cervical nystagmus and related disorders. *Brain* 1969;**92**:437–458.

89. De Jong PTVM, De Jong JMBV, Cohen B, Jongkees LBW. Ataxia and nystagmus induced by injection of local anaesthetics in the neck. *Ann Neurol* 1977;**1**:240–246.

90. Lund S. Postural effects of neck muscle vibration. *Experientia* 1980;**36**:1398.

91. Popov K, Lekhel H, Bronstein A, Gresty M. Postural responses to vibration of neck muscles

in patients with unilateral vestibular lesions. *Neurosci Lett* 1996;**214**:202–204.

92. Biguer B, Donaldson IML, Hein, A., Jeannerod M. Neck muscle vibration modifies the representation of visual motion and direction in man. *Brain* 1988;**111**:1405–1424.

93. Roll R, Velay JL, Roll JP. Eye and neck proprioceptive messages contribute to the spatial coding of retinal input in visually oriented activities. *Exp Brain Res* 1991;**85**:423–431.

94. Karnath H-O, Sievering D, Fetter M. The interactive contribution of neck muscle proprioception and vestibular stimulation to subjective "straight ahead" orientation in man. *Exp Brain Res* 1994;**101**:140–146.

95. Han Y, Lennerstrand G. Eye movements in normal subjects induced by vibratory activation of neck muscle proprioceptors. *Acta Ophthalmol Scand* 1995;**73**:414–416.

96. Taylor JL, McCloskey DI. Illusions of head and visual target displacement induced by vibration of neck muscles. *Brain* 1991;**114**:755–759.

97. Loudon JK, Ruhl M, Field E. Ability to reproduce head position after whiplash injury. *Spine* 1997;**22**:865–868.

98. Heikkilä HV, Wenngren BI. Cervicocephalic kinesthetic sensibility, active range of cervical motion, and oculomotor function in patients with whiplash injury. *Arch Phys Med Rehabil* 1998;**79**:1089–1094.

99. Karlberg M, Persson L, Magnusson M. Impaired postural control in patients with cervico-brachial pain. *Acta Oto-Laryngol* 1995;**520** (pt 2):440–442.

100. Richmond FJR, Liinamaa TL, Keane J. Morphometry, histochemistry, and innervation of cervical shoulder muscles in the cat. *J Morphol* 1999;**239**:255–269.

101. Coggeshall RE, Maynard CW, Langford LA. Unmyelinated sensory and preganglionic fibers in rat L6 and S1 ventral spinal roots. *J Comp Neurol* 1980;**193**:41–47.

102. Scheurer S, Gottschall J, Groh V. Afferent projections of the rat major occipital nerve studied by transganglionic transport of HRP. *Anat Embryol* 1983;**167**:425–438.

103. Abrahams VC, Keane J. Contralateral, midline, and commissural motoneurons of neck muscles: A retrograde HRP study in the cat. *J Comp Neurol* 1984;**223**:448–456.

104. Ammann B, Gottschall J, Zenker W. Afferent projections from the rat longus capitis muscle studied by transganglionic transport of HRP. *Anat Embryol* 1983;**166**:275–289.

105. Bakker DA, Richmond FJR, Abrahams VC. Central projections from cat suboccipital muscles: A study using transganglionic transport of horseradish peroxidase. *J Compar Neurol* 1984;**228**:409–421.

106. Hirai N, Hongo T, Sasaki S, Yamashita M, *et al*. Neck muscle afferent input to spinocerebellar tract cells of the central cervical nucleus of cat. *Exp Brain Res* 1984;**55**:286–300.

107. Richmond FJR, Courville J, Saint-Cyr JA. Spino-olivary projections from the upper cervical spinal cord: an experimental study using autoradiography and horseradish peroxidase. *Exp Brain Res* 1982;**47**:239–251.

108. Anderson ME. Segmental reflex inputs to motoneurons innervating dorsal neck musculature in the cat. *Exp Brain Res* 1977;**28**:175–187.

109. Rapoport S. Reflex connexions of motoneurones of muscles involved in head movement in the cat. *J Physiol* 1979;311–327.

110. Rose PK, Keirstead SA. Segmental projection from muscle spindles: A perspective from the upper cervical spinal cord. *Can J Physiol Pharmacol* 1986;**64**:505–507.

111. Abrahams VC, Richmond FJR, Rose PK. Absence of monosynaptic reflex in dorsal neck muscles in the cat. *Brain Res* 1975;**92**:130–131.

112. Richmond FJR, Loeb GE. Electromyographic studies of neck muscles in the intact cat. II. Reflexes evoked by muscle nerve stimulation. *Exp Brain Res* 1992;**88**:59–66.

113. Bakker DA, Abrahams VC. Central projections from nuchal afferent systems. In *Control of Head Movement* (eds. BW Peterson, FJR Richmond), New York: Oxford University Press, pp.63–75, 1988.

114. Corvaja N, Mergner T, Pompeiano O. Organization of reticular projections to the vestibular nuclei in the cat. *Prog Brain Res* 1979; **50**:631–644.

115. Coulter JD, Mergner T, Pompeiano O. Integration of afferent inputs from neck muscles and macular labyrinthine receptors within the lateral reticular nucleus. *Arch Ital Biol* 1977;**115**:332–354.

116. Kubin L, Magherini PC, Manzoni D, Pompeiano O. Responses of lateral reticular neurons to sinusoidal rotation of neck in the decerebrate cat. *Neurosci* 1981;**6**:1277–1290.

117. Kubin L, Manzoni D, Pompeiano O. Responses of lateral reticular neurons to convergent neck and macular vestibular inputs. *J Neurophysiol* 1981;**46**:48–64.

118. Manzoni D, Pompeiano O, Stampaccia G. Tonic cervical influences on posture and reflex movements. *Arch Ital Biol* 1979;**117**:81–110.

119. Berthoz A, Llinás R. Afferent neck projections to the cat cerebellar cortex. *Exp Brain Res* 1974;**20**:385–401.

120. Wilson VJ, Maeda M, Franck JI. Input from neck afferents to the cat flocculus. *Brain Res* 1975;**89**:133–138.

121. Wilson VJ, Maeda M, Franck JI. Inhibitory interaction between labyrinthine, visual and neck inputs to the cat flocculus. *Brain Res* 1975;**96**:357–360.

122. Wilson VJ, Maeda M, Franck JI, Shimazu H. Mossy fiber neck and second order labyrinthine projections to cat flocculus. *J Neurophysiol* 1976;**39**:301–310.

123. Erway LC, Ghelarducci B, Pompeiano O, Stanojevic M. Responses of cerebellar fastigial neurons to afferent inputs from neck muscles and macular labyrinthine receptors. *Arch Ital Biol* 1978;**116**:173–224.

124. Denoth F, Magherini PC, Pompeiano O, Stanojevic M. Responses of Purkinje cells of the cerebellar vermis to neck and macular vestibular inputs. *Pflugers Arch* 1979;**381**:87–98.

125. Denoth F, Magherini PC, Pompeiano O, Stanojevic M. Neck and macular labyrinthine influences on the Purkinje cell of the cerebellar vermis. In *Reflex Control of Posture and Movement* (eds. R Granit, O Pompeiano), Amsterdam: Elsevier/North-Holland: Biomedical Press, pp. 515–527, 1979

126. Denoth F, Magherini PC, Pompeiano O, Stanojevic M. Responses of Purkinje cells of cerebellar vermis to sinusoidal rotation of neck. *Exp Brain Res* 1980;**18**:548–562.

127. Boyle R, Pompeiano O. Response characteristics of cerebellar interpositus and intermediate cortex neurons to sinusoidal stimulation of neck and labyrinth receptors. *Neurosci* 1980;**5**:357–372.

128. Chan YS, Manzoni D, Pompeiano O. Response characteristics of cerebellar dentate and lateral cortex neurons to sinusoidal stimulation of neck and labyrinth receptors. *Neurosci* 1982;**7**:2993–3011.

129. Kenins P, Kikillus H, Schomburg ED. Short and long-latency reflex pathways from neck afferents to hindlimb motoneurones in the cat. *Brain Res* 1978;**149**:235–238.

Chapter 3

Neurophysiological mechanisms of head, face and neck pain

James W. Hu

PAIN: BIOLOGICAL SIGNIFICANCE

Pain in humans is defined as 'an unpleasant sensory and emotional experience associated with actual or potential tissue damage, or described in terms of such damage' [1]. It is a uniquely human experience; in fact, the word 'nociception' is used for pain behaviour or experience associated with animals. According to the preceding definition, pain has two essential qualities: a sensory, discriminative aspect and an emotional, affective or suffering aspect. The McGill Pain Questionnaire (MPQ) uses two sets of words to measure pain quality [2]. For example, the words used to describe the sensory aspect of pain are 'sharp, cutting, and lacerating', while the words 'fearful, frightful and terrifying' are used for the affective aspect.

There are also two types of pain. The first type is transient pain, which is protective; it warns us of impending tissue damage and forces us to rest the injured part and avoid further damage. The stimulus can be identified. It usually resolves in a short period – hours or days. The second type is chronic pain; it persists a long time after the injury or inflammation has apparently healed, possibly for months or years. Sometimes, this pain has no apparent origin, or is stimulus independent. Chronic pain is non-protective and is considered to be a disease, the treatment of which is paramount to one's health. This chapter will deal with both types of pain and will review the information concerning mainly the head and neck region.

The major nerves in the head and neck region are the cranial nerve V, also called the trigeminal nerve, and the upper cervical spinal nerves. The trigeminal nerve innervates the intraoral structures, face, masticatory muscles, temporomandibular joint (TMJ), and intracranial vessels, while the upper cervical spinal nerves innervate the scalp and neck region (also see chapter 2 by Richmond and Corneil). As reviewed below, central pain processing concerning these two areas involves what is really a continuous unit. This is why the manifestation of injuries in the head and neck region can overlap and become widespread in both regions. For example, whiplash can result in symptoms such as headache, temporomandibular joint disorders, stiff neck, etc. Accordingly, this review will cover pain processing and pathways in both the trigeminal and upper cervical nerves.

CUTANEOUS PRIMARY AFFERENT FIBRES INNERVATE CRANIOFACIAL AND NECK REGIONS

Somatosensory receptors can be classified as mechanoreceptors, thermoreceptors or nociceptors. A free nerve ending or specialized structure is associated with these receptors. Conventionally, the nerve conduction velocities are the most important attribute for classification of these different primary afferent fibres, i.e., A-beta (80–40 m/s), A-delta (40–2.5 m/s) and C-fibres (less than 2.5 m/s). The A-fibres are myelinated nerve fibres and C fibres are unmyelinated. Mechanoreceptors have many types, including a fast-conducting, fast-adapting type (FA) and a fast-conducting, slow-adapting type (SA). Mechanoreceptors have conduction velocities in the A-beta to C-fibre range; however, the majority of them are in the A-beta range. Some mechanoreceptors have a high threshold of activation and, as a result, are termed mechanonociceptors, with conduction velocity in the A-delta range. The thermal and mechanical nociceptors are associated with a small fibre population (A-delta and C-fibre range) because their conduction velocities are relatively slower than the majority of low-threshold mechanoreceptors of the A-beta fibre population. The most extensively studied C-fibre type is the polymodal C-nociceptor that responds to noxious mechanical, heat and chemical stimulation.

Recently it has been shown that C-fibre afferent nociceptors can be divided into two major subpopulations: IB-4-positive and CGRP-positive [3]. The former are sensitive to mechanical stimuli but not to heat stimuli. The latter contain the neuropeptides, such as CGRP, substance P and other neurokinins, and are heat sensitive. The functional significance of this division is still to be elucidated. Through the use of receptor cloning techniques [4] at least five different nociceptive receptor types have been identified: VR-1 receptors (a capsaicin-sensitive, heat-sensitive type), two types of acid-sensitive (proton) receptors, P2X3 (ATP-sensitive) receptors, and TTX-insensitive sodium channel receptors (assumed to play a part in neuropathic pain) [5]. It is too early to associate these cloned receptors with a particular defined function of known nociceptors, such as heat, high threshold mechanoreceptors or polymodal nociceptors at different conductive velocities definitively, but a solution is near.

When a brief noxious electrical or heat stimulus is applied to the remote part of an extremity, human subjects can feel two distinct and separate painful sensations: a well localized, sharp 'first pain' which is mediated by A-delta fibre afferents, and a poorly localized, diffuse 'second pain,' which is mediated by C-fibre afferents [6]. Since the conductive distance of the neck and facial region is relatively short, it is difficult to detect first and second pain separately.

FUNCTIONAL SIGNIFICANCE OF THE NERVE FIBRE TYPES IN DEEP TISSUES

Free nerve endings in the craniofacial and neck region provide the peripheral basis for pain; many free nerve endings act as nociceptors, i.e., they are the sense organs that respond to noxious stimulation of peripheral tissues [7]. Their activation may result in the excitation of the small-diameter (A-delta or C) afferent nerve fibres with which they are associated and which provide sensory, discriminative information to the brain about the location, quality, intensity and duration of the noxious stimulus. One important feature of these afferent fibres that innervate deep tissues, which is also true for those which innervate visceral organs, is the so-called 'silent nociceptor'. These afferent fibres have an extremely high threshold of activation; they are thus silent during normal motor action and do not become activated until an organ or tissue is inflamed, whereupon their activating thresholds reduce dramatically [7]. The inflammatory mediators (see Table 3.1) are crucial for the activation of these silent nociceptors.

The temporomandibular joint (TMJ) contains numerous free nerve endings, but there is not an abundance of the more specialized endings. Most of the afferents supplying these specialized and non-specialized receptors are less than 10 μm in diameter (i.e. Groups II, III and IV), especially in those species lacking specialized receptors [8–10]. Many of these small-diameter afferents contain substance P and other neuropeptides involved in nociception and neurogenic inflammation, and some of the innervating fibres are not afferents but efferents of the sympathetic nervous system. These afferents as well as smaller diameter sensory nerve fibres and sympathetic afferents also supply the masticatory muscles. Little information exists on the functional properties of the smaller diameter afferents that supply these muscles and the TMJ, many of which appear to be nociceptive (for review, see Hannam and Sessle [11]).

Table 3.1 Neuroactive substances related to peripheral and central pain processing

Substances	Natural ligands/actions	Receptors	Functions
Peripherally activated substance/receptors/actions			
Bradykinin	Bradykinin	Bk1, BK2	Inflammatory mediator/sensitized afferents
Histamine	Histamine	H1, H2	Inflammatory mediator/sensitized afferents
PGE$_2$	PGE$_2$		Inflammatory mediator/sensitized afferents
5HT	5HT	5HT1B	Inflammatory mediator/sensitized afferents
ATP	ATP	P2X3	Mechanonociceptive
Nerve growth factors	Nerve growth factors		Wide range of sensitization, especially to deep tissues
Ka+	Ka+	Wide range of receptors	Generalized activation/sensitize afferents
H+ (proton)	Mechanical deformation?	Acid-sensing proton-gated	Mechanosensitive/sensitized afferents
CGRP	CGRP	?	Sensory/neurotrophic function
Substance P	Substance P	NK-1	Vasodilatation/sensitized afferents
Neurokinin A	Neurokinin A	NK-2	Vasodilatation/sensitized afferents
Capsaicin	Heat	VR-1	Acts on C-fibre afferents
Acetylcholine	?	?	Modulators
Opioids	enkephalins, endorphins Dynorphin, etc.	mu, kappa, delta	Inhibitory action
Glutamate	glutamate	Ionotropic, NMDA, AMPA, KA	Small nociceptive afferents/sensitized afferents
Noradrenaline	noradrenaline	Ionotropic, alpha, beta	Activate small injured afferents/neuropathic pain
Cholecystokinin	cholecystokinin		?
Bombesin	bombesin		?
Cannabinoid	Anandamide	CB1	Antinociception
Centrally activated substance/receptors/actions			
Glutamate	Glutamate/aspartate	Ionotropic, NMDA, AMPA, KA	Central sensitization and activation of neurons
5HT	5HT	5HT-1A, 5HT1D and others	Nociceptive neurons, related to migraine
Adenosin	ATP, ADP	P2X3, IB-4 positive neurons	Mechanical nociception
CGRP	CGRP	?	Central sensitization
Substance P	Substance P	NK-1	Central sensitization
Neurokinin A	Neurokinin A	NK-2	Central sensitization
Acetylcholine	Acetylcholine	Nicotinic, Muscarinic	Central nociceptive neurons
Opioids	enkephalins, endorphins etc. Dynorphin, etc.	mu, kappa, delta Kappa	Mainly inhibitory action on central neurons Excitatory
Noradrenaline	noradrenaline	Ionotropic, alpha 2	Activate small injured afferents/pain modulation
Cholecystokinin	cholecystokinin	CCK	Anti-opioid action
Cannabinoid	Anandamide	CB1, CB2	Antinociception plus psychoactive actions
Galanin	Galanin	?	Up-regulated after deafferentation

In most muscles, some of the large, fast-conducting afferents are associated with specialized receptors, e.g., muscle spindles and Golgi tendon organs. These various low-threshold receptors are considered to have a role in perceptual and reflex responses related to muscular and articular stimuli. Chapter 2 has described in detail the innervation patterns of deep tissues in the neck region.

SENSITIZATION AND LOCAL INTERACTION AT THE DEEP PRIMARY AFFERENT RECEPTORS

Repeated noxious stimuli or exposure to so-called inflammatory mediators, such as bradykinin and serotonin, and prostaglandins, such as PGE2 (see Table 3.1), reduces the threshold of these nociceptors and increases their response magnitude. These changes define the state of 'primary afferent sensitization' (in contrast with central sensitization occurring in the central neurons, see below). In the case of deep afferents, this sensitization process is critical to the change from silent nociceptors to active ones (see above).

Recent advances from studying the primary afferents from deep craniofacial and spinal structures indicate the existence of several excitatory and inhibitory receptor types, including glutamate, an excitatory amino acid (EAA), [12], opioid [13] and γ-aminobutyric acid (GABA) [14] receptors. Glutamate, as well as receptor subtypes NMDA, AMPA and kainate, applied to craniofacial tissues evokes the reflex expression of neuroplasticity that can be blocked by peripheral co-administration of specific receptor subtype antagonists [12,15]. There are marked differences between male and female rats in terms of the magnitude of glutamate-evoked jaw muscle electromyographic (EMG) activity. These differences appear to be mediated, in part, by oestrogen levels, since female gonadectomy eliminates these sex-related differences, while oestrogen replacement therapy restores them. These findings open up new perspectives on the mechanisms underlying nociceptive processing and pain and, in addition, point to peripheral as well as central neurochemical features that may prove to be of clinical significance in the development of additional therapeutic approaches to managing craniofacial pain.

The opioid [16] and GABA-A [14] receptors are inhibitory types that can suppress the nociceptive reflex behaviour if these algesic compounds are applied directly to temporomandibular tissue. There exists a possibility of complex interactions in the peripheral environment. These local interactions are theoretically possible, but the source of these ligands, i.e., active endogenous substances that can activate these receptor mechanisms, is uncertain. For example, direct application of morphine or other opiates at the relative higher concentration than the one existing in the normal tissue into the knee during a knee joint operation can produce an analgesic action [17], but no-one can be sure that these concentrations can be achieved via an endogenous process (or processes) such as the release of enkephalins from macrophages or mast cell degranulation. Discoveries of these functional receptor types in the periphery may provide a basis for novel therapeutic treatments. However, such potential has yet to be fulfilled. This author speculates that manipulation or massage within the deep tissues could lead to a release or a redistribution of the inhibitory receptor ligands, such as GABA, which are ubiquitously distributed in the whole body, and possible endogenous opioids, which may be released by mast cells. This redistribution could reduce the excitability of already activated nociceptive afferents as a result of muscular soreness, stiffness or localized pain.

SECOND-ORDER NEURONS IN THE UPPER CERVICAL SPINAL DORSAL HORN (UCDH) AND TRIGEMINAL BRAINSTEM COMPLEX:

Both the central projection sites within the trigeminal (V) brainstem complex of TMJ and the craniofacial muscle nociceptive afferents have also received limited attention. In spinal afferents, the projection of Group III deep afferents to laminae I, IV and V has been documented, although the laminar projection of Group IV deep nociceptive afferents is not yet resolved [18–20]. Similarly, anatomical studies have shown that craniofacial deep afferents project to one or more subdivisions of the

V brainstem complex including both the superficial and deeper laminae of the V subnucleus caudalis (Vc) as well as the UCDH [21,22]. The close functional similarity, as well as the parallels in morphological and immunohistochemical features between the subnucleus caudalis and the spinal dorsal horn have led to the former's designation as the medullary dorsal horn (see Dubner and Bennett [23], Gobel *et al.* [24] and Sessle *et al.* [25] and below). These include the laminar structure (i.e., at least five or six laminae), substantia gelatinosa, specific primary afferent terminal patterns associated with specific afferent types, and the presence of nociceptive neurons. In fact, there is no dividing line between the UCDH and Vc; it is an anatomical and functional continuum (see below). In rats, Molander *et al.* [26] have delineated each UCDH and Vc with anatomical landmarks. In additional to the criteria mentioned by Molander *et al.*, this author has made additional observations which show three important anatomical points separating the UCDH and Vc: (1) deep bundles, a landmark structure for internuclear communications within the V brainstem complex [24], are present in C1 but not C2; (2) the Lissauer tract appears at C2 dorsal horn, and not in C1 dorsal horn; (3) ventral horn or motor neurons appear at the C1DH level. Thus, the transition from the medullary dorsal horn to the spinal dorsal horn is gradual without any marked anatomical separation.

The afferents innervating craniofacial deep structures (e.g. joint, muscle) as well as cutaneous, intraoral, deep cerebrovascular tissues project to the V brainstem complex. The V brainstem complex can be subdivided into the main or principal sensory nucleus and the spinal tract nucleus, which comprises three subnuclei – oralis, interpolaris and caudalis (Figure 3.1). Based on anatomical, clinical and electrophysiological observations, the subnucleus caudalis is usually viewed as the principal brainstem relay site of V nociceptive information ([27–29], and see Sessle [30]). For example, anatomical studies have revealed that the small-diameter afferents carrying nociceptive information from the various craniofacial tissues terminate predominantly in the caudalis laminae I, II and V/VI. Moreover, recent immunocytochemical studies of the expression of proto-oncogene, c-fos (a marker associated with noxious activation) have revealed that increased c-fos expression occurs in the caudalis neurons, and in some cases the UCDH as well, following noxious stimulation of craniofacial tissues including skin, TMJ, cornea and cerebrovascular tissues [31–33]. These findings are consistent with observations that V tractotomy near the obex in humans or analogous lesions in experimental animals may produce a profound facial analgesia (and thermoanaesthesia) to stimulation of certain parts of the craniofacial region (but ineffective in producing anaesthesia for intraoral structures), without the loss of tactile sensibility. Craniofacial noxious stimulation of deep tissues also reflexly evokes autonomic responses (e.g., blood pressure, respiration) as well as muscle activities. Recent studies here revealed that many of these are dependent on a relay in the subnucleus caudalis and the UCDH [12] (see Hu *et al.* [34]). However, studies show the inputs from neck region are more complex with neuron distribution overlapping in both the caudalis and the UCDH region (see below).

Electrophysiological studies have revealed that many neurons, in both the caudalis and the UCDH, respond to cutaneous nociceptive inputs; these nociceptive neurons have been categorized as either 'nociceptive-specific (NS) neurons' or 'wide dynamic range (WDR) neurons' [27–29] (see Sessle [30]). The NS neurons respond only to noxious stimuli (e.g., pinching and heat) applied to a localized craniofacial receptive field (RF) and receive small-diameter afferent inputs from A-delta and/or C fibres. WDR neurons are excited by non-noxious (e.g., tactile) stimuli as well as by noxious stimuli, and may receive large-diameter and small-diameter A-fibre inputs as well as C-fibre inputs. Many NS and WDR neurons in the subnucleus caudalis and the UCDH can be excited only by natural stimulation of cutaneous or mucosal tissues and have properties consistent with a role in the detection, localization and discrimination of superficial noxious stimuli [27,28,35] (see Table 3.2). These nociceptive neurons have properties indicating a role in localization and intensity coding of noxious thermal facial, cornea or tooth-pulp stimuli [28,29,35]. The majority of NS and WDR neurons can, none the less, also be excited by other types of peripheral afferent inputs such as those from TMJ, masticatory muscle nerves or C1/C2 nerves [25,27,36–38].

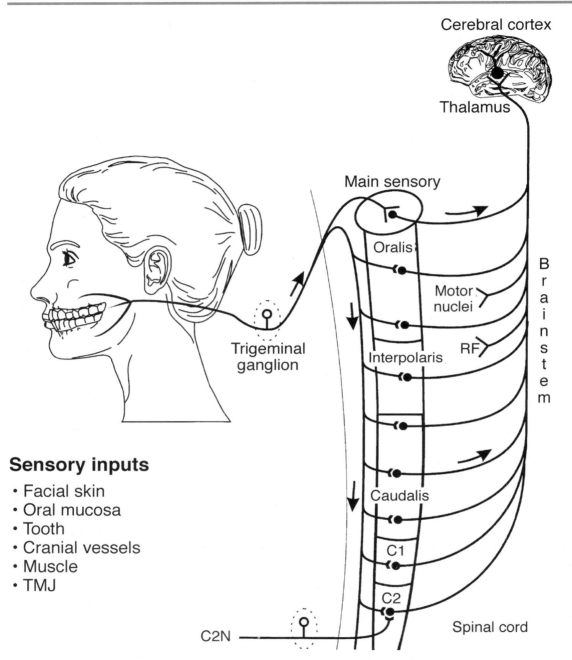

Sensory inputs

- Facial skin
- Oral mucosa
- Tooth
- Cranial vessels
- Muscle
- TMJ

Figure 3.1 *Major somatosensory pathways from the face and mouth. Note that trigeminal primary afferents project via the trigeminal (V) ganglion to second-order neurons in the V brainstem complex. These neurons may project to neurons in brainstem regions such cranial nerve nuclei or the reticular formation (RF) or in higher levels of the brain (e.g., in the thalamus). Not shown are the projections of some cervical nerve afferents and cranial nerve VII, IX, X, XII and the first few cervical spinal nerves to the V complex and the projection of many VII, IX and X afferents to the solitary tract nucleus. Further input via C2N nerve of the second cervical nerve is detailed in the previous chapters (From Sessle, 1999, with modifications, reprinted from* Journal of Orofacial Pain, *with permission).*

The subnucleus caudalis is considered as a rostral extension of the UCDH. Interesting studies in rats, cats and monkeys [39–45] indicate that these nociceptive neurons with receptive fields mainly in the face, neck and upper arm are indicative of normal innervation for these upper cervical dermatomes. Except for the receptive field location/organization, the nociceptive neurons from Vc and UCDH both have their afferent inputs; the response properties, laminal distribution and projection status of nociceptive neurons for both Vc and UCDH are very similar. In addition, these neurons also receive very wide-ranging input from various visceral and autonomic inputs, such as cardial, phrenic and sympathetic nerves if either electrical or algesic chemical stimuli are used for testing. Further evidence to support this view has been provided by c-fos expression experiments when the vaga or hypoglossal nerves were stimulated electrically [46,47]. Fos-positive neurons were observed at the same location at the superficial laminae of the caudal Vc and C1/C2 DH in addition to the transition zone of Vi/Vc, similar to those found with TMJ-fos expression experiments (see above).

In a rat study from a different vantage point, Sun *et al.* [38] (see Table 3.1) showed that the same population of nociceptive neurons in the C1 and C2 DH received wide facial cutaneous input along with input from one of the jaw muscles (i.e., hypoglossal nerve or tongue musculature). There is a trend that the more caudal the location (of relative anterior and posterior position) in the DH, the more the mechanoreceptive field shows a posterior location, gradually moving from the facial into the neck region. Foreman [45] argues these particular convergent patterns, especially via vagal input, and neuronal mechanoreceptive fields, are critically important for referral of pain to the neck and jaw during angina pectoris. Chandler *et al.* [39,40] showed that vagal stimulation serves as a more potent stimulus to activate UCDH neurons (with their RF either in face or neck) than the input from sympathetic cardiopulmonary afferent input. Furthermore, they also showed a wide range of visceral inputs to C1and C2 DH [40].

The projection status of the UCDH is important to discuss in detail. In three species, i.e., the rat, cat and monkey, over half of the spinothalamic neurons were found to be located in the deeper lamina (lamina IV to VII) of the UCDH (see Willis and Coggeshall [48]). The UCDH is known for heavy projection to the ventroposterior lateral (VPL: for body representation) or medial (VPM: for face representation) nuclei of thalamus ([49], and see Willis and Coggeshall [48]). These spinothalamic neurons are considered to be the critical element for the sensory discriminative aspect of pain. The trigeminal subnucleus caudalis (so-called trigeminothalamic projection) as well as the other DHs did not have such a high concentration of the thalamic projection neurons. The location of projection neurons are those which received heavy convergent inputs from vagal, phrenic, neck as well as a wide range of craniofacial inputs (see above). On the contrary, there are heavy projections from the marginal layer (or lamina I) of Vc and UCDH to the parabrachial area (PBA) which is one of the integral centres for autonomic function [50,51].

The functional significance of the organization of the caudalis and the UCDH is unclear at the present. However, there are two possible explanations to account for the above-discussed neural organization regarding this highly convergent pattern. The first explanation argues that each region in the caudalis and UCDH has a different degree of convergence and represents different functions. The high degree of spinothalamic projection and the unusual convergent pattern makes this explanation less likely. Foreman [45] also reviewed evidence that there are distinct influences on the cardiopulmonary function from different spinal regions, such as excitatory thorax inputs versus inhibitory lumbar inputs. Thus, the unique characteristics of the neural organization of the caudal Vc and the UCDH favours the alternative explanation. The second explanation argues the caudal Vc and the first two cervical dorsal horns are the site of significant and special sensory processing with a high incidence of thalamic projection as well as a site receiving special sensory convergence (i.e., muscular and visceral) from the head and body. According to this explanation, the UCDH and caudal Vc represent a previously undiscovered integral centre for these visceral/deep inputs. Indeed, Villanueva *et al.* [52] proposed that subnucleus reticularis dorsalis neurons in the rat medulla are the critical relay and integrative centre for 'diffuse

Table 3.2 Comparison of properties of the nociceptive neurons recorded from rostral subnucleus caudalis (RVc, data from Hu, 1990), caudal Vc and C1 dorsal horn (CVc/Cl DH) and C2 dorsal horn (C2DH)

Location (Cell number)	Wide dynamic range neurons (%)			Nociceptive-specific neurons (%)		
	RVc (51)	CVc/C1DH (10)	C2DH (15)	RVc (27)	CVc/C1DH (16)	C2DH (23)
Peripheral afferent inputs:						
Response to noxious heat	90	70	93 / 71	81	79	
C-afferent from skin (electrical)	80	100	92 / 33	50	56	
XII nerve (electrical)	51	70	80 / 65	24	50	
Mechanoreceptive field (RF):						
Involving V RF	100	100	100 / 100	100	100	
Involving intraoral component	51	28	46 / 39	50	62	
Involving neck, occiput or back of ear (C1/C2 RF)	N/A	50	73	N/A	25	43
Involving TMJ deep component	N/A	33	71	N/A	67	57

noxious inhibitory controls' (DNIC) (see below for detail). These subnucleus reticularis dorsalis neurons have very wide mechanoreceptive fields with wide convergence from many parts of the body. Indeed, the subnucleus reticularis dorsalis is located in the caudal and ventral to the Vc, and Hu [27] argued that this structure was located below the Vc and possessed a different functional entity. At present, further research is needed to clarify the relationship between the subnucleus reticularis dorsalis and either the Vc/C1 DH because these share the same exact brainstem/spinal position but are located at different depths [27]. None the less, the caudal Vc and UCDH could be a very important area for sensory integration, not only critical to the craniofacial and neck region but also to a wide range of convergence from many internal organs and many parts of the body, including visceral and deep structures. Therapeutic treatments in the neck and facial region may have more profound effects than previously conceived (see below: 'Afferent and descending modulation').

The properties of nociceptive neurons in the brain (spinal/brainstem and supraspinal sites) can also be modified as a consequence of peripheral nerve injuries as well as by peripheral tissue trauma and inflammatory conditions. They appear to be due to mechanisms that reflect a 'functional plasticity' or 'central sensitization' of nociceptive neurons and involvement of the extensive pattern (see below) of convergent afferent inputs to these neurons [53,54]. For example, in both the Vc and the UCDH, the injection of the inflammatory irritant and small-fibre excitant, mustard oil, into deep tissues (such as the TMJ, masticatory or neck muscles) can lead to expansion of the RF and enhancement of the responses to cutaneous stimuli in the NS and WDR neurons [55,56] (Hu, Sun and Vernon, unpublished data). Chemical stimulation of cerebrovascular or corneal afferents may also induce comparable neuroplastic changes in Vc/UCDH brainstem neurons [57,58]. Recently, similar hyperexcitability of Vc nociceptive neurons was also observed 24 hours after long-acting inflammatory stimuli, using complete Freund's adjuvant [59]. These irritant-induced changes in the craniofacial and neck tissues may evoke hyperexcitability in Vc/UCDH neurons and may be accompanied by reflexly induced activity in jaw and neck muscles ([15,60], and see Hu *et al.* [34]).

These neuroplastic changes are remarkable since, depending on the stimulus or form of injury or inflammation, they can last for hours or days, even weeks, and are associated clinically with behavioural changes in pain sensitivity.

REFLEXES EVOKED BY NECK AND CRANIOFACIAL NOCICEPTIVE INPUTS

Craniofacial somatosensory inputs into the CNS may access brainstem motor and autonomic systems as well as ascending sensory systems. Reflex activity in the craniofacial muscles and autonomic reflex changes (e.g., in blood pressure, respiration, salivation) have been studied extensively by stimulating cutaneous, mucosal, dental pulp and periodontal afferent inputs (see Hannam and Sessle [11]). In contrast, reflex responses specifically evoked by applying nociceptive stimuli to articular and muscle receptors have not been investigated to any great extent until recently, although a jaw-opening reflex (transient jaw-closing muscle inhibition and jaw-opening muscle activation) as well as a tongue protrusive reflex can be elicited by stimulation of these receptors. In 1993, Hu *et al.* [60] reported that a prolonged inflammatory stimulus, MO, injected into the neck paraspinal region provoked muscle activity not only in the neck bilateral superficial and deep muscles but also in the jaw muscles. This study and other craniofacial studies have shown that sustained noxious stimulation of high-threshold craniofacial articular and muscle receptors can produce jaw reflex effects which are longer lasting, and perhaps more clinically relevant than the transient responses employed in previous studies (see Hannam and Sessle [11]). For example, in the rat, significant and reversible increases in electromyographic (EMG) activity in jaw-closing as well as jaw-opening muscles, which lasted 3–15 minutes, occurred when MO was injected into the TMJ region [15] or neck [60]. There is evidence indicating TMJ-evoked reflex activity is dependent on the intactness of the subnucleus caudalis (see Hu *et al.* [34]) and the involvement of NMDA mechanisms, similar to the neuroplasticity induced by inflammation (see above).

Recently, evidence has also shown the involvement of central opioid mechanisms in neuroplastic changes in Vc nociceptive neurons and associated jaw-muscle activity. Systemic administration of the opiate antagonist naloxone 30 minutes after MO injection into the tongue muscle enhances the excitability of nociceptive Vc neurons [61]. Likewise, systemic or central administration of naloxone 30 minutes after the MO injection to the TMJ region significantly increases (i.e. 're-kindles') jaw-muscle activity after it has returned to baseline levels [62–64]. That naloxone induced the rekindling effect was also demonstrated in a dose-dependent process when MO was injected into the neck to evoke neck muscle activity. These findings suggest the recruitment of a central opioid inhibitory mechanism evoked by a nociceptive afferent input, which evokes Vc and UCDH nociceptive neuronal activity and associated neuromuscular changes. In turn, this opioid inhibitory mechanism could limit the central neural changes associated with the nociceptive afferent input related to the central sensitization/hyperexcitability process [34,61,62].

AFFERENT AND DESCENDING MODULATION

Afferent or segmental inhibition of tactile transmission has been extensively studied within LTM neurons in the V brainstem nuclei, spinal, dorsal column nuclei and neurons at higher levels of the CNS. This inhibitory influence appears to reflect mechanisms necessary for 'sharpening' the coding properties of LTM neurons and to contribute to spatial acuity of touch sensation. For nociceptive neurons, investigations of the effects of peripherally evoked afferent inputs on craniofacial nociceptive processes have primarily involved the efficacy of noxious or non-noxious stimuli, or therapeutic procedures such as acupuncture and transcutaneous electrical nerve stimulation (TENS) ([30,65–67], for review see Melzack [68] and Woolf and Thompson [69]). These studies have shown that acupuncture and TENS may inhibit, for example, the jaw-opening reflex and trigeminal neuronal responses elicited by tooth-pulp stimulation in animals, and may also raise the threshold of pulp-evoked sensations in humans. The responses of neurons to small-diameter afferent inputs evoked by pulp, TMJ, muscle or cutaneous noxious stimuli can also be suppressed by non-noxious stimuli (e.g., vibratory or tactile) that excite large afferent nerve fibres. Vagal afferent stimulation may also be effective [70].

Noxious stimulation applied to various spatially dispersed regions of the body may also inhibit V neuronal, reflex or perceptual responses to small-fibre craniofacial nociceptive afferent inputs. Le Bars and colleagues called this inhibitory action 'diffuse noxious inhibitory controls' (DNIC). In simple words, pain can inhibit pain since small-diameter (A-delta and C-fibres) afferents appear responsible for the inhibitory effects (see Le Bars *et al.* [71,72] and Villanueva *et al.* [73]). This mechanism may be related to findings in humans that thermal pain perception can be decreased by noxious counterirritants (and non-noxious stimuli), and that noxious forearm ischaemia is very effective in reducing the intensity, unpleasantness and spatial referral of pulpal pain (for review, see Maixner *et al.* [66], Melzack [68] and Woolf and Thompson [69]). Hu [27] demonstrated that the cutaneous as well as deep input of nociceptive Vc neurons can be modulated with noxious heat from a rat's tail. It is also possible that DNIC or analogous mechanisms can contribute to the analgesia induced by acupuncture and TENS. These procedures elicit afferent inputs that could bring about suppression of nociceptive transmission by segmental processes or by recruitment of descending influences from higher brain structures. Since the UCDH may possess an unusual pattern of convergence from a very wide visceral and deep structures (see above), the manipulation of neck structures, such as muscle and joints, may potentially interact with these organs/structures from the face to the gut to obtain therapeutic effects. This is definitely a promising future research direction.

Recently, our laboratory has provided evidence of the involvement of central opioid mechanisms in neuroplastic changes in Vc and UCDH nociceptive neurons [61] and associated jaw/neck-muscle activity [62,64] (see below: 'Short-term neuroplasticity: inflammation'). Systemic administration of the opiate antagonist naloxone 30 minutes after MO injection into tongue muscle enhances the excitability of nociceptive Vc neurons [61]. Likewise, systemic or intracaudalis application of naloxone 30 minutes after the MO injection into the TMJ region or neck-tongue musculature significantly increases (i.e., 're-kindling effect') jaw [63,64] or neck muscle activity [62] after it has returned to baseline levels. This centrally based 'rekindling' effect is dose dependent, stereoselective and appears to be mediated mainly via mu opioid receptor subtypes [74] (and see Hu *et al.* [34]). These findings suggest that a nociceptive afferent input triggered by the application of a noxious stimulus to the TMJ or neck region evokes Vc and UCDH nociceptive neuronal activity and associated neuromusular changes, but that these central neural changes are limited by the recruitment of a central opioid inhibitory mechanism (see Hu *et al.* [61]). This central opioid inhibitory mechanism may be segmental or involved with descending modulation (see below). This endogenous modulatory process could be the basis for the analgesic action after certain types of manipulative treatment.

Modification of somatosensory transmission can occur at thalamic and cortical neuronal levels, although the modification of ascending somatosensory messages may in fact largely occur earlier in the V pathway – namely, in the brainstem [35,75,76]. The intricate organization of each subdivision of the V brainstem complex and the variety of inputs to each of them from peripheral tissues or from intrinsic brain regions provide the substrate for numerous interactions between the various inputs. For example, the activity of V nociceptive brainstem neurons to deep noxious stimuli can be modulated (e.g. suppressed) by influences derived from structures within the V brainstem complex itself (e.g. substantia gelatinosa) as well as from other parts of the brainstem and higher centres (e.g., periaqueductal grey, somatosensory cortex) which utilize endogenous neurochemicals such as opioids, 5-HT or GABA. These modulatory influences are of clinical significance since they have been implicated as intrinsic mechanisms contributing to the analgesic effects of several therapeutic approaches, e.g., deep brain stimulation, acupuncture, and opiate-related drugs [77,78].

SHORT-TERM NEURO-PLASTICITY: INFLAMMATION

Central sensitization takes place within the dorsal horn of the spinal cord, the brainstem, and the brain (see Figures 3.2 and 3.3) [34,53,61]. Amplification of nociceptive input in the spinal cord produces secondary hyperalgesia around the site of injury. Mechanical hypersensitivity and allodynia to light touch after central sensitization are pathological in that they are evoked by A-beta low-threshold mechanoreceptors, which normally do not produce painful sensations. Peripheral sensitization allows low-intensity stimuli to produce pain by activating A-delta and C nociceptors. Central sensitization allows non-noxious low-threshold A-beta mechanoreceptors to produce pain as a result of changes in sensory processing in the spinal cord. For example, Chiang *et al.* [79] have shown that an NS neuron can become tactile-sensitive after the application of mustard oil into the pulp in rats. This could provide the neural basis for allodynia. Central sensitization involves a variety of transmitters and postsynaptic mechanisms (see Table 3.1 and Figure 3.3). It is initiated by slow synaptic potentials that A-delta and C fibres evoke in the dorsal horn (see Urban *et al.* [80]). The long duration of these slow potentials permits summation of potentials during repetitive nociceptor input (wind-up) and generates progressively greater and longer-lasting depolarization in dorsal horn neurons. Several seconds of C-fibre input results in several minutes of postsynaptic depolarization. This cumulative depolarization results from the activation of N-methyl-D-aspartic acid (NMDA) receptors by glutamate, and activation of the NK-1 tachykinin receptor by substance P and neurokinin A. Activation of these receptors allows an in-rush of calcium through ligand and voltage-gated ion channels and activation of guanosine triphosphate (GTP)-binding proteins. These second messengers, in turn, stimulate protein kinase C activity, which enhances the function of ion channels and intracellular enzymes by phosphorylating proteins. Second messengers can also indirectly alter proteins by regulating the activation of immediate-early gene products. Substance P and neurokinin A, released in superficial layers, diffuse well into the dorsal horn [81]. The importance of gluta-

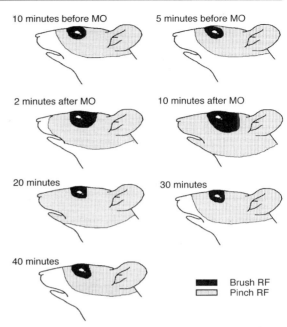

Figure 3.2 *This represents an example of a nociceptive (wide-dynamic-range) neuron in which the mechanoreceptive field has shown an increase of excitability after an injection of mustard oil into the neck muscles. This neuron was recorded under the conditions where the microelectrode was introduced through a long pathway, via cortex and other structures, to avoid the injury of neck skin/muscle and reach the subnucleus caudalis. At different times (zero is the time when the mustard oil was injected into neck muscle structure), the mechanoreceptive fields were outlined according to the observation assessed by the experimenter. These mechanoreceptive field expansions are the result of central sensitization process described in the text. (From Vernon and Hu, 1999, reprinted by permission of the* Journal of the Neuromusculoskeletal System)

mate, substance P and neurokinin A for central sensitization has been demonstrated by the capacity of antagonists at the NMDA and tachykinin receptors to prevent it. Further, mice lacking the gene for an isoform of protein kinase C have normal acute pain responses but minimal allodynia after sciatic nerve injury (see Basbaum [82]). Another mechanism of central sensitization involves the production of intracellular nitric oxide. It has been proposed that activation of the NMDA receptor leads to an influx of calcium ions, which activates the

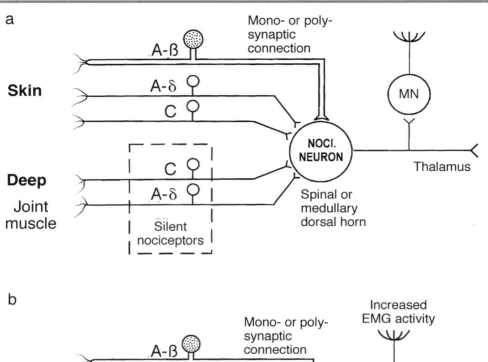

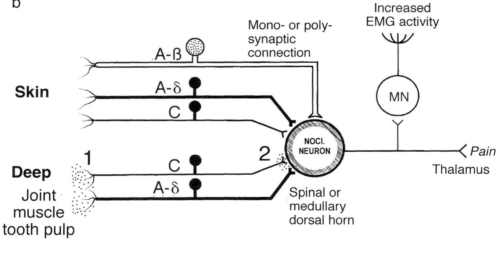

Figure 3.3 *Normal and centrally sensitized nociceptive transmission mechanisms with the subnucleus caudalis and dorsal horn. Central sensory neurons, such as wide-dynamic-range neurons, are designated by large circle and arrow. In normal conditions, the A-delta and C-fibre afferents from the deep structures are of the silent-nociceptor type (Schmidt et al. [7]). However, with inflammation/injury induced by the peripheral factors, indicated as '1' (listed in Table 3.1), peripherally activated substances sensitize peripheral primary afferents. This leads to a central sensitization that is shown in (B). This results in the release of substances, indicated as '2', which are also listed in Table 3.1 (centrally activated substances/transmitters). The central sensitization results in the change of properties of these central sensory neurons, such as enlargement of the receptive field, reduction of activation thresholds, increase of response magnitude and spontaneous activity. Changes in the shading of central nociceptive neurons indicate this change. Furthermore, this central sensitization process may lead a number of other changes, such as an increase in muscle activity and other central pathway activation. (Modified from Hu, 1994.)*

enzyme nitric oxide synthetase. Intracellular nitric oxide release stimulates transduction of protein kinase C, increases the effects of glutamate, and may interfere with release of inhibitory neurotransmitters from inhibitory neurons. Nitric oxide antagonism is therefore another strategy to prevent central sensitization [83]. In the craniofacial region, experiments have been performed to demonstrate this central sensitization process and involvement of NMDA process [54,60,75,84] (see above), but there is a lack of experiments dealing with the aforementioned intracellular and molecular mechanisms.

LONG-TERM NEUROPLASTICITY: DEAFFERENTATION AND NEUROPATHIC PAIN

The simple logic for the treatment of pain would be blocking the pain source, namely the cut off of the input, usually the peripheral nerve. Local anaesthetics are very effective for this short-term solution, and sometimes the analgesic effect outlasts the duration of drug effects. For a longer effect, a surgical disruption of the nerve innervating the painful area would be the next step, but this procedure can lead to disastrous consequences. A peripheral nerve usually contains large as well as small diameter nerve fibres. Many of the latter type also contain neuropeptides, which may have a trophic function to maintain the wellbeing of both peripheral and central nervous structures (i.e., dorsal horn/caudalis). In addition, the activity of the large diameter afferent fibres may have an important balancing function to the pain-mediated small diameter afferent fibres as Wall and Melzack's gate control theory of pain indicated. In general, a deprivation of inputs in nervous system will result in a neuroplastic and compensatory reaction. Anatomically, degeneration of higher-order neurons, especially the inhibitory interneurons in the substantia gelatinosa of the dorsal horn or caudalis, and sprouting have resulted in new and different nerve fibres being created in a chaotic fashion for the connectivity of neural pathways (see Ren and Dubner [85]). For example, denervation of spinal nerve may result in the large afferents terminating in unusual loci, such as the substantia gelatinosa, instead of lamina IV (see Dubner and Ruda

[53]). Functionally, the signal becomes chaotic, and the enlargement of the neuronal receptive field similar to those described above with central sensitization after inflammation, changes the activation thresholds [54,64,79]. This pathology is chronic and is similar to the neuropathic pain, i.e., abnormal sensation such as allodynia, i.e., touch evoked pain. The best example of this is trigeminal neuralgia, or tic douloureux. Damage of peripheral nerves also leads to deafferentation and neuropathic pain conditions [86]. However, this particular type research has not been studied extensively in either the craniofacial or neck region (c.f., Vos *et al.* [87]).

ORGANIZATION OF THE CENTRAL ASCENDING PAIN PATHWAY

There are two major ascending pathways from second order neurons to higher level ones. The first one involves low-threshold mechanoreceptor synapses in the dorsal column nuclei (gracile and cuneate nuclei and the trigeminal equivalent principalis nucleus) which project via the medial lemniscus to the ventrobasal thalamus (VPL or VPM). The other pathway is the dorsal horn or trigeminal subnucleus caudalis, which contains or relays pain and thermal information processes. This pathway projects via the spino- and trigemino-thalamic pathway to the VPL or VPM. The classic distinction between these two pathways has recently been challenged. The dorsal column (DC) pathway was found to be responsible for processing visceral nociceptive information via the so-called post-synaptic DC pathway (see Willis *et al* [88]).

Unlike the peripheral nerve and dorsal horn (including Vc second order neurons), the thalamic, cortical and other higher CNS pain-related structures have a rather ambiguous and diffused pain processing organization. For example, during exploratory brain surgery for control of motor disorders, such as Parkinson's disease, electrical stimulation of ventroposterior thalamic nucleus in conscious humans (i.e., the target of the spinothalamic pathway) yields very few sites (<2%) with pain reaction [89]. In animal studies, this structure does contain some nociceptive neurons, indicative of the involvement of pain processing (see

Willis and Westlund [90]). In animal studies, very few nociceptive neurons were found in the primary sensory cortex. The scarcity of pain-related sites within the pain processing relays does not imply their non-involvement, but rather that many different structures all contribute to different aspects of pain sensation and experience, including the emotional/affective, autonomic, reflexive and, most importantly, the modulation of pain.

Neurons at all levels of the V brainstem complex project to other brainstem regions including the reticular formation and cranial nerve motor nuclei; their connectivity to these particular regions provides the central substrate underlying the autonomic and muscle reflex responses to craniofacial stimuli that were mentioned above. Many V brainstem neurons may project to the contralateral thalamus via direct or multisynaptic paths [28,29,35]. The regions of the thalamus that are well known to receive and relay somatosensory information from the craniofacial region are the VPM as well as the so-called posterior group of nuclei, and the medial thalamus. These thalamic regions contain NS and WDR neurons having properties that are generally similar to those described for comparable neurons in the subthalamic relays, such as the subnucleus caudalis. The ventrobasal nociceptive neurons have properties and connections with the overlying somatosensory cerebral cortex indicative of a role for most of them in the sensory-discriminative dimension of pain. In contrast, nociceptive neurons in the more medial nuclei (e.g., intralaminar nuclei; parafascicular nucleus) are generally considered to have properties and connections (e.g., with the anterior cingulate cortex; see below) suggestive of a role more in the affective or motivational dimensions of pain. Neurons have been described in the somatosensory cortex with properties indicating a role in localization and intensity coding of noxious thermal facial, muscular or tooth-pulp stimuli [91–94]. Nociceptive neurons also occur in other cortical regions, such as the anterior cingulate cortex, which has been implicated in the affective dimension of pain [95]. The significance of these mechanisms to human pain processes is underscored by recent brain imaging findings in humans of activation by noxious stimuli of several cortical regions, including the somatosensory cortex and

anterior cingulate cortex [95]. The UCDH is known for heavy projection to the VPL/VPM thalamus [46,47]. Up to now, no specific thalamic and cortical study has been designed to study the central pain processing for the neck region.

CONCLUSIONS

The upper cervical dorsal horn has received limited attention before; however, new data gradually have shed light on its importance in the sensory-discrimination aspects of pain processing. The lack of data, especially in term of deafferentation and neuropathic pain, impedes our understanding of its function. However, the understanding gained from both trigeminal and spinal studies has shown the way for future studies. Further research effort will be needed to clarify many unsolved issues, but the clinical implications from these future studies may bring a new therapeutic approach for pain in the neck region.

REFERENCES

1. Mersky H (Chairman). Pain terms: a list with definitions and notes on usage. *Pain* 1979;**6**:249–252.
2. Melzack R. The McGill pain questionnaire: major properties and scoring methods. *Pain* 1975;**1**:277–299.
3. Stucky CL, Lewin GR. Isolectin B(4)-positive and -negative nociceptors are functionally distinct. *J Neurosci* 1999;**19**:6497–6505.
4. McClesky EW, Gold MS. Ion channels of nociception. *Ann Rev Physiol* 1999;**61**:835–856.
5. Waxman SG, Dib-Hajj S, Cummins TR, Black JA. Sodium channels and pain. *Proc Natl Acad Sci* 1999;**96**:7675–7679.
6. Price DD, Hu JW, Dubner R, Gracely R. Peripheral suppression of first pain and central summation of second pain evoked by noxious heat pulses. *Pain* 1977;**3**:57–68.
7. Schmidt RF, Schaible H-G, Messlinger K, Heppelmann B, *et al*. Silent and active nociceptors: Structure, functions, and clinical Implications. In *Proceedings of the 7th World Congress on Pain* (eds. GF Gebhart, DL Hammond, TS Jensen), Seattle: IASP Press, pp.325–366, 1994.
8. Capra NF, Dessem D. Central connections of trigeminal primary afferent neurons: topographical and functional considerations. *Crit Rev Oral Biol Med* 1992;**4**:1–52.

9. Kido MA, Kiyoshima T, Ibuki T, Shimizu S, *et al*. A topographical and ultrastructural study of sensory trigeminal nerve endings in the rat temporomandibular joint as demonstrated by anterograde transport of wheat germ agglutinin-horseradish peroxidase (WGA-HRP) *J Dent Res* 1995;**74**:1353–1359.

10. Widenfalk B, Wiberg M. Origin of sympathetic and sensory innervation of the temporo-mandibular joint. A retrograde axonal tracing study in the rat. *Neurosci Lett* 1990;**109**:30–35.

11. Hannam AG, Sessle BJ. Temporomandibular neurosensory and neuromuscular physiology. In *Temporomandibular joint and masticatory muscle disorders*. (eds. GE Zarb, G Carlsson, BJ Sessle, ND Mohl), Munksgaard, pp. 67–100, 1994

12. Cairns BE, Sessle BJ, Hu JW. Evidence that excitatory amino acid receptors within the temporomandibular joint region are involved in the reflex activation of the jaw muscles. *J Neurosci* 1998;**16**:8052–8060.

13. Carlton SM, Coggeshall RE. Nociceptive integration: Does it have a peripheral component? *Pain Forum* 1998;**7**:71–78.

14. Cairns BE, Sessle BJ, Hu JW. Activation of peripheral GABAA receptors inhibits jaw muscle activity reflexly evoked by application of glutamate to the temporomandibular joint region. *J Neurophysiol* 1999;**81**:1966–1969.

15. Yu X-M, Hu JW, Sessle BJ. Effects of inflammatory irritant application to the rat temporo-mandibular joint on jaw and neck muscle activity. *Pain* 1995;**60**:143–149.

16. Bakke M, Sessle BJ, Hu JW. Morphine application to peripheral tissues modulates nociceptive jaw reflex. *Neuroreport* 1998;**9**:3315–3319.

17. Stein C. The control of pain in peripheral tissue by opioids. *New Engl J Med* 1995;**332**:1685–1690.

18. Craig AD, Heppelmann B, Schaible HG. Projection of the medial and posterior articular nerves of the cat's knee to the spinal cord. *J Comp Neurol* 1988;**276**:279–288.

19. Mense S. Nociception from skeletal muscle in relation to clinical muscle pain. *Pain* 1993;**54**:241–289.

20. Schaible H-G, Grubb BD. Afferent and spinal mechanisms of joint pain. *Pain* 1993;**55**:241–289.

21. Nazruddin S, Uemune S, Shirana Y, Yamauchi K, *et al*. The cells of origin of the hypoglossal afferent nerves and central projections in the cat. *Brain Res* 1989;**490**:219–235.

22. Shigenaga Y, Sera M, Nishimori T, Suemune S, *et al*. The central projection of masticatory afferent fibers to the trigeminal sensory nuclear complex and upper cervical spinal cord. *J Comp Neurol* 1988;**268**:489–507.

23. Dubner R, Bennett GJ. Spinal and trigeminal mechanisms of nociception. *Ann Rev Neurosci* 1983;**6**:381–418.

24. Gobel S, Hockfield S, Ruda MA. Anatomical similarities between medullary and spinal dorsal horns. In *Oral-facial sensory and motor functions* (eds. Y Kawamura, R Dubner), Quintessence, pp. 211–223, 1981.

25. Sessle BJ, Hu JW, Amano N, Zhong G. Convergence of cutaneous, tooth pulp, visceral, neck and muscle afferents onto nociceptive and non-nociceptive neurones in trigeminal subnucleus caudalis (medullary dorsal horn) and its implications for referred pain. *Pain* 1986;**27**:219–235.

26. Molander C, Xu Q, Rivero-Melian C, Grant G. Cytoarchitectonic organization of the spinal cord in the rat: II. The cervical and upper thoracic cord. *J Comp Neurol* 1989;**289**:375–385.

27. Hu JW. Response properties of nociceptive and nonnociceptive neurons in the rat's trigeminal subnucleus caudalis (medullary dorsal horn) related to cutaneous and deep craniofacial afferent stimulation and modulation by diffuse noxious inhibitory controls. *Pain* 1990;**41**:331–345.

28. Hu JW, Dostrovsky JO, Sessle BJ. Functional properties of neurons in cat trigeminal subnucleus caudalis (medullary dorsal horn) I. Response to oral-facial noxious and non-noxious stimuli and projections to thalamus and subnucleus oralis. *J Neurophysiol* 1981;**45**:173–192.

29. Price DD, Dubner R, Hu JW. Trigeminothalamic neurons in nucleus caudalis responsive to tactile, thermal, and nociceptive stimulation of the monkey's face. *J Neurophysiol* 1976;**39**:936–953.

30. Sessle BJ. Mechanisms of trigeminal and occipital pain. *Pain Rev* 1996;**3**:91–116.

31. Hathaway CB, Hu JW, Bereiter DA. Distribution of Fos-like immunoreactivity in the caudal brain stem of the rat following noxious chemical stimulation of the temporomandibular joint. *J Comp Neurol* 1995;**356**:444–456.

32. Meng ID, Bereiter DA. Differential distribution of Fos-like immunoreactivity in the spinal trigeminal nucleus after noxious and innocuous thermal and chemical stimulation of rat cornea. *Neurosci* 1996;**72**:243–254.

33. Strassman AM, Vos BP. Somatotopic and laminar organization of Fos-like immunoreactivity in the medullary and cervical dorsal hron induced by noxious facial stimulation in the rat. *J Comp Neurol* 1993;**331**:495–516.

34. Hu JW, Tsai CM, Bakke M, Seo K, *et al*. Deep Craniofacial Pain: Involvement of trigeminal subnucleus caudalis and its modulation. In *Proceedings of the 8th World Congress on Pain* (eds. TS Jensen, JA Turner, Z Wiesenfeld-

Hallin), Seattle, WA: IASP Press, pp. 497–506, 1997.

35. Meng ID, Hu JW, Bereiter D. Encoding of corneal input in two distinct regions of the spinal trigeminal nucleus in the rat: cutaneous receptive field properties, responses to thermal and chemical stimulation, modulation by diffuse noxious inhibitory controls, and projections. *J Neurophysiol* 1997;**77**:43–56.

36. Amano N, Hu JW, Sessle BJ. Responses of neurons in feline trigeminal subnucleus caudalis (medullary dorsal horn) to cutaneous, intraoral and muscle afferent stimuli. *J Neurophysiol* 1986;**55**:227–243.

37. Broton JG, Hu JW, Sessle BJ. Effects of temporomandibular joint stimulation on nociceptive and non-nociceptive neurons of the cat's trigeminal (V) subnucleus caudalis (medullary dorsal horn) *J Neurophysiol* 1988;**59**:1575–1589.

38. Sun KQ, Vernon H, Sessle BJ, Hu JW. Responses of nociceptive neurones in rat trigeminal subnucleus caudalis and C2 dorsal horn to cutaneous and deep afferent inputs. *Neurosci Abstr* 1997;**23**:2351.

39. Chandler MJ, Zhang J, Foreman RD. Vagal, sympathetic and somatic sensory inputs to upper cervical (C1–C3) spinothalamic tract neurons in monkeys. *J Neurophysiol* 1996;**76**:2555–2567.

40. Chandler MJ, Qin C, Yuan Y, Foreman RD. Convergence of trigeminal input with visceral and phrenic inputs on primate C1–C2 spinothalamic tract neurons. *Brain Res* 1999;**829**:204–208.

41. Razook JC, Chandler MJ, Foreman RD. Phrenic afferent input excites C1–C2 spinal neurons in rats. *Pain* 1995;**63**:117–125.

42. Smith MV, Apkarian AV, Hodge CJ. Somatosensory response properties of contralaterallly projecting spinothalmic and non-spinothalmic neurons in the second cervical segment of the cat. *J Neurophysiol* 1991;**66**:83–102.

43. Yezierski RP, Broton JG. Functional properties of spinomesencephalic tract cells in the upper cervical spinal cord of the cat. *Pain* 1991;**45**:187–196.

44. Zhang J, Chandler MJ, Miller KE, Foreman RD. Cardiopulmonary sympathetic afferent input does not require dorsal column pathways to excite C1–C3 spinal cells in rats. *Brain Res* 1997;**771**:25–30

45. Foreman RD. Mechanisms of cardiac pain. *Ann Rev Physiol* 1999;**61**:143–167.

46. Bereiter DA, Berieter DF, Benetti AP, Hu JW. Sex differences in morphine sensitivity and amino acid release in spinal trigeminal nucleus after injury to TMJ region. *Neurosci Abst* 1998;**24**:389.

47. Bereiter DA, Bereiter DF, Hu JW, Hirata H. Hypoglossal nerve-evoked c-fos expression in spinal trigeminal nucleus of the rat. *Neurosci Abst* 1997;**23**:2351.

48. Willis WD, Coggeshall RE (eds.) *Sensory Mechanisms of the Spinal Cord*. Plenum, 1991.

49. Apkarian AV, Hodge CJ. Primate spinothalamic pathways I. A quantitative study of the cells of origin of the spinothalamic pathway. *J Comp Neurol* 1989;**288**:447–473.

50. Bernard JF, Huang GF, Besson JM. The parabrachial area: Electrophysiological evidence for an involvement in visceral nociceptive processes. *J Neurophysiol* 1994;**71**:1646–1660.

51. Feil K, Herbert H. Topographic organization of spinal and trigeminal somatosensory pathways to the rat parabrachial and Kolliker-Fuse nuclei. *J Comp Neurol* 1995;**353**:506–528

52. Villanueva L, Bouhassira D, Bing Z, Le Bars D. Convergence of heterotopic nociceptive information onto subnucleus reticularis dorsalis neurons in the rat medulla. *J Neurophysiol* 1988;**60**:980–1009.

53. Dubner R, Ruda MA. Activity-dependent neuronal plasticity following tissue injury and inflammation. *Trends Neurosci* 1993;**15**:96–103.

54. Woolf CJ, Mannion RJ. Neuropathic pain: aetiology, symptoms, mechanisms, and management. *Lancet* 1999;**353**:1959–1964.

55. Hu JW, Sessle BJ, Raboisson P, Dallel R, *et al.* Stimulation of craniofacial muscle afferents induces prolonged facilitatory effects in trigeminal nociceptive brainstem neurones. *Pain* 1992;**48**:53–60.

56. Yu X-M, Sessle BJ, Hu JW. Differential effects of cutaneous and deep application of inflammatory irritant on mechanoreceptive field properties of trigeminal brain stem neurones. *J Neurophysiol* 1993;**70**:1704–1707.

57. Burstein R, Yamamura H, Malick A, Strassman AM. Chemical stimulation of the intracranial dura induces enhanced responses to facial stimulation in brain stem trigeminal neurons. *J Neurophysiol* 1998;**79**:964–982.

58. Pozo MA, Cervero F. Neurons in the rat spinal trigeminal complex driven by corneal nociceptors: receptive-field properties and effects of noxious stimulation of the cornea. *J Neurophysiol* 1993;**70**:2370–2378

59. Iwata K, Tashiro A, Tsuboi Y, Takao I, *et al.* Medullary dorsal horn neuronal activity in rats with persistent temporomandibular joint and perioral inflammation. *J Neurophysiol* 1999;**82**:1244–1253.

60. Hu JW, Yu X-M, Vernon H, Sessle BJ. Excitatory effects on neck and jaw muscle activity of inflammatory irritant injections into cervical paraspinal tissues. *Pain* 1993;**55**:243–350.

61. Hu JW, Yu X-M, Sunakawa M, Chiang CY, *et al*. Electromyographic and trigeminal brainstem neuronal changes associated with inflammatory irritation of superficial and deep craniofacial tissues in rats. In *Proceedings of the 7th World Congress on Pain* (eds. GF Gebhart, DL Hammond, TS Jensen), Seattle, WA: IASP Press, pp. 325–366, 1994.

62. Hu JW, Tatourian I, Vernon H. Opioid involvement in electromyographic (EMG) responses induced by injection of inflammatory irritant into deep neck tissues. *Somatosens Motor Res* 1996;**13**:139–146.

63. Seo K, Sessle BJ, Haas DA, Hu JW. "Rekindling" effect of intrathecal injection of naloxone on jaw muscle activity evoked by mustard oil application to temporomandibular joint in rat: possible involvement of trigeminal subnucleus caudalis (Vc). *Neurosci Abstr* 1995;**21**:1168.

64. Yu X-M, Sessle BJ, Vernon H, Hu JW. Administration of opiate antagonist naloxone induces recurrence of increased jaw muscle activities related to inflammatory irritant application to rat temporomandubular joint region. *J Neurophysiol* 1994;**72**:1430–1433.

65. Maillou P, Cadden SW. Effects of remote deep somatic noxious stimuli on a jaw reflex in man. *Arch Oral Biol* 1997;**42**:323–327.

66. Maixner W, Sigurdsson A, Fillingim RB, Lundeen T, *et al*. Regulation of acute and chronic orofacial pain. In *Orofacial Pain and Temporomandibular Disorders. Advances in Pain Research and Therapy* (eds. JR Fricton and R Dubner), Vol 21. New York: Raven Press, pp. 85–102, 1995.

67. Okada K, Oshima M, Kawakita K. Examination of the afferent fiber responsible for the suppression of jaw-opening reflex in heat, cold, and manual acupuncture stimulation in rats. *Brain Res* 1996;**740**:201–207.

68. Melzack R. Folk medicine and the sensory modulation of pain. In *Textbook of Pain*, 3rd edn (eds. PD Wall, R Melzack), London: Churchill Livingstone, pp. 1209–1217, 1994.

69. Woolf CJ, Thompson JW. Stimulation fibre-induced analgesia: transcutaneous electrical nerve stimulation (TENS) and vibration. In *Textbook of Pain*, 3rd edn (eds. PD Wall, R Melzack), London: Churchill Livingstone, pp. 1191–1208, 1994.

70. Aicher SA, Lewis SJ, Randich A. Antinociception produced by electrical stimulation of vagal afferents: independence of cervical and subdiaphragmatic branches. *Brain Res* 1991; **542**:63–70.

71. Le Bars D, Dickenson AH, Besson JM. Diffuse noxious inhibitory controls (DNIC). I. Effects on dorsal horn convergent neurons in the rat. *Pain* 1997;**6**:283–304.

72. Le Bars D, Dickenson AH, Besson JM. Diffuse noxious inhibitory controls (DNIC). II. Lack of effect on non-convergent neurons, supraspinal involvement and theoretical implications. *Pain* 1997;**6**:305–327.

73. Villanueva L, Bouhassira D, Le Bars D. The medullary subnucleus reticularis dorsalis (SRD) as a key link in both the transmission and modulation of pain signals. *Pain* 1996; **67**:231–240.

74. Tambeli CH, Sessle BJ, Hu JW. Central opioid modulation of mustard oil-evoked jaw muscle activity involves mu and kappa but not delta opioid receptor mechanisms. *Neurosci Abstr* 1997;**23**:1018.

75. Chiang CY, Hu JW, Sessle BJ. Parabrachial area and nucleus raphe magnus-induced modulation of nociceptive and non-nociceptive trigeminal subnucleus caudalis neurones activated by cutaneous or deep inputs. *J Neurophysiol* 1994;**71**:2430–2445.

76. Sessle BJ, Hu JW, Dubner A, Lucier GE. Functional properties of neurons in cat trigeminal subnucleus caudalis (medullary dorsal horn) II. Modulation of responses to noxious and non-noxious stimuli by periaqueductal grey, nucleus raphe magnus, cerebral cortex and afferent influences, and effect of naloxone. *J Neurophysiol* 1981;**45**:193–207.

77. Yaksh TL, Malmberg AB. Central pharmacology of nociceptive transmission. In *Textbook of Pain*, 3rd edn (eds. PD Wall, R Melzack), London: Churchill Livingstone, pp. 165–200, 1994

78. Fields HL, Basbaum AI. Central nervous system mechanisms of pain modulation. In *Textbook of Pain*, 3rd edn (eds. PD Wall, R Melzack), London: Churchill Livingstone, pp. 243–257, 1994.

79. Chiang CY, Hu JW, Sessle BJ. NMDA receptor involvement in neuroplastic changes induced by neonatal C-fiber depletion in trigeminal (V) brainstem nociceptive neurons of adult rats. *J Neurophysiol* 1998;**99**:2803.

80. Urban L, Thompson SWN, Dray A. Modulation of spinal excitability: co-operation between neurokinin and excitatory amino acid neurotransmitters. *Trends Neurosci* 1994;**17**:432–438.

81. Honore P, Menning PM, Rogers SD, Nichols ML, *et al*. Spinal substance P receptor expression and internalization in acute, short-term, and long-term inflammatory pain states. *J Neurosci* 1999;**19**:7670–7678.

82. Basbaum AI. Distinct neurochemical features of acute and persistent pain. *Proc Natl Acad Sci* 1999;**96**:7675–7679.

83. Meller ST, Gebhart GF. Nitric oxide (NO) and nociceptive processing in the spinal cord. *Pain* 1993;**52**:235–240.

84. Yu X-M, Sessle BJ, Haas DA, Izzo A, *et al.* Involvement of NMDA receptor mechanisms in the jaw electromyographic activity and plasma extravasation induced by inflammatory irritant injection into the temporomandibular joint region. *Pain* 1996;**68**:169–178.

85. Ren K, Dubner R. Central nervous system plasticity and persistent pain. *J Orofacial Pain* 1999;**13**:155–163.

86. Bennett GJ. Neuropathic pain. In *Textbook of Pain*, 3rd edn (eds. PD Wall, R Melzack), London: Churchill Livingstone, pp. 201–224, 1994.

87. Vos BP, Strassman AM, Maciewicz RJ. Behavioral evidence of trigeminal neuropathic pain following chronic constriction injury to the rat's infraorbital nerve. *J Neurosci* 1994;**14**:2708–2723.

88. Willis WD, Al-Chaer ED, Quast MJ, Westlund KN. A visceral pain pathway in the dorsal column of the spinal cord. *Proc Natl Acad Sci* 1999;**96**:7675–7679.

89. Davis KD, Lozano RM, Manduch M, Tasker RR, *et al.* Thalamic relay site for cold perception in humans. *J Neurophysiol* 1999;**81**:1970–1973.

90. Willis WD, Westlund KN. Neuranatomy of the pain system and of the pathways that modulate pain. *J Clin Neurophysiol* 1997;**14**:2–31.

91. Iwata K, Tsuboi Y, Sumino R. Primary somatosensory cortical neuronal activity during monkey's detection of perceived change in tooth-pulp stimulus intensity. *J Neurophysiol* 1998;**79**:1717–1725

92. Kenshalo DR, Isensee O. Responses of primate SI cortical neurons to noxious stimuli. *J Neurophysiol* 1983;**50**:1479–1496.

93. Kenshalo DR, Chudler EH, Anton F, Dubner R. SI nociceptive neurons participate in the encoding process by which monkeys perceive the intensity of noxious thermal stimulation. *Brain Res* 1988;**5**:378–382.

94. Tsuboi Y, Iwata K, Muramatsu H, Yagi J, *et al.* Response properties of primary somatosensory cortical neurons responsive to cold stimulation of the facial skin and oral mucous membrane. *Brain Res* 1993;**613**:93–202.

95. Hsieh JC, Stone-Elander S, Ingvar M. Anticipatory coping of pain expressed in the human anterior cingulate cortex: a positron emission tomography study. *Neurosci Lett* 1999; **262**:61–64.

Further reading

Hu JW. Cephalic myofascial pain pathways. In *Tension-type Headache: Classification, Mechanisms, and Treatment* (eds. J Olesen, J Schoenen), New York: Raven Press, p. 69–77, 1994.

Sessle BJ. The neural basis of temporomandibular joint and masticatory muscle pain. *J Orofac Pain* 1999;**13**:238–245.

Vernon H, Hu JW. Neuroplasticity of neck/craniofacial pain mechanisms: A review of basic science studies. *J Neuromusculoskel Sys* 1999; **7**:51–64.

Chapter 4

Diagnostic imaging of the cranio-cervical region

Marshall N. Deltoff

INTRODUCTION

Diagnostic imaging today embodies a variety of modalities that may be used individually or in combination to provide the clinician with information helpful in making a diagnosis and choosing a therapeutic regimen. These modalities include plain film radiography, contrast-enhanced radiography, computed tomography (CT), magnetic resonance imaging (MRI), nuclear scans and diagnostic ultrasound.

Radiographic examinations are typically requisitioned for one or both of two predominant reasons: pathological screening and postural evaluation/biomechanical assessment [1].

Pathological screening

The various imaging procedures frequently provide diagnostic confirmation of the presence of bony, articular and soft tissue abnormality and/or pathology. In this respect, radiology functions to assist in the primary diagnostic exercise. Secondly, the appropriateness of various therapeutic measures, such as spinal manipulation, can also be assessed via *X-ray* examination.

Throughout the various categories of osteopathology there are certain conditions, often demonstrable radiographically, in which spinal manipulation may be contraindicated,

referral to another practitioner may be necessary or a modification of therapeutic procedure should be considered. Examples include a wide assortment of anomalies, arthritides, malignancies, infection, fractures, dislocations and systemic disease.

Postural evaluation and biomechanical assessment

Radiographic examination can assist in the analysis of biomechanical factors relevant to cervical spinal dysfunction. Static postural alignment of both the regional as well as the segmental anatomy is easily afforded by the standard plain film views of the upper and lower cervical spine. Dynamic function can be assessed with end-motion views such as flexion/extension and lateral bending. These studies can assist in establishing the segmental levels at which to concentrate therapy and in ascertaining how, optimally, to perform manipulative procedures.

A detailed presentation of the varied chiropractic interpretive procedures for the radiographic evaluation of spinal posture and biomechanics is beyond the scope of this chapter. A thorough discussion of the categories of osteopathology will also not be attempted.

It must be remembered that a radiographic postural or biomechanical evaluation requires consideration of the geometric magnification and projectional distortion inherent in the practice of diagnostic radiology [1]. Thus, optimal patient positioning is paramount in securing the best images for assessing the cervical spine.

This chapter will, therefore, begin with optimum *X-ray* positioning and technology considerations followed by a brief overview of advanced imaging options. A synopsis of cervical roentgenometrics is then presented. The chapter concludes with an imaging atlas of cervical spine cases consisting of a varied selection from the categories of skeletal disease.

RADIOGRAPHIC EXAMINATION OF THE CERVICAL SPINE [2–7]

With the continuing improvement in films, screens, *X-ray* generators and automatic exposure control devices, plain film radiographic examinations continue to become easier, more efficient and safer, as well as remaining the most accessible and cost-effective imaging modality at our disposal. These increasing technical advances do not obviate the ordering of the proper study and suitable number of views, and it remains the responsibility of the technologist or doctor performing the examination to ensure that neither radiographic quality nor patient and examiner safety are compromised.

With respect to cervical spine radiology, and especially in cases of trauma, the radiologist must be satisfied that every region, from occiput to T1, is satisfactorily visualized.

The basic radiographic examination of the cervical spine should include the A/P open

mouth, A/P lower cervical and neutral lateral projections. Oblique views can be added, as they are deemed to be clinically warranted, in order to visualize the intervertebral foramina. Furthermore, flexion and extension views, when indicated, complete the seven-view Davis series. Flexion and extension views may provide additional information regarding intersegmental spinal relationships which may be a clue to disc disease, ligamentous damage and facet injury. Additional supplementary projections, the pillar views, allow visualization of the articular masses *en face*, and can be utilized when further imaging of the articular pillars is required.

The patient can be seated or standing. Apron-type gonadal shielding should be utilized. All jewellery in the radiographic field is removed, e.g., earrings, necklaces, hairpins, and barrettes, as well as wigs, eyeglasses, hearing aids and, if possible, dentures.

Optimum KVp with variable mAs technique is recommended. Always attempt to reduce the object-film distance; this will minimize effects of magnification. Where tube tilt is required, remember to reduce the actual tube-film distance by 1 inch for every 5 degrees of tube tilt; this will maintain a uniform effective focal-film distance. (Table 4.1)

Anteroposterior open mouth view (Fig. 4.1)

This view visualizes the odontoid, axis body, atlas lateral masses and periodontal interspaces in the coronal plane.

The patient stands or is seated facing the *X-ray* tube, with the cervical spine centred to the midline of the bucky or grid cabinet. The head

Table 4.1 Technical considerations for cervical spine radiographs

	Kvp	Bucky	Focal-film distance	Film size	Tube angulation
AP open mouth	70	yes	40″	8″ × 10″	–
AP lower cervical	70	yes	40″	8″ × 10″	15 degrees cephalad
Lateral (neutral, flexion, extension)	70	no	72″	8″ × 10″	–
Obliques: anterior	70	no	72″	8″ × 10″	15 degrees caudad
posterior	70	no	72″	8″ × 10″	15 degrees cephalad
Pillar	70	yes	40″	8″ × 10″	35 degrees caudad
Base posterior	75–85	yes (angled 45 degrees)	40″	8″ × 10″	–

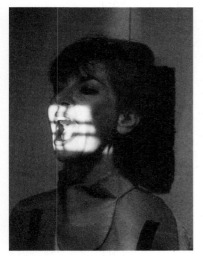

(a)

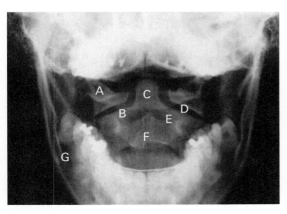

(b)

Figure 4.1 *Anteroposterior open mouth. (a) Positioning. (b) Normal radiograph: A, lateral mass of atlas, B, atlas posterior arch, C, dens (odontoid process), D, atlanto-axial joint space, E, body of axis, F, spinous process of axis, G, mandibular ramus.*

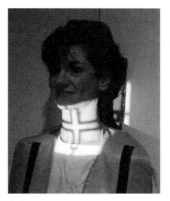

(a)

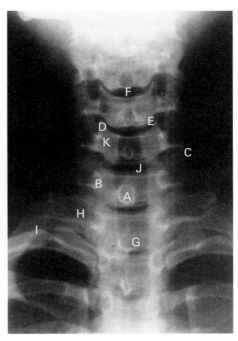

(b)

Figure 4.2 *Anteroposterior lower cervical. (a) Positioning. (b) Normal radiograph: A, C7 spinous process, B, C7 pedicle, C, C7 transverse process, D, uncinate process, E, joint of von Luschka, F, intervertebral disc, G, T1 spinous process, H, T1 transverse process, I, first rib, J, air-filled trachea, K, C6 vertebral body.*

is then positioned so that the inferior margin of the upper incisors and the base of the occiput, or the mastoid processes, are in the same plane, perpendicular to the film. Make sure the face is not rotated. The patient's mouth is opened as wide as possible. This clears the teeth from the field of view, allowing C1–C2 to be visualized through the open jaws. If the head is tilted back, then the base of the occiput may superimpose over the cervical vertebrae; if the head is tilted forward, then

the upper incisors can superimpose over the cervical vertebrae. Only when the upper teeth and occiput are exactly superimposed (in the same plane) will the upper cervical vertebrae be optimally visualized. The central ray is through the uvula. Collimate to just below the nose, and laterally, to the skin of the cheeks. The mAs should be double the value for the A/P lower cervical view.

A/P lower cervical view (Fig. 4.2)

The cervical vertebral bodies from C3 through the upper thoracic segments are visualized in the coronal plane. The uncinate processes comprising the joints of von Luschka can be evaluated for degenerative alterations.

The cervical spine is centred to the midline of the bucky. Raise the chin slightly to clear the mandible from superimposition over the mid-cervical spine. Angle the tube 15 degrees cephalad; this facilitates a central ray that more optimally visualizes the joints of von Luschka. The central ray is at the mid-thyroid cartilage, approximately at the C4 level. Collimate to the angle of the mandible; include the lung apices.

Lateral – neutral view (Fig. 4.3)

Atlas to C7 is visualized in the sagittal plane; disc status is evaluated. Soft tissue anterior to the spine can also be examined.

The patient's sagittal plane is parallel to the film, with the skull in a true lateral position. The patient's shoulder is in contact with the cassette holder. Since the patient's shoulder will not allow the spine to be as close to the film as in the A/P view, the tube is moved from a 40 inch to a 72 inch focal-film distance to compensate ('air-gap' technique), so that magnification is avoided. For large shoulders, it is helpful to place weights in the hands, in order to pull the shoulders down, so that the lower cervical vertebrae are not superimposed by the shoulders. The central ray is at the C4–C5 disc level. Collimate behind the eyes, and superiorly, to just above the ear.

Lateral – flexion and extension view

These two views are routine for any cervical trauma such as whiplash since they allow assessment of ligamentous damage; overlay studies utilizing the neutral lateral provide information on intersegmental motion at each level.

Flexion (Fig. 4.4): From the neutral lateral position, get the patient to tuck in his or her

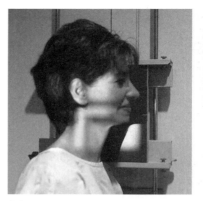

(a)

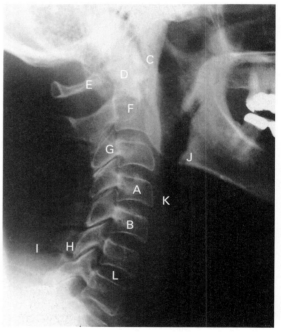

(b)

Figure 4.3 *Lateral cervical (neutral). (a) Positioning. (b) Normal radiograph: A, C4 vertebral body, B, C5 transverse process, C, atlas anterior tubercle, D, dens, E, atlas posterior arch, F, axis body, G, C3 articular process, H, C6 lamina, I, C6 spinous process, J, mandibular ramus, K, trachea, L, C6–C7 intervertebral disc space.*

chin, and then flex his or her neck as far forward as is comfortably possible. Tucking the chin in before maximum forward flexion will help to emphasize subtle aberrant intersegmental biomechanics.

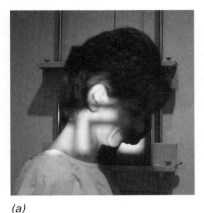

(a)

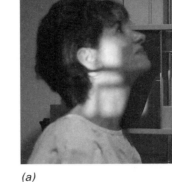

(a)

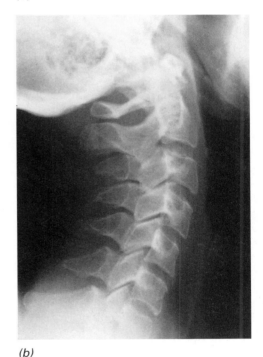

(b)

(b)

Figure 4.4 *Flexion lateral cervical. (a) Positioning. (b) Normal radiograph.*

Figure 4.5 *Extension lateral cervical. (a) Positioning. (b) Normal radiograph.*

Extension (Fig.4.5): From the neutral lateral position, get the patient to lift the chin, tilting the head back as far as is comfortably possible to look up at the ceiling.

Oblique views (Fig. 4.6) – anterior or posterior

The primary purpose of these views is to assess the patency of the intervertebral foramina (IVF).

Osteoarthritic spurs (osteophytes) may encroach on the IVFs to varying degrees in cases of degenerative disc disease, uncinate arthrosis or facet arthrosis. Patients may present with shoulder, arm or hand paraesthesias or radiations.

Anterior obliques (Fig. 4.6a): The patient is standing or seated, facing the cassette. Angle the patient's body 45 degrees from the cassette, first to the left, for a left anterior oblique (LAO) view, and then to the right, for

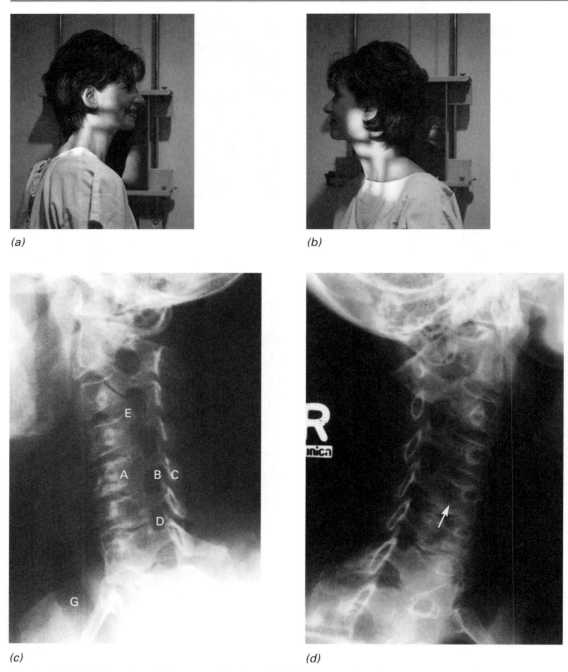

(a)

(b)

(c)

(d)

Figure 4.6 *(a) Anterior oblique positioning. This left anterior oblique view will demonstrate the left intervertebral foramina. (b) Posterior oblique positioning. This right posterior oblique view will also demonstrate the left intervertebral foramina. (c) Normal radiograph: A, C5 vertebral body. B, C5 pedicle. C, C5 lamina. D, C6–C7 intervertebral foramen. E, C3–C4 joint of von Luschka. F, first rib. G, trachea. (d) Right anterior oblique projection of a 58-year-old woman demonstrates osteophytic spur encroachment into the IVF at the C5–C6 level (arrow), due to osteoarthritis of the ipsilateral joint of von Luschka (courtesy Arnie B Deltoff, DC, FATA, Toronto, Ontario, Canada).*

a right anterior oblique (RAO) view. In each case, the face should then be turned away from the anterior shoulder so that the head is parallel to the cassette. Place the appropriate marker behind the spine. The tube is angled 15 degrees caudally. Remember, on a LAO film, the left intervertebral foramina are visualized. The central ray enters at C3–C4.

Posterior obliques (Fig. 4.6b): The patient is standing or seated, facing the tube. The patient is turned 45 degrees, first to the left for a left posterior oblique (LPO) view, then to the right to produce a right posterior oblique (RPO) view. In each case, the face should then be turned away from the anterior shoulder so that the head is parallel to the cassette. Place the appropriate marker in front of the spine. The tube is angled 15 degrees cephalad. Remember, on a LPO film, the right intervertebral foramina are visualized.

Pillar views (Fig. 4.7)

These projections (left and right) optimally visualize the facet joints comprising each articular pillar.

The patient is standing or seated, facing the tube. The face is turned 45 degrees away from the side being examined. The tube is angled 35 degrees caudally. The central ray enters approximately 3 inches below the external auditory meatus, at the C4 level.

Base posterior views (Fig. 4.8)

This specialized projection is utilized for Palmer technique upper cervical analysis. The atlas, axis and nasal septum are the primary structures visualized. Atlas rotation is assessed.

The patient is seated with head in neutral position, facing the tube. The skull vertex is centred to the bucky, which is angled 45 degrees. Filtration is used over the orbits. The central ray is tilted cephalad so that it enters 1 inch below the chin, passing half an inch anterior to the external auditory meatus.

Supplementary imaging

Additional imaging options, such as those outlined below, may be of assistance in certain cases where the use of plain film radiography,

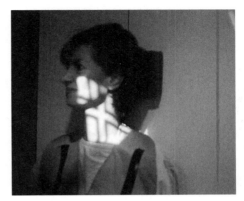

(a)

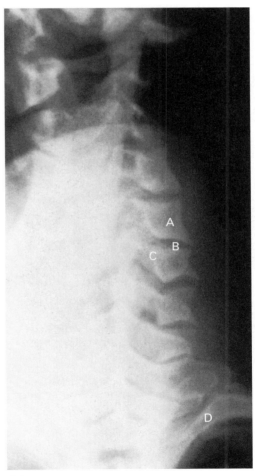

(b)

Figure 4.7 *Pillar projection. (a) Left pillar positioning. (b) Normal radiograph: A, C4 articular process. B, C4–C5 apophyseal joint. C, C5 lamina. D, first rib.*

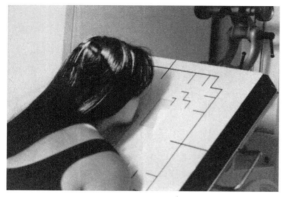

(a)

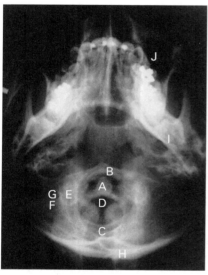

(b)

Figure 4.8 *Base posterior projection. (a) Positioning (from Marchiori D.: Clinical Imaging with Skeletal, Chest and Abdomen Pattern Differentials, St Louis: Mosby, 1999). (b) Normal radiograph: A, odontoid. B, anterior arch of atlas. C, posterior arch of atlas. D, spinal canal. E, articulating surface of atlas lateral mass. F, atlas transverse process. G, foramen transversarium. H, occiput. I, mandibular ramus. J, maxillary sinus (courtesy Robert C Tatum, DC, DACBR, Davenport, Iowa, USA).*

clinical history and examination findings, does not provide sufficient information to allow the formulation of a specific therapeutic approach to a particular patient's problem.

It is established practice that plain film *X-rays* be taken before advanced imaging is performed [8]. (Skull trauma evaluation would be a notable exception to this rule.) Following plain film studies, the clinician often decides between CT and MRI as the next step in imaging the patient's spine. MRI today is considered the imaging modality of choice for most regions of the body. The advantages of MRI over CT scanning include the lack of ionizing radiation, improved contrast resolution allowing for superior soft tissue differentiation and the capability of multiplanar imaging without loss of image quality. Generally, MRI is requested when there is suspicion of soft tissue lesions of the spinal column and cord. CT is indicated for optimal evaluation of cortical bone, osseous detail and small calcified lesions.

The typically longer examination times in MRI may be a consideration, as traditional units may foster claustrophobic anxiety in some patients; newer 'open' or 'C-shaped' systems have helped to reduce this occurrence. Availability and cost of each procedure must also be weighed.

(i) Computed tomography

Undoubtedly, computed tomography (CT) has been the most notable and prominent development in *X-ray* imaging since Roentgen's original discovery of *X-rays*. While conventional radiography is limited in its depiction of distinct soft tissues, CT enables direct imaging and differentiation of soft tissue structures, in addition to its depiction of osseous detail.

Transaxial images of the spine are obtained. However, computer reformatting of the collected data images in sagittal, coronal or oblique planes can be assembled without additional patient radiation exposure. Reconstructions can provide a three-dimensional perspective that is impossible with traditional radiography. The data can also be manipulated in the computer to produce images that selectively optimize visualization of either skeletal structures or the various soft tissues.

Superior contrast resolution, which is at least 100 times better than plain film [9], and a capacity to provide quantitative measurements of tissue, are among the features of CT. The ability of CT to image in the axial plain allows a more precise localization of anatomical structures and pathological processes. For example, CT is a valuable tool in the contemporary comprehensive assessment and management of acute cervical spinal trauma. Indications for CT in cervical spine trauma include plain films that are suggestive of, or suspicious for, vertebral fracture, further evaluation of a fracture or dislocation visualized on plain film, and situations when plain films and neurological symptoms do not correlate. CT is very accurate in determining whether neurological compression is due to bone or soft tissue [10]. With regard to neoplasm, CT scans demonstrate the size, spatial location and extent of a tumour. The images are used to plan radiotherapy and surgical protocols as well as assisting in determining how a tumour is responding to treatment. Cortical integrity and fine periosteal reactions are best visualized on CT. CT is also used to measure bone mineral density for the detection of osteoporosis. Adjunctive introduction of metrizamide contrast before CT examination enhances visualization of the subarachnoid space and is frequently used in cervical spine examination [5]. CT demonstrates a high effectiveness in the detection and evaluation of degenerative osseous changes, particularly of the facet joints, and correlates well with symptomatology and surgical findings [8].

Notwithstanding that CT is generally a valuable and reliable diagnostic technique, there are some drawbacks to consider. First, as *X-rays* are used to produce the CT image, consideration must be given to the patient's radiation exposure. Second, although the conventional axial images can be reconstructed into other planes, these resultant reformatted images have not typically possessed distinctly sharp detail. Improvements in this area are being made.

Additionally, the fixed gantry size of 55–70 cm prevents CT examination of particularly large patients who may not be able to physically fit into the gantry. Additionally, the patient table has a weight limit tolerance of approximately 300 lb (approx. 136 kg) [9].

Advances in CT imaging include the development of the spiral CT scanner. Through the use of an innovation called a power slip ring, this 'spiral' or 'helical' scanning allows the collection of a volume of data all in one position, rather than the original CT method of acquiring a stack of individual incremental slices. The spiral technique minimizes the potential for the slices to be misaligned on reformatting because of slight patient motion or breathing in between each slice acquisition. The result is a much quicker, more accurate and clearer scan. Faster scanning times will reduce patient movement artefacts. The newest machines are utilizing 'multislice' spiral CT scanning, and can collect up to four slices of data in 250–350 ms.

The data can even be computer-reconstructed to provide three-dimensional pictures. New software and advanced computer systems are being developed that enable creation of 3D 'virtual reality' images. These images are excellent surgical aids.

CT scanning has had a remarkable effect on the way patients are evaluated and subsequently treated. This exciting cutting edge technology continues to grow.

(ii) Magnetic resonance imaging

MRI, as applied to examination of the musculoskeletal system, has proved extremely useful owing to its distinctive ability to obtain direct images in the axial, coronal and sagittal planes. This multiplanar formatting capability, without the use of ionizing radiation or the need for patient repositioning, distinguishes MRI as an extremely flexible imaging modality. The excellent anatomical display and the sensitivity to early pathological changes make MRI a preferred imaging choice.

Because of the ability of MRI to provide superior contrast detail between different tissues possessing similar densities, it can distinguish between cortical bone, epidural fat, cerebrospinal fluid and the spinal cord. Therefore, MRI provides an unparalleled ability to assess cartilaginous, ligamentous, tendinous, synovial and osseous integrity.

MRI is an invaluable aid in diagnosing disorders of the brainstem, medulla, upper cervical cord and spinal canal. Congenital lesions, intramedullary and extramedullary intradural disease, including tumours, infection, ischaemia and demyelination can be assessed [10]. MRI also provides valuable information about the encompassing bony and ligamentous structures of the cranio-vertebral junction and cervical spine.

There is still debate over whether CT or MRI is the best modality for spinal imaging.

MRI is recommended by some for evaluation of patients with cervical myelopathy, as plain CT frequently does not optimally image cervical intervertebral discs [11]. However, there is more difficulty differentiating herniated disc from posterior osteophyte in the cervical spine than in the lumbar spine using MRI [8]. Evaluation of facet joint disease is less efficient with MRI. Disc herniation is probably better depicted by MRI than by other more conventional modalities. The clear distinction between annulus fibrosis and nucleus pulposus, and the visualization of the outer annulus and posterior longitudinal ligament complex can assist in characterizing the type of herniation (protrusion, extrusion or sequestration) [12]. Owing to loss of disc water content, disc degeneration can actually be ascertained much earlier with MRI than with plain film examination [4].

Owing to its use of a strong static magnetic field, contraindications for MRI include patients with cardiac pacemakers, certain ferromagnetic surgical clips, insulin infusion and chemotherapy pumps, other implants or prostheses, shrapnel and other metallic foreign bodies. Some metals are completely safe for MRI, such as non-ferromagnetic clips, dental amalgam, gold and silver. The safety of MRI for pregnant patients has not been determined. There are no known detrimental side effects to MRI; however, it is still a relatively new procedure.

With constant improvement in technology, new potentials for MRI continue to be realized. Studies are becoming shorter in duration, more comfortable and more affordable. These changes ensure MRI's future as the imaging modality of choice in a wide variety of clinical scenarios.

(iii) Spinal videofluoroscopy

Videofluoroscopy (VF), or cineradiography, involves the fluoroscopic examination of the cervical spine as it performs throughout its ranges of motion, including nodding, flexion and extension in the lateral and oblique projections, lateral bending, rotation and lateral bending in the open mouth projection. The examination is videotaped for detection and analysis of abnormal motion, including hypermobility or hypomobility, anterolisthesis, retrolisthesis, widening of the facet joints and lateral translation of atlas on axis.

Although it is a frequently employed modality, VF has been and continues to be somewhat controversial. Supporters claim that reliable, valid and therapeutically significant data are obtained from a VF study [13]. Critics point to research investigations failing to properly demonstrate efficacy, accuracy, positive or negative predictive value or reliability.

Additionally, and very importantly, there is no universally accepted terminology for the various phenomena visualized on VF, particularly as to what constitutes 'normal' motion. Other definitions, including abnormal motion, subluxation, hypermobility, hypomobility and instability, have also not been standardized

While VF certainly visualizes joint motion, drawing conclusions about the normality or abnormality of that motion is unreliable and unvalidated [14].

VF is excellent for visualizing real-time spinal motion. However, two problems become evident. The first is a reliability issue; attempts to quantify the findings of a videofluoroscopic examination seem to lack a solid foundation at this time. [8] Without digitization, accuracy in measurement with videofluoroscopy, i.e., numeric quantification, becomes essentially impossible to achieve. Reliability studies in peer review journals are needed. Some early evidence suggests that high resolution digital videofluoroscopy may prove a reliable method of measuring spinal motion [15–17].

The second problem remains. Once acceptable quantification of results with VF is achievable, clinical correlation to the demonstrated reliability still remains as an entirely separate issue [14]. There has been some preliminary testing regarding clinical correlation [18,19].

An important question to be addressed by advocates of videofluoroscopy is whether therapy will be altered by the additional information of abnormal 'within-range' motion when abnormal intersegmental motion has already been determined with plain film radiography; that is, how will the utilization of VF as a supplement to plain film affect the treatment protocol of the doctor?

Proponents claim that there is additional information gained, i.e., abnormal within-range motion, facilitating a better understanding of the mechanisms of hyper- and hypomobility following trauma. Furthermore, they contend that these joint motion studies provide hard medico-legal evidence, allowing follow-up studies to evaluate effectiveness of treatment as well as assisting in the assessment of the permanence of a disability [20].

Contemporary recommended protocols and position papers for spinal application of video-fluoroscopy do not appear to have a strong foundation in the current literature and may be motivated by financial, personal or political bias [8].

Although VF may have a future place in the biomechanical assessment of the cervical spine, much basic research must be completed before the confident clinical application of this modality to broad patient populations.

(iv) Radionuclide imaging

Radionuclide imaging of a chosen organ system depends on the selective concentration of specific radioactive pharmaceuticals that have been introduced into the patient, usually by injection into the venous system. Gamma rays are emitted by the patient, detected by a gamma camera and a radiographic image is produced. Tissue commonly evaluated via this method include the skeleton, brain, lungs, liver, thyroid and heart [4,21]. Different pharmaceuticals are used depending on the desired tissue to be examined.

Skeletal radionuclide imaging, also referred to as bone scintigraphy or a bone scan, utilizes technetium-99m methylene diphosphonate (99^{m}Tc-MDP). This radionuclide is incorporated into the hydroxyapatite crystal of bone by the osteoblasts. Increased uptake of the isotope is observed as a dark region or 'hot spot' in conditions that cause an increased metabolic activity in osseous tissue, as well as an increased blood supply. This includes tumours, infections, healing fractures, some systemic metabolic conditions and joint diseases. Therefore, function and physiology, as well as anatomy, are being assessed in bone scintigraphy. The isotope is excreted by the kidneys, providing an examination of renal function as well. Only 3–5% bone destruction is necessary to be visible on a bone scan. Although scintigraphy is highly sensitive, up to 10 times more sensitive than plain film examinations [4], it is not as specific. The image is quantitative, as a measure of metabolic activity

[4]; the underlying cause is not specifically discernible. Therefore, for example, a scan of a neoplasm may appear identical to that of osteomyelitis; the ultimate diagnosis lies in the integration and correlation of other radiographic examinations, clinical data and possibly a biopsy. The sensitivity of scintigraphy makes it ideal for the detection of subtle or occult fractures. A bone scan will determine whether a vertebral body compression fracture seen on plain film is old or new, when the history and clinical presentation are equivocal. Bone scans do have the advantage of permitting the entire skeleton to be imaged at one time, and thus are very useful in the detection of multiple metastatic foci. Pregnancy and breastfeeding are contraindications for all radionuclide imaging [21].

SELECTED CERVICAL SPINE ROENTGENOMETRICS

While the use of radiography as an aid in the biomechanical and postural evaluation of a patient is well accepted, the various specific systems of line-drawing and spinographic analysis are not as universally acknowledged. For example, upper cervical practitioners utilize the radiographic measurement of static vertebral misalignment to help determine on which side and at what angle the adjustment should be given. Results may be used to demonstrate correction of the occipital-atlanto-axial misalignment on pre- and post-*X*-ray*s* [22]. Few research studies have been published that examine the accuracy of the upper cervical marking procedures and the studies that do exist offer conflicting conclusions. The findings of Sigler and Howe suggest that the ranges of error of any measured differences using this system are just as likely to be from marking error as from actual atlas positioning change [22]. Rochester and others have found that all aspects of the upper cervical marking procedures are very reliable [23]. One must recognize, however, that there exists inherent error in any attempt to measure and quantify aspects of the human body radiographically, including image blurring, projectional distortion, variability in patient positioning, anatomical variation, location of standard reference points and observer error. Regarding the extent that spinal structural asymmetry affects the accuracy of these techniques, Howe states, 'Any method of spinographic interpretation which utilizes millimetric measurements from any set of preselected points is very likely to be faulty because structural asymmetry is universal in all vertebrae' [24].

Normal cervical spine flexion and extension in the sagittal plane involve a rotational or angular component (tilting) and a translational component (gliding). The superior cervical segments tend to have a larger glide component, while the inferior segments exhibit a larger tilting component. Many methods measure the change in angle between positions of adjacent vertebrae on flexion and extension; this is the tilt component. An attempt to quantify the translational aspect of cervical vertebral segment motion was undertaken by Henderson and Dorman [25].

The reader is invited to decide on the merits of the abundant available measurements and their methodologies for her/himself, and is therefore advised to consult any of a plethora of manuscripts and manuals of these various systems for their individual approaches to film analysis and explanations of their advocated potential significance to spinal manipulation. A selection of chiropractic and orthopaedic roentgenometrics follows [4,26,27].

McGregor's line (Fig. 4.9)

On a lateral cervical film, taken at a 72-inch focal-film distance, a line is drawn joining the posterior margin of the hard palate to the inferior aspect of the occiput. The apex of the odontoid should not project above this line more than 8 mm in men and 10 mm in women. Under 18 years of age, these maximum values diminish with decreasing chronological age. An abnormal superior migration of the dens indicates basilar impression (invagination). Common aetiologies for basilar impression include bone softening diseases such as Paget's disease, osteomalacia and fibrous dysplasia. McGregor's line is considered to be the most optimal method for assessing basilar impression.

Chamberlain's line (Fig. 4.10)

On a lateral cervical film, taken at a 72-inch focal-film distance, a line is drawn joining the

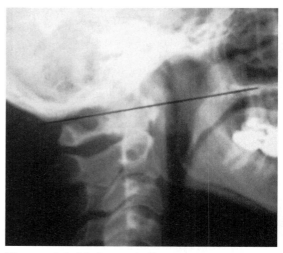

Figure 4.9 *McGregor's line (courtesy Arnie B Deltoff, DC, FATA, Toronto, Ontario, Canada).*

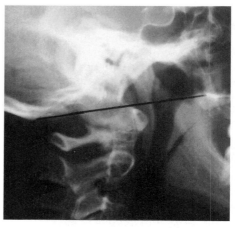

Figure 4.10 *Chamberlain's line (courtesy Robert J Bacon, DC, FATA, Toronto, Ontario, Canada).*

posterior margin of the hard palate to the posterior margin of the foramen magnum (opisthion). Basilar impression is present if the odontoid apex projects 7 mm above this line.

MacRae's line (foramen magnum line) (Fig. 4.11)

On a lateral cervical or lateral skull film a line is drawn to join the anterior margin (basion)

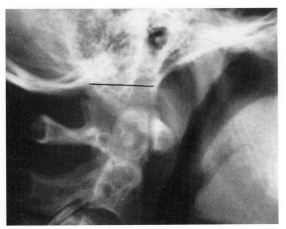

Figure 4.11 *MacRae's line and the effective foramen magnum distance.*

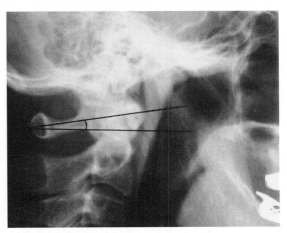

Figure 4.12 *Horizontal line of atlas.*

and the posterior margin (opisthion) of the foramen magnum. Basilar invagination, secondary to acquired or congenital bone softening diseases, is present if the inferior margin of the posterior occiput is convex upward, or extends above the line. Additionally, a perpendicular line drawn through the odontoid apex should intersect MacRae's line in its anterior quarter; if not, fracture, dislocation or dysplasia of the dens may be present.

Effective foramen magnum distance (Fig. 4.11)

On a neutral lateral cervical film, taken at a 72-inch focal-film distance, MacRae's line is drawn to assess the sagittal diameter of the foramen magnum; it should not measure less than 19 mm for an adult. A lesser value is highly indicative that the patient will demonstrate signs and symptoms of lower medulla or upper cord involvement. A higher value may indicate a congenitally large foramen magnum, which may be seen in an Arnold-Chiari malformation.

Horizontal line of atlas (Fig. 4.12)

On a neutral lateral cervical film, a line is drawn joining the middle of C1's anterior tubercle to the middle of its posterior tubercle. This line should normally form an angle within the range of 7–20 degrees to a true horizontal line.

If the angle measures greater than 20 degrees, a hyperextension malposition of atlas is demonstrated; an angle less than 7 degrees indicates a hyperflexion malposition.

Horizontal line of axis (Fig. 4.13)

On a neutral lateral cervical film, a line is drawn joining the middle of the anterior body margin of C2 (not including the dens) with the middle of its spinous process. This line should ideally be parallel to Chamberlain's line.

Deviance from parallel indicates the presence of a hyperflexion or hyperextension malposition of axis.

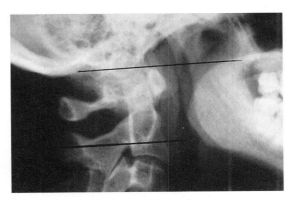

Figure 4.13 *Horizontal line of axis.*

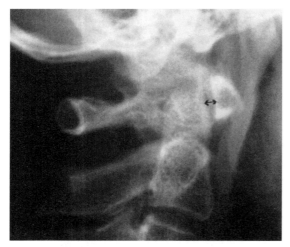

Figure 4.14 *Atlanto-dental interspace.*

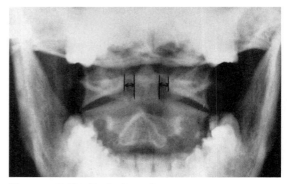

Figure 4.15 *Periodontal space.*

and an inverted 'V'-shape in extension; in such cases the measurement is made at the narrowest portion of the joint.

Atlanto-dental interval (ADI) (Fig. 4.14)

A neutral lateral cervical spine film is utilized, taken at a 72-inch focal-film distance. Flexion and extension views can be used for comparison. The distance between the midpoint of the posterior margin of the anterior tubercle of atlas and the anterior surface of the odontoid process is measured. One to 2 mm is the normal adult value. This distance should not exceed 3 mm for adults and 5 mm for children. An increase in this measurement is indicative of damage to, or absence of, the transverse ligament of atlas.

Flexion is the most optimum view to assess this interspace, since in this position the most stress is placed on the transverse ligament. An increased measurement noted on the flexion view compared with the neutral is strongly indicative of transverse ligament insufficiency and will confirm a borderline diagnosis from a neutral film. A decreased space may be noted due to degenerative arthritis.

Some causes of increased ADI include rheumatoid arthritis and its variants such as ankylosing spondylitis, psoriatic arthritis, Reiter's syndrome (all due to hyperaemic inflammatory resorption of the tubercles of attachment of the transverse ligament), trauma (tearing of the transverse ligament), Down's syndrome, and post-streptococcal pharyngeal infection (Grisel's disease). It is not uncommon for the normal ADI to acquire a 'V'-shaped configuration in flexion,

Periodontal space (Fig. 4.15)

On an anteroposterior open-mouth view, the distance between the medial margin of each lateral mass and the odontoid is assessed. The space on either side of the dens should be identical in width and have parallel margins.

A difference between left and right measurements indicates a lateral shift of atlas on axis. This may be due to subluxation, axis fracture or alar ligament insufficiency. If the axis spinous process is not in the midline, there is a possible rotational component to the malposition.

Atlanto-axial alignment (Fig. 4.16)

On an anteroposterior open-mouth view, a line is drawn along the lateral border of each lateral mass. Another line is drawn along the lateral margins of the axis body. The lateral margin of the atlas's lateral mass is compared to the ipsilateral lateral aspect of the axis vertebral body. Normally, these two landmarks should be in complete alignment bilaterally. Bilateral lateral displacement of the C1 lateral masses suggests Jefferson's fracture of atlas; bilateral lateral displacement of C2 body margins suggests axis fracture.

Unilateral nonalignment may be seen in an atlas-axis rotatory subluxation, odontoid fracture or alar ligament damage. In children, a mild degree of 'overhanging' of atlas may be a normal variant.

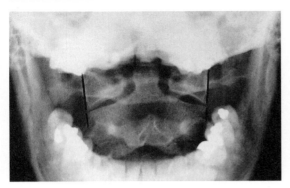

Figure 4.16 *Atlanto-axial alignment.*

George's line (Fig. 4.17)

On a lateral cervical film, the posterior body surfaces from C2 through C7 are connected with a continuous curved line, which traverses the disc spaces. It is important to utilize the mid-body of each segment as a guide in the construction of the line, as the presence of degenerative spurs at the vertebral body endplates and uncinate processes can result in interpreting a false positive break in the line. Flexion and extension views are especially useful to determine disruptions in George's line. Care should be taken to eliminate positional rotation, since this may create a projectional disruption. In normal younger patients who are particularly flexible, mild disruptions at multiple consecutive levels may occur in flexion and extension; this should not be misinterpreted as pathological. Adjacent posterior body margins should not translate more than 3 mm in these patients on comparison of the flexion and extension views.

A true break in the continuous smooth contour of the line, manifesting as an anterolisthesis or retrolisthesis, may be a radiographic sign of instability due to fracture, dislocation, degenerative joint disease or inflammatory joint disease.

Spinolaminar junction line (posterior cervical line) (Fig. 4.18)

On a lateral cervical spine film, the lamina-spinous process junction, seen as a distinct cortical white line, is identified at each level from atlas to C7. (This white line will be absent at any level possessing spina bifida.)

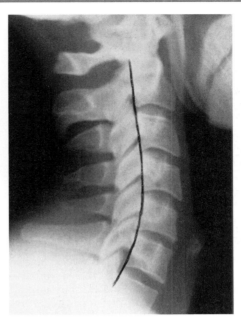

Figure 4.17 *George's line (courtesy Robert J Bacon, DC, FATA, Toronto, Ontario, Canada).*

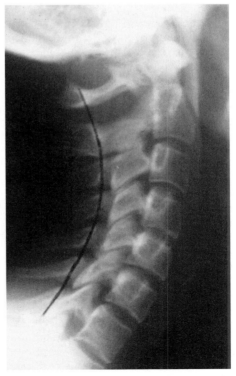

Figure 4.18 *Spinolaminar junction line (courtesy Robert J Bacon, DC, FATA, Toronto, Ontario, Canada).*

Each spinolaminar junction demonstrates an anterior convexity. A curved line is drawn joining atlas to C7 using the most anterior aspect of each spinolaminar junction. This line should form a smooth, continuous curve. If the curve is discontinuous at any level, anterior or posterior vertebral displacement is likely present. This line is especially useful to detect subtle fractures of the dens and atlanto-axial subluxation, which otherwise may be overlooked. Disruption in the mid to lower cervical spine may indicate anterolisthesis, retrolisthesis or frank dislocation.

This line is used primarily as a check to confirm an abnormal George's line finding, or to replace George's line if exuberant pathology of the posterior vertebral bodies or poor quality film makes landmark identification difficult. In children, the spinolaminar junction line of axis should not appear greater than 2 mm anterior to the other levels.

Sagittal dimension of spinal canal (Fig. 4.19)

A neutral lateral cervical spine film is used, taken at a 72-inch focal film distance. Measurements are made at each level between the posterior surface of the mid-vertebral body and the nearest surface of the same segmental spinolaminar junction line. For adults, the minimum dimensions are: C1–16 mm; C2–14 mm; C3–13 mm; C4 through C7–12 mm.

Canal stenosis is suggested when the measurement is less than these values. If degenerative posterior osteophytes are present, the measurement is taken from the tip of the osteophyte, in order to examine the magnitude of its stenotic effect; this is best accomplished with an extension film. MRI or CT are more accurate modalities for assessing spinal stenosis.

A widened canal may indicate intradural, extramedullary or extradural lesions, including spinal neoplasm, such as a meningioma, or syringomyelia. Pathological erosion of the posterior vertebral body may also increase the canal diameter. For adults, the maximum normal measurements are: C1–31 mm; C2–27 mm; C3–23 mm; C4 through C7–22 mm. Other entities that may alter this measurement include achondroplastic dwarfism and neurofibromatosis.

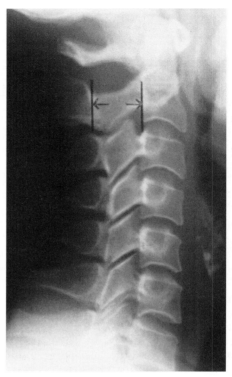

Figure 4.19 *Sagittal dimension of spinal canal (courtesy Robert J Bacon, DC, FATA, Toronto, Ontario, Canada).*

Cervical gravitational line (Fig. 4.20)

On a neutral lateral cervical spine film, a vertical line is drawn through the odontoid apex, perpendicular to the bottom edge of the film. The distance between this line and the anterosuperior corner of the C7 vertebral body is evaluated. Ideally, the gravitational line should intersect the anterosuperior margin of C7. If the line descends anteriorly to the anterosuperior margin of C7, this indicates the presence of an anterior gravitational line with resultant anterior head carriage. This line allows a gross assessment of where gravitational forces or stresses are acting. An anterior gravitational line denotes an anterior weight-bearing posture, and is suggestive of an inordinate amount of gravitational forces acting on the discs, whereas a posterior gravitational line suggests that an inordinate amount of gravitational forces are acting on the facet joints. An abnormal cervical lordosis often accompanies a shift in the gravitational line.

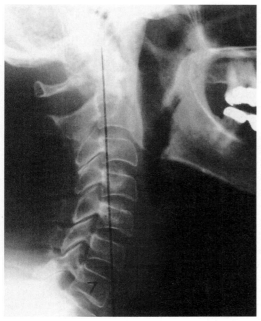

(a)

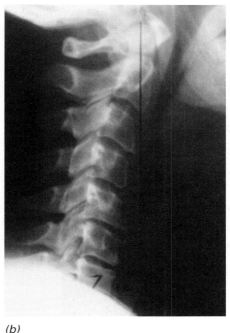

(b)

Figure 4.20 *(a) Cervical gravitational line (courtesy Don R Leck, BSc, DC, Toronto, Ontario, Canada). (b) This 47-year-old man demonstrates cervical kyphosis with a 12-mm anterior shift in the gravitational line (courtesy Leo Slivka, DC, FATA, Toronto, Ontario, Canada).*

Cervical lordosis

(i) Angle of cervical curve (Fig. 4.21)

On a lateral cervical spine film, a line is drawn through the midpoints of the C1 anterior and posterior tubercles; another line is drawn along the inferior surface of the C7 vertebral body. Perpendiculars are constructed from these lines to the point of intersection, and the resultant acute angle is measured. The average lordosis is 40 degrees. Angles less than 35 degrees are considered hypolordotic, while angles greater than 45 degrees are considered hyperlordotic. Reduced curves may be observed due to trauma, osteoarthritic changes, muscle spasm and aberrant intersegmental mechanics. A kyphotic cervical spine will produce an obtuse angle.

The cervical lordosis angle may provide an objective value that does not appear to coincide with the observer's subjective assessment of the curve. This is because only the positions of atlas and C7 are considered. Therefore, while a spine may present an objectively normal lordotic measurement, it may

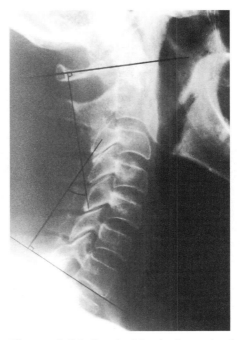

Figure 4.21 *Cervical lordosis evaluation: angle of cervical curve.*

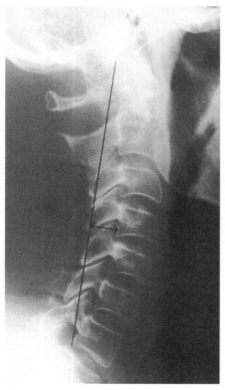

Figure 4.22 *Cervical lordosis evaluation: depth method.*

visually appear to be hyper or hypolordotic. This is usually due to a partial abnormality in the curve, with some degree of compensation. For example, C1 and C7 may be normal but the mid-portion of the curve is flattened.

Position of the head is critical; if the chin is lowered or retracted, its effect is to straighten the lordosis. Yochum states that many authors have stressed the lack of correlation between altered cervical curvature and clinical symptomatology.

(ii) Depth method (Fig. 4.22)

This is a more accurate but less commonly used evaluation of cervical lordosis. On a lateral cervical spine film, taken at a 72-inch focal-film distance, a line is drawn from the posterosuperior aspect of the dens to the posteroinferior corner of the C7 vertebral body. The largest transverse distance between this line and the posterior vertebral body margins is measured; this is usually at C4. The normal curve range is from 7 to 17 mm, with an average depth of 12 mm.

Ruth Jackson's cervical stress lines

Cervical flexion (Fig. 4.23b) and extension (Fig. 4.23a) views are used. Two lines are

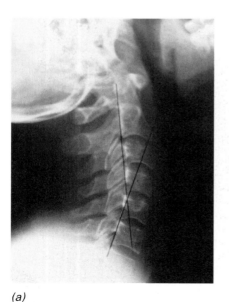

(a)

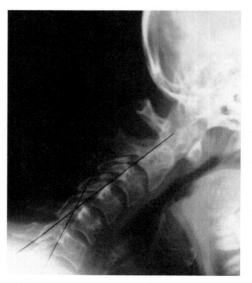

(b)

Figure 4.23 *Ruth Jackson's cervical stress lines. (a) Extension (courtesy Robert J Bacon, DC, FATA, Toronto, Ontario, Canada). (b) Flexion (courtesy Don R Leck, BSc, DC, Toronto, Ontario, Canada).*

drawn on each film. The first is drawn along the posterior surface of the C2 body; the second line is drawn along the posterior surface of the C7 body, until it intersects with the first line. Normally, these lines should intersect at the level of the C5–C6 disc space or facet joints in flexion, and at the level of the C4–C5 disc space or facet joints in extension.

It has been proposed that the lines intersect at the level of greatest stress when the cervical spine is placed in flexion and extension. Osteoarthritic changes, muscle spasm and aberrant kinematics may alter the stress point.

Prevertebral soft tissues (Fig. 4.24)

On a neutral lateral cervical film, taken at a 72-inch focal-film distance, the soft tissue thickness at two levels are most frequently evaluated:

(a) The retropharyngeal interspace
The distance between the anteroinferior corner of C2 and the posterior border of the pharyngeal air shadow is measured, and should not exceed 7 mm.

(b) The retrotracheal interspace
The distance between the anteroinferior corner of C6 and the posterior border of the tracheal air shadow is measured, and should not exceed 20 mm.

The significance of these measurements is to determine if any soft tissue swelling is present. Care must be taken to measure at the true vertebral body border and not to include any degenerative changes in the bone such as osteophytes that may alter the value. Examples of pathologies which can increase these measurements include precervical neoplasia, metastasis, retropharyngeal and retrotracheal abscesses (tonsils and adenoids), and traumatic oedema or haemorrhage. For increases in retrotracheal interspace especially, consider the presence of haematoma, spinal fracture, goitre, chordoma, Zenker's diverticulum, postcricoid carcinoma, and inflammatory disease.

ATLAS OF CERVICAL SPINE IMAGING

Examples of a variety of conditions affecting the cervical spine are presented in Figures 4.25–4.85

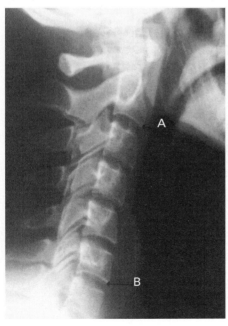

Figure 4.24 *Prevertebral soft tissues: A, Retropharyngeal interspace. B, Retrotracheal interspace.*

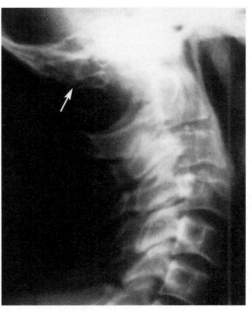

Figure 4.25 *Occipitalization. Note the complete fusion of atlas to occiput (arrow) (from Deltoff MN, Kogon PK: The Portable Skeletal X-ray Library, St Louis, Mosby, 1997).*

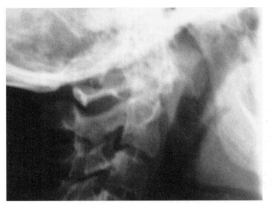

Figure 4.26 *Markedly hypoplastic posterior arch of atlas in a 29-year-old woman. (courtesy Lorne Greenspan, MD, Toronto, Ontario, Canada).*

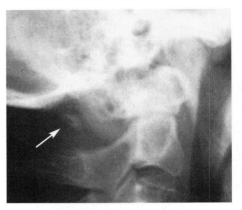

Figure 4.27 *This 32-year-old woman demonstrates agenesis of the posterior arch of atlas. Only the posterior tubercle is ossified (arrow).*

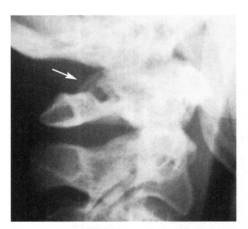

Figure 4.28 *Pons posticus of atlas (arrow) forming an arcuate foramen in this 47-year-old man. (courtesy Leo Slivka, DC, FATA, Toronto, Ontario, Canada).*

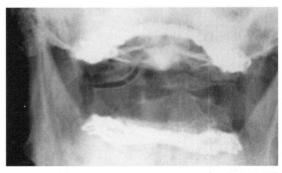

Figure 4.29 *Asymmetrical articular surfaces are observed at atlas-axis in this 55-year-old man (courtesy Catherine Straus, DC, Kitchener, Ontario, Canada).*

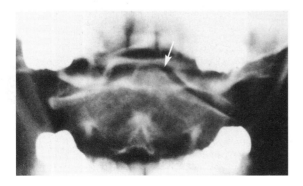

Figure 4.30 *Congenitally hypoplastic odontoid. The dens has not fully ossified, and manifests as an osseous mound (arrow) in this 52-year-old woman.*

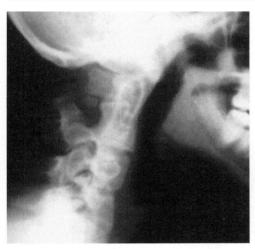

Figure 4.31 *Marked upper cervical congenital anomalies in this patient include occipitalization and abnormal segmentation of atlas and axis.*

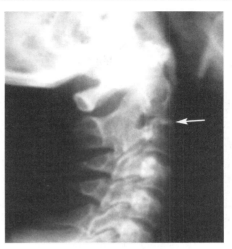

Figure 4.33 *Congenital synostosis of C2–C3. Note the 'wasp-waist' deformity (arrow) anterior to the rudimentary disc, fusion of the posterior vertebral elements, and visualization of the intervertebral foramen at this level in the lateral projection (from Deltoff MN, Kogon PK: The Portable Skeletal X-ray Library, St Louis, Mosby, 1997).*

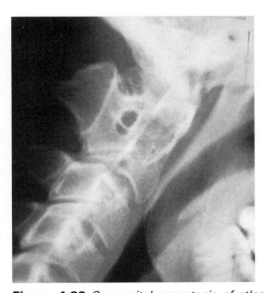

Figure 4.32 *Congenital synostosis of atlas-axis in a 31-year-old man. Note the complete fusion of both the anterior and posterior vertebral elements, with clear depiction of an intervertebral foramen (courtesy Sheldon Hershkop, MD, Toronto, Ontario, Canada) (from Deltoff MN, Kogon PK: The Portable Skeletal X-ray Library, St Louis, Mosby, 1997).*

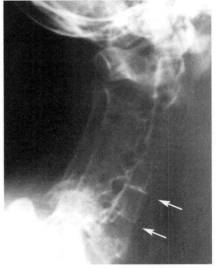

Figure 4.34 *Multiple congenital block vertebrae in a 47-year-old man with Klippel-Feil syndrome. C2–C7 demonstrates complete fusion of the vertebral bodies as well as the posterior elements. Rudimentary discs are evident (arrows), and the intervertebral foramina are visualized on this lateral projection. These radiographic signs indicate congenital synostosis (courtesy Patricia McCord, DC, Scarborough, Ontario, Canada).*

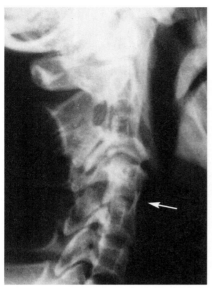

Figure 4.35 *Multiple congenital block vertebrae, C2–C3 and C4–C5, in a 41-year-old woman. Observe the anterior concavity or 'wasp waist' deformity (arrow) at the site of the C4–C5 rudimentary disc. Secondary degenerative disc disease has resulted at the remaining mobile segments, C3–C4 and C5–C6 (courtesy Keith Thomson, DC, Peterborough, Ontario, Canada).*

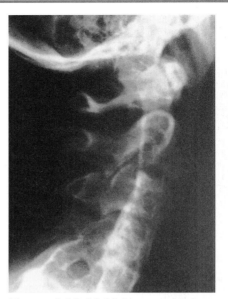

Figure 4.36 *Multiple congenital synostosis from C3–C4 caudad in a 19-year-old woman with Klippel-Feil syndrome (courtesy Mark Binsted, DC, Fernie, British Columbia, Canada).*

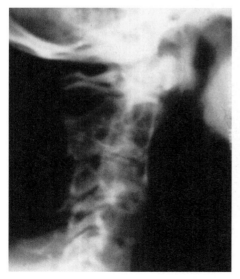

Figure 4.37 *C2–C5 multiple congenital block vertebrae, with non-fusion of the atlas posterior arch. (courtesy of Jacinthe Demarais, DC, Greenfield Park, Quebec, Canada). (from Deltoff MN, Kogon PK: The Portable Skeletal X-ray Library, St Louis, Mosby, 1997).*

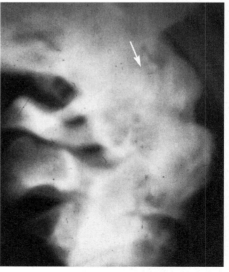

Figure 4.38 *Os odontoideum. The entire atlas and the odontoid tip (arrow) demonstrate posterior translation. (from Deltoff MN, Kogon PK: The Portable Skeletal X-ray Library, St Louis, Mosby, 1997).*

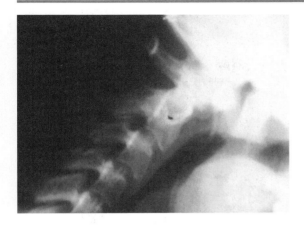

Figure 4.39 *Os odontoideum. Note the marked anterior translation of the odontoid and atlas on forward flexion (from Deltoff MN, Kogon PK: The Portable Skeletal X-ray Library, St Louis, Mosby, 1997).*

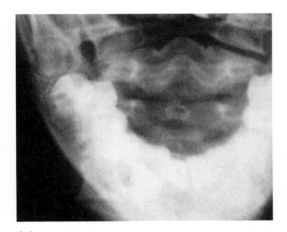

(a)

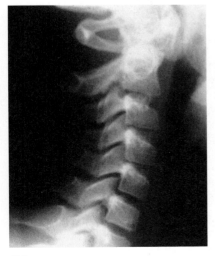

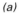
(b)

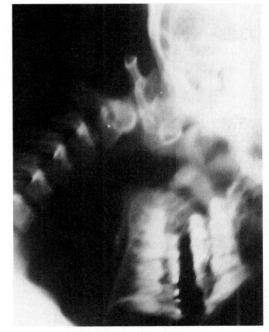

(c)

Figure 4.40 *Os odontoideum in a 9-year-old boy. (a) AP open mouth. (b) Neutral lateral. (c) Flexion. Note the extensive anterior translation of atlas. This patient required posterior surgical stabilization (courtesy Patrick G Bickert, DC, Kelowna, British Columbia, Canada).*

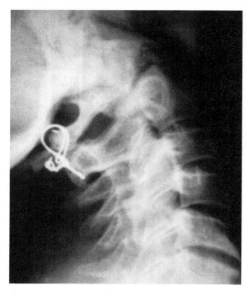

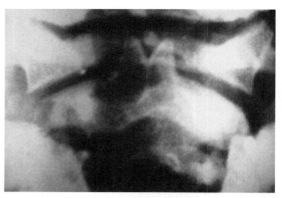

Figure 4.42 *Ossiculum terminale of Bergmann. Observe the non-fusion of the odontoid tip, separated from the remainder of the dens by a characteristic 'V'-shaped cleft. (from Deltoff MN, Kogon PK: The Portable Skeletal X-ray Library, St Louis, Mosby, 1997).*

Figure 4.41 *Surgical wires have been used to reduce instability in this patient with os odontoideum.*

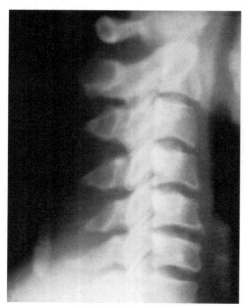

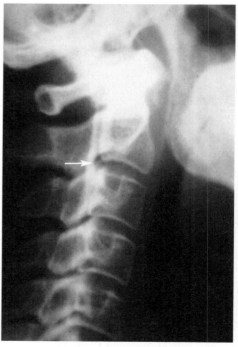

Figure 4.43 *A large nuchal bone is incidentally observed in the nuchal ligament.*

Figure 4.44 *Note the linear calcific density (arrow) in the anterior spinal canal, representing ossification of the posterior longitudinal ligament (OPLL).*

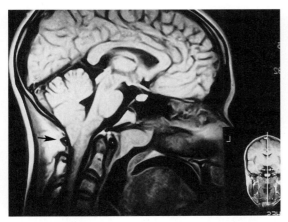

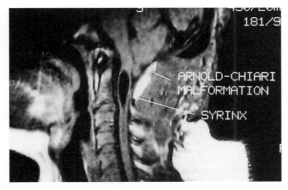

(a)

Figure 4.45 *MRI demonstrating Arnold-Chiari malformation. Note the cerebellar herniation (arrow) through the foramen magnum (courtesy Ray N Conley, DC, DACBR, Overland Park, Kansas, USA).*

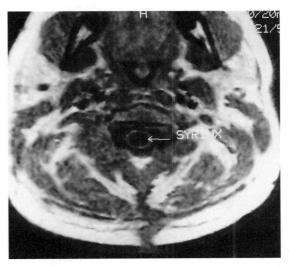

(b)

Figure 4.46 *(a) MRI demonstrating Arnold-Chiari malformation and a syrinx at the C2 level in a 31-year-old man. (b) Axial view depicting syrinx (courtesy David L Berens, MD, Buffalo MRI, Amherst, New York, USA).*

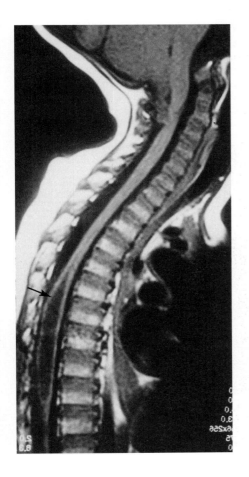

Figure 4.47 *Paediatric thoracic syrinx (arrow) accompanied by an Arnold-Chiari malformation (courtesy Picker International Inc., Cleveland, Ohio, USA).*

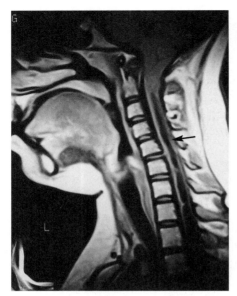

Figure 4.48 *Syringomyelia. Note the extensive irregular longitudinal fluid-filled cavity (syrinx) running longitudinally throughout the length of the spinal cord (arrow) (courtesy Ray N Conley, DC, DACBR, Overland Park, Kansas, USA).*

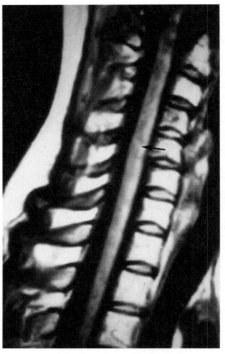

Figure 4.49 *Note the plaques of demyelination (arrow) disseminated throughout the length of the spinal cord in this patient with multiple sclerosis (courtesy Richard A Leverone, DC, DACBR, St Petersburg, Florida, USA).*

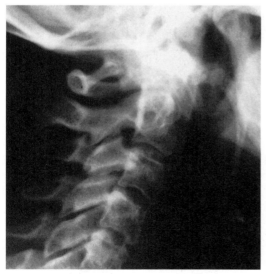

Figure 4.50 *Bilateral ossification of the stylohyoid ligaments in a 43-year-old woman. When symptoms occur, which may include dysphagia, the condition is referred to as Eagle syndrome (courtesy Shane Fainman, MD, Toronto, Ontario, Canada).*

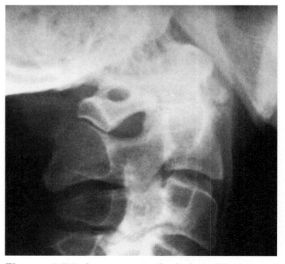

Figure 4.51 *Accessory articulation, 'kissing spinouses,' at atlas-axis, in a 63-year-old man. A pons posticus is incidentally noted (courtesy George D Gale, MD, Toronto, Ontario, Canada).*

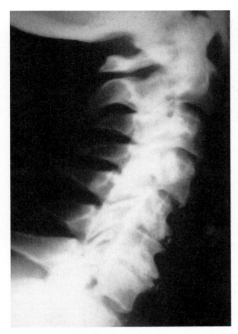

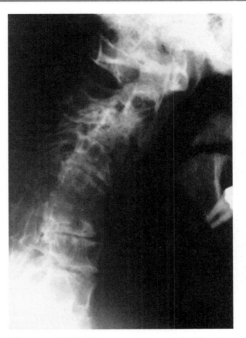

Figure 4.52 *Advanced degenerative disc disease at C5–C6 and C6–C7. Note the loss of disc height, subarticular sclerosis and osteophyte formation. Also note the alordosis from C4 caudad, which has probably contributed to, and accelerated, the osteoarthritic process (from Deltoff MN, Kogon PK: The Portable Skeletal X-ray Library, St Louis, Mosby, 1997).*

Figure 4.53 *Severe osteoarthritic changes are observed at all levels. Degenerative anterolistheses are noted at C2 and C3. Complete fusion across the C5–C6 disc space is present owing to the markedly advanced longstanding degenerative process.*

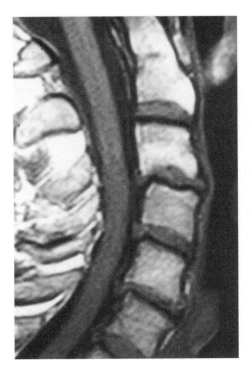

Figure 4.54 *Multiple disc herniations, from C3–C4 through C6–C7, are demonstrated with MRI (courtesy Picker International Inc., Cleveland, Ohio, USA).*

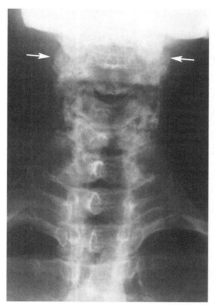

Figure 4.55 *Osteoarthritis of the joints of von Luschka in a 63-year-old woman. Marked blunting and moderate sclerosis of the uncinate processes are observed at C6–C7 bilaterally, and at C5–C6 on the reading left. Additionally, sclerotic osseous hypertrophic spurring is evident bilaterally at the C3–C4 level (arrows), indicating advanced facet arthrosis (courtesy Howard Jacobs, MD, Toronto, Ontario, Canada).*

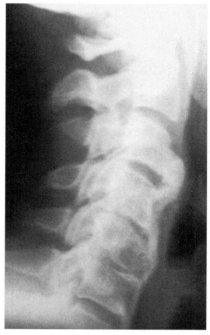

Figure 4.56 *Diffuse idiopathic skeletal hyperostosis (DISH) in a 51-year-old man. Note the marked 'flowing' osseous bridging of the anterior vertebral bodies from C3–C4 caudad. Aside from overlying degenerative disc disease at C4–C5 and C5–C6, the remaining disc spaces are well maintained.*

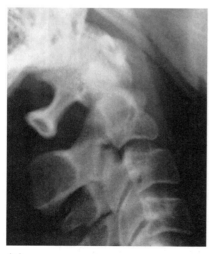

(a)

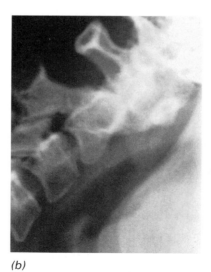

(b)

Figure 4.57 *52-year-old woman with rheumatoid arthritis. (a) Extension. (b) Flexion. Atlanto-axial instability due to transverse ligament rupture manifests as a marked increase in the atlantodental interspace (ADI). The ADI measured 3 mm on extension and increases to 9 mm on flexion (courtesy Lisette A Logan, MRT, Brampton, Ontario, Canada).*

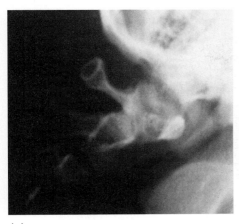

(a)

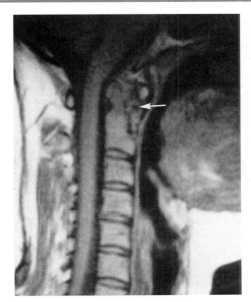

(b)

Figure 4.58 *Rheumatoid arthritis in a 25-year-old woman. (a) Flexion demonstrates increased atlantodental interspace due to transverse ligament rupture. The odontoid is not visualized. (b) MRI demonstrates marked destruction of the odontoid by pannus (arrow) (courtesy Michael T Buehler, DC, DACBR, Lake Zurich, Illinois, USA).*

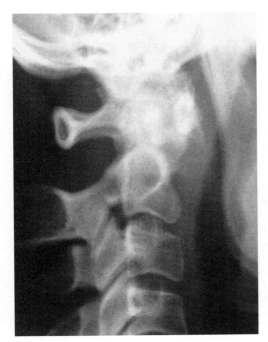

Figure 4.59 *A widened ADI (4 mm), secondary to rupture of the transverse ligament, is observed in this 40-year-old woman with psoriatic arthritis (courtesy Ernest Perry, DC, Toronto, Ontario, Canada).*

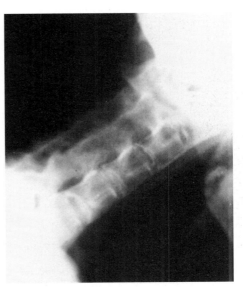

Figure 4.60 *Ankylosing spondylitis. Note the total anterior and posterior fusion, with marked anterior head carriage.*

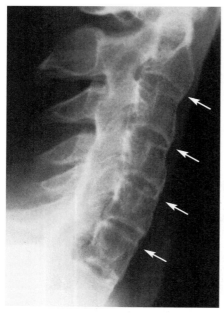

Figure 4.61 *Ankylosing spondylitis. Note the very thin, vertical, inflammatory syndesmophytes (arrows) resulting in vertebral body fusion throughout. Disc spaces are totally maintained. Facetal fusion from C2–C3 caudad completes the total cervical spine ankylosis.*

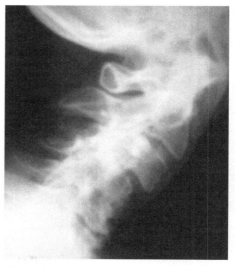

Figure 4.62 *C4–C5 advanced infectious discitis. Note the complete destruction of the C4 inferior endplate and C5 superior endplate, with eradication of the disc space, and marked increase in the prevertebral soft tissue. Also observe the advanced facet arthrosis throughout and the incidentally noted nuchal bone.*

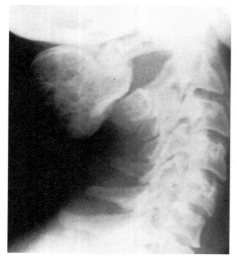

Figure 4.63 *A 43-year-old woman with an osteoblastoma demonstrating marked expansion of the posterior atlas tubercle, with prolific internal septation and amorphous calcification. The neural arch is a preferred site for osteoblastoma (courtesy Howard W Fisher, DC, Toronto, Ontario, Canada).*

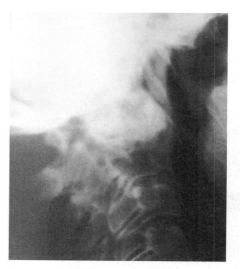

Figure 4.64 *Complete destruction of the C2 vertebral body due to metastatic disease in a 73-year-old woman.*

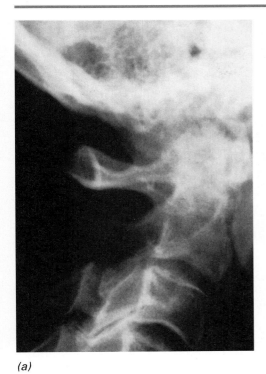

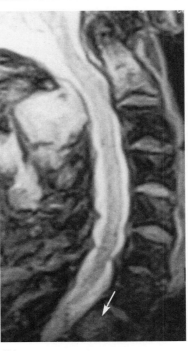

(a)

(b)

Figure 4.65 *Lytic metastasis to C2 in a 60-year-old man. (a) Note the complete destruction of the axis posterior arch. (b) MRI demonstrates involvement of the C2 body as well as the posterior elements, as denoted by the brighter signal. In addition, the T1 body is also affected (arrow) (courtesy Michael T Buehler, DC, DACBR, Lake Zurich, Illinois, USA).*

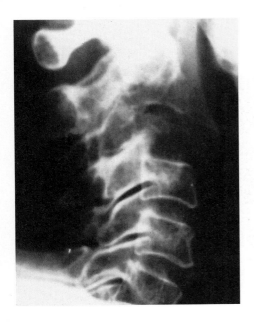

Figure 4.66 *Lytic metastatic disease has resulted in obliteration of the C3 vertebral body (courtesy Peter L Kogon, DC, DACBR, FCCR(C), FICC, Trois-Rivieres, Quebec, Canada).*

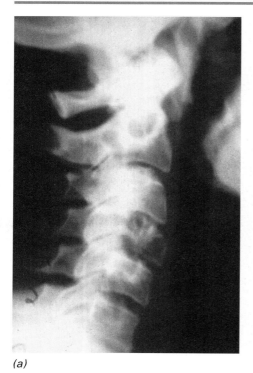

(a)

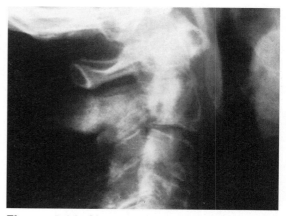

(b)

Figure 4.67 *Lytic metastasis to the C4 vertebral body in a 45-year-old man. (a) The plain film demonstrates lytic destruction of the C4 body. (b) Retropulsion of the affected body has resulted in ventral cord compression as demonstrated on MRI (courtesy Richard A Leverone, DC, DACBR, St Petersburg, Florida, Canada).*

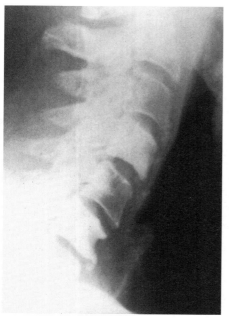

Figure 4.68 *Blastic metastasis from a primary prostate carcinoma in a 74-year-old man. Note the homogeneously radiodense 'ivory' vertebral bodies at C4 and C6.*

Figure 4.69 *Observe the blastic metastasis in the posterior arch of axis from a primary prostate carcinoma (courtesy Douglas G Sandwell, DC, Toronto, Ontario, Canada).*

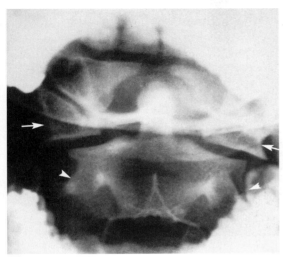

(a)

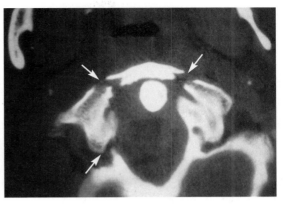

(b)

Figure 4.70 *Jefferson fracture of the atlas. (a) The outer margins of the lateral masses of atlas (arrows) overhang the lateral aspect of the axis body (arrowheads), signifying a 'bursting ring' fracture of the atlas (from Deltoff MN, Kogon PK: The Portable Skeletal X-ray Library, St Louis, Mosby, 1997). (b) Multiple fracture sites (arrows) through the atlas ring are clearly demonstrated on CT (courtesy Richard A Leverone, DC, DACBR, St Petersburg, Florida, USA).*

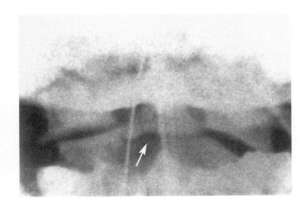

Figure 4.71 *A Jefferson fracture of the atlas, demonstrated by bilateral overhanging of the lateral masses, is accompanied by a fracture through the base of the odontoid (arrow) (courtesy Michael T Buehler, DC, DACBR, Lake Zurich, Illinois, USA).*

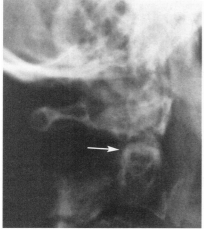

(a)

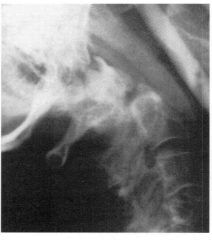

(b)

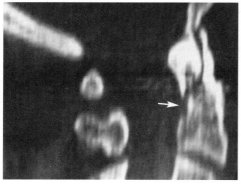

(c)

Figure 4.72 *This 66-year-old man has a Type 2 fracture of the odontoid. This is a common but unstable fracture running through the base of the dens (courtesy Hartley B Bressler, DC, MD, CCFP, Toronto, Ontario, Canada) (a) An oblique radiolucent line traverses the dens (arrow). (b) Extension demonstrates marked retrolisthesis of the atlas and the dens. (c) CT sagittal reconstruction clearly delineates the fracture (arrow). (d and e) Surgical fixation of the upper cervical complex.*

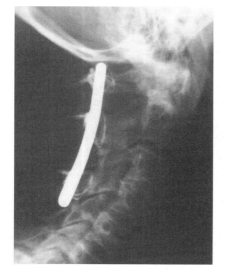

(d)

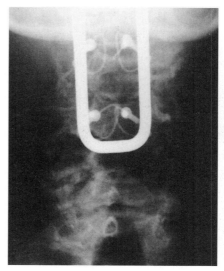

(e)

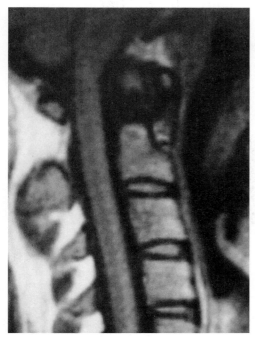

Figure 4.73 *MRI demonstrates a fracture through the odontoid and anterior aspect of the C2 body in this 39-year-old man (courtesy Michael T Buehler, DC, DACBR, Lake Zurich, Illinois, USA).*

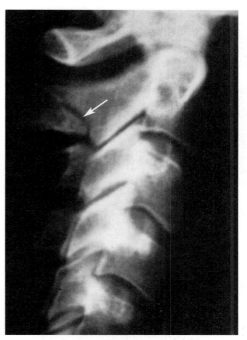

Figure 4.74 *Hangman's fracture. Observe the jagged, oblique, lucent fracture line (arrow) through the posterior elements of axis.*

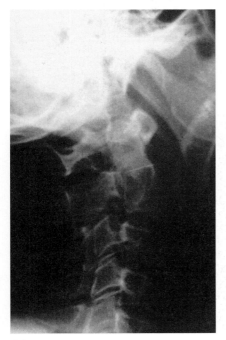

(a)

(b)

Figure 4.75 *Axis fracture. (a) Misalignment of the posterior elements of C2 and C3 with visualization of both C3 facets is observed. (b) CT demonstrates a complete transverse fracture separating the neural arch from the body at C2 (courtesy Michael T Buehler, DC, DACBR, Lake Zurich, Illinois, USA).*

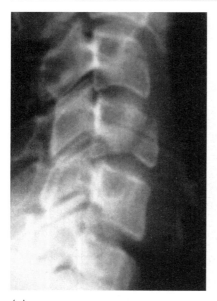

(a)

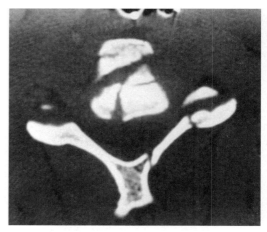

(b)

Figure 4.76 *(a) A comminuted fracture of the C4 body is observed following a motor vehicle accident. (b) CT demonstrates the extensive involvement of the C4 vertebra more clearly (courtesy Michael T Buehler, DC, DACBR, Lake Zurich, Illinois, USA).*

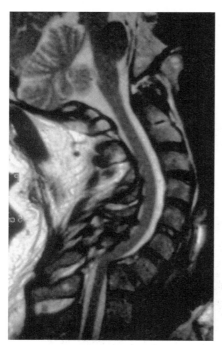

Figure 4.77 *This 37-year-old man was thrown head first into the boards while playing hockey. A traumatic grade 5 spondylolisthesis of C7 accompanies compression of the anterosuperior endplate of T1 with severe distortion of the spinal cord (courtesy Philips Medical Systems Canada, Calgary, Alberta, Canada).*

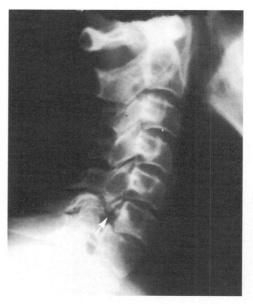

Figure 4.78 *Grade 1 spondylolisthesis of C6, with posterior element defects (arrow) (from Deltoff MN, Kogon PK: The Portable Skeletal X-ray Library, St Louis, Mosby, 1997).*

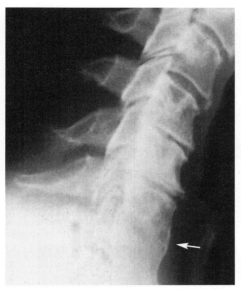

Figure 4.79 *Surgical synostosis at C6–C7. Note the anterior convexity (arrow) at the former site of the C6–C7 disc. No rudimentary disc is evident, and there is complete osseous vertebral body fusion. Marked degenerative disc disease is observed at multiple cephalad levels (courtesy Jerry Cott, DC, Toronto, Ontario, Canada).*

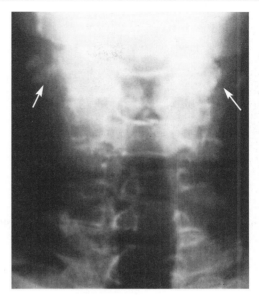

Figure 4.80 *Carotid sinus calcification. Observe the bilateral, flocculent calcification in the lateral soft tissue of the neck (arrows).*

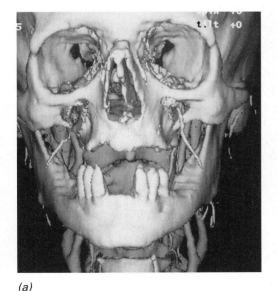

(a)

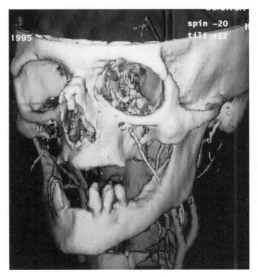

(b)

Figure 4.81 *(a and b) Three-dimensional MRI reconstructions demonstrating carotid artery and cranial vascular anatomy in a post-brain infarct patient (courtesy Siemens Electric Limited, Pointe Claire, Quebec, Canada).*

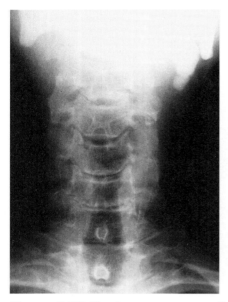

Figure 4.82 *The homogeneous radiodensity inferomedial to the mandibular ramus on the reading right represents calcification of the submandibular gland in this 49-year-old man (courtesy Ron Gitelman, DC, FCCS(C), Toronto, Ontario, Canada).*

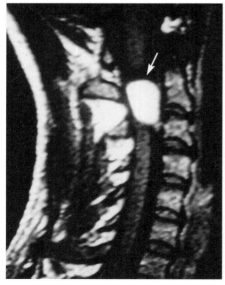

Figure 4.83 *A malignant spinal cord tumour (arrow), likely an astrocytoma, appears at the C2–C3 level on this MRI study (courtesy Richard A Leverone, DC, DACBR, St Petersburg, Florida, USA).*

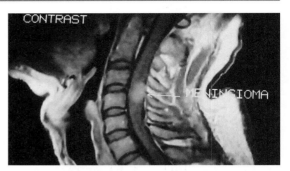

Figure 4.84 *A 55-year-old man with a meningioma at the C3–C4 level as visualized with MRI (courtesy David L Berens, MD, Buffalo MRI, Amherst, New York, USA).*

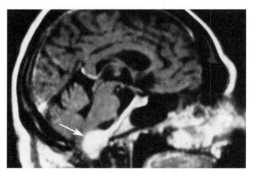

(a)

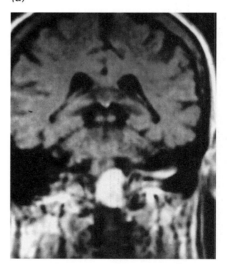

(b)

Figure 4.85 *A large meningioma (arrow) at the anterior foramen magnum is observed on MRI. (a) Sagittal plane. (b) Coronal plane (courtesy Richard A Leverone, DC, DACBR, St Petersburg, Florida, USA).*

REFERENCES

1. Phillips RB. The Use of X-rays in Spinal Manipulative Therapy. In *Modern Developments in the Principles and Practice of Chiropractic* (ed. S Haldeman), pp. 189–208, Appleton-Century-Crofts, 1980.
2. Jaeger SA. *Atlas of Radiographic Positioning*, Appleton & Lange, 1988.
3. De Bono V. Radiographic Positioning. In *Clinical Imaging* (ed. D Marchiori), St Louis: Mosby, pp. 109–115, 1999.
4. Yochum TR, Rowe LJ. *Essentials of Skeletal Radiology*, Williams & Wilkins, 1987.
5. Sandman TD. Improving patient positioning in routine radiography. *Today's Chiropractic* 1994;**23**:46–47.
6. Harris JH, Edeiken-Moore B. *The Radiology of Acute Cervical Spine Trauma*, St Louis: Mosby, 1987.
7. Berlin L. The importance of proper radiographic positioning and technique. *Am J Roentgenol* 1996;**166**:769–771.
8. Schultz GD, Phillips RB, Cooley J, et al. Diagnostic imaging of the spine in chiropractic practice: recommendations for utilization. *Chiro J Aust* 1992;**22**:141–152.
9. Guebert GM, Pirtle OL, Yochum TR. *Essentials of Diagnostic Imaging*, St Louis: Mosby, 1995.
10. Quencer RM. *MRI of the Spine*, New York: Raven Press, 1991.
11. Reinke TS, Jahn WT. Spinal diagnostic imaging; computerized axial tomography vs. magnetic resonance imaging. *Am J Chiro Med*. 1988; **1**:181–184.
12. Modic MT, Masaryk TJ, Ross JS. *Magnetic Resonance Imaging of the Spine*. Chicago: Year Book Medical Publishers, 1989.
13. Bailey DN. Plain film vs. videofluoroscopy: comparison of clinical value in the cervical spine: a retrospective study. *JACA* 1991;**28**:20–23.
14. Schultz GD. A literature review of spinal videofluoroscopy. *Proceedings of the 8th annual conference on research and education*, sponsored by the Consortium for Spinal Research, 1993.
15. Breen AC, Allen R, Morris A. Spine kinematics: a digital videofluoroscopic technique. *J Biomed Eng* 1989;**11**:224–228.
16. Breen AC, Allen R, Morris A. A digital fluoroscopic technique for spine kinematics. *J Mech Technol* 1989;**13**:109–113.
17. Wallace HL, Pierce WV, Wagnon RJ. Cervical flexion and extension analysis using digitized videofluoroscopy. *J Chiro Research Clin Invest* 1992;**7**:94–97.
18. Brodeur RR, Wallace HL. Cervical spine intervertebral kinematics for females suffering from headaches: a preliminary study. *J Chiro Res Clin Invest* 1993;**8**:3–77.
19. Wallace HL, Jahner S, Buckle K, *et al*. The relationship of changes in cervical curvature to visual analog scale, neck disability index scores and pressure algometry in patients with neck pain. In *Proceedings of the World Congress on Chiropractic*, London, UK, May 27–31, 1993.
20. Phillips RB. Radiological and magnetic resonance imaging of cervical spine instability. (Letter). *J Manipulative Physiol Ther* 1988;**11**:446–452.
21. McLean ID. Specialized imaging. In *Clinical Imaging* (ed. D Marchiori), pp. 43–53, Mosby, 1999.
22. Sigler DC, Howe JW. Inter- and intra-examiner reliability of the upper cervical X-ray marking system. *J Manipulative Physiol Ther* 1985;**8**:75–80.
23. Rochester RP. Inter- and intra-examiner reliability of the upper cervical X-ray marking system; a third and expanded look. *Chiropractic Res J* 1994;**3**:23–31.
24. Howe JW. Some considerations in spinal X-ray interpretations. *J Clin Chiro Arch* 1971;**1**:75.
25. Henderson DJ, Dorman TM. Functional roentgenometric evaluation of the cervical spine in the sagittal plane. *JMPT* 1985;**8**:219–227.
26. MacRae J. *Roentgenometrics in Chiropractic*, Canadian Memorial Chiropractic College, 1983.
27. Peterson C. Radiographic positioning. In *Clinical Imaging*. (ed. D Marchiori), pp. 71–82, St Louis: Mosby, 1999.

Chapter 5

Biomechanics of the upper cervical spine

Raymond R. Brodeur

INTRODUCTION

The upper cervical spine contains one of the most complex series of joints in the human body, allowing extensive motion while simultaneously protecting the spinal cord. The motions require the coordination of bony structure, joints and ligaments, and are orchestrated via an array of muscles ranging from the large and powerful trapezius to the delicate suboccipital muscles. Research on cervical spine biomechanics is growing but is by no means complete. Past research has concentrated on gross joint motions, using cadavers to study kinematics and to investigate the mechanisms of major trauma and its effects on joint stability and neurological integrity. It is only now that the effects of minor trauma are being studied. The use of magnetic resonance imaging (MRI) to determine muscle function [1–3], and the advent of new tools such as motion MRI [4], will probably greatly improve our understanding of cervical spine biomechanics. In this chapter we will describe our current knowledge of the kinematics of the cervical spine and the role of bone, cartilage, ligaments and muscle in guiding and constraining the motion. We begin by reviewing basic terminology.

TERMS AND DEFINITIONS

Orthogonal coordinate system

In order to standardize spinal kinematic studies, there has been an effort to use a consistent three-dimensional, orthogonal coordinate system for describing vertebral displacements and motions. An orthogonal coordinate system simply means that the axes are all at right angles (perpendicular) to each other. Figure 5.1 shows a coordinate system standard proposed by White and Panjabi [5]. The origin (zero point) of the coordinate system is located in the trunk of the body at the intersections of the sagittal, frontal and horizontal planes. The X-axis points from the origin to the left, the Y-axis is positive in the cephalad direction and the Z-axis is positive towards the anterior of the body.

Translation

Translation is defined as a motion where all parts of a rigid body move parallel to each other, so that there is no rotation. The movements along the X, Y and Z-axes can be used to describe the motion of any body segment with respect to either the whole body or with respect to an adjacent body segment. For example, a +Z translation of the head means the head translates forward, without any rotation (Table 5.1).

Rotation

Rotations are defined as a motion such that all points along a line have zero displacement. As shown in Figure 5.2a, there is no motion at the axis of rotation while points further away from the axis have a displacement that is proportional to the distance from the axis. Rotations are described using the 'right-hand rule'. For

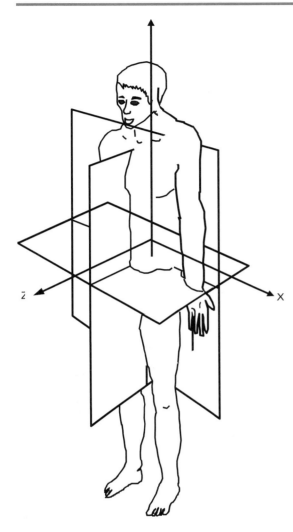

Table 5.1 Comparison between standard antomical definitions of movement with descriptions based on an orthogonal coordinate system. Standard anatomical definitions for translational and rotational motions are listed next to the same motions described relative to an orthogonal coordinate system

Standard anatomical description	Orthogonal coordinate system description
P-A translation	$+Z$
A-P translation	$-Z$
Right to left translation	$+X$
Left to right translation	$-X$
Inferior to superior translation	$+Y$
Superior to inferior translation	$-Y$
Flexion	$+\theta_X$
Extension	$-\theta_X$
Right lateral flexion	$+\theta_Z$
Left lateral flexion	$-\theta_Z$
Left axial rotation	$+\theta_Y$
Right axial rotation	$-\theta_Y$

Figure 5.1 *Orthogonal coordinate system compared to anatomical descriptions. An orthogonal coordinate system can be used to describe locations of body parts as well as motion of each body part. Translations can be described as components parallel to each axis. For example, moving the head forward (protrusion) is a complex motion for the cervical spine, but in terms of the actual head motion, it can be described as a translation along the +Z direction. Rotations can also be described as components of rotation about each axis (this is true if the rotations are small). The symbol θ is used to denote a rotation. For example, flexion about the X axis is termed $+\theta_X$ while $-\theta_X$ is used to denote extension. (Modified from White AA, Panjabi MM.: Clinical biomechanics of the spine. 2nd edn, Philadelphia: JB Lippincott Co., 1990.)*

example, in Figure 5.2b, if you place your right hand on the X-axis so that your thumb points in the positive X-direction, a positive rotation is the direction your fingers 'curl' around the axis. Thus, using the White and Panjabi coordinate system, a positive rotation about the X-axis is flexion, or X. The relationship between standard anatomical definitions and rotations about specific axes are listed in Table 5.1.

Kinematics

Kinematics is the study of the motion of rigid bodies, described without taking into account the forces required to maintain the motion. To date, most information on the spine describes end-motion, with little detail available regarding the path required to move from end-point to end-point. As a result, in this chapter, most motion descriptions are of the end-point positions. Full paths are given where available.

Planar motion

Planar motion describes movements limited to one plane. For example, flexion-extension of

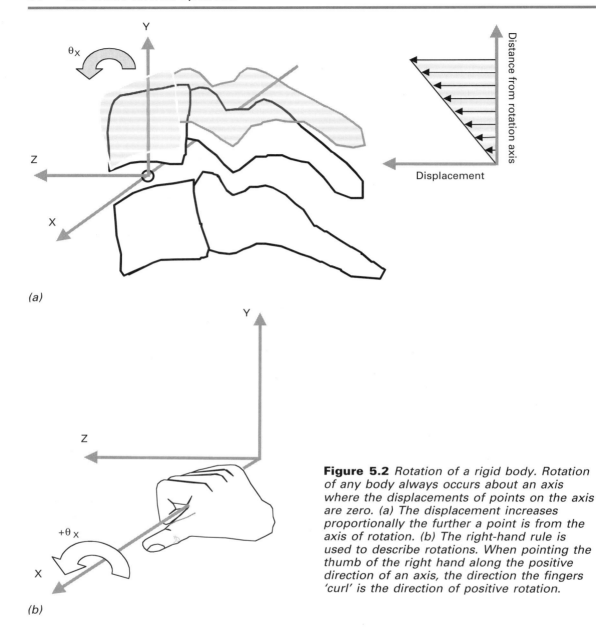

(a)

(b)

Figure 5.2 *Rotation of a rigid body. Rotation of any body always occurs about an axis where the displacements of points on the axis are zero. (a) The displacement increases proportionally the further a point is from the axis of rotation. (b) The right-hand rule is used to describe rotations. When pointing the thumb of the right hand along the positive direction of an axis, the direction the fingers 'curl' is the direction of positive rotation.*

the cervical spine is motion that occurs in a single plane. To describe planar motion of a rigid body requires describing both the translation of the body as well as its rotation in space. The translations of most joints are small and so, for clinical purposes, the joint motion can be adequately described by the angle alone. For example, vertebral translations are small and thus the flexion/extension of such a joint can be described by the angular range of motion.

Centre of rotation

The centre of rotation (COR) (also called the axis of rotation) is used to describe the point about which a rigid body is rotating when the motion of that body is limited to a single plane

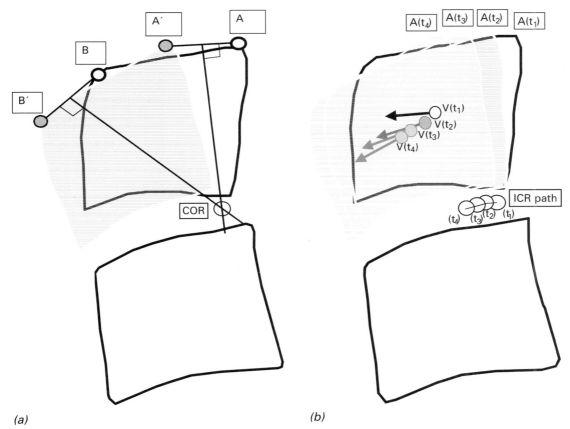

(a) *(b)*

Figure 5.3 *Centre of rotation (COR) and instantaneous centre of rotation (ICR). The centre of rotation is the point about which a rigid body rotates to move from an initial position to a final position. (a) The COR can be calculated if the position of two points are known for each position of the body. In the initial position, points A and B are on the upper surface of the upper vertebra. After moving to the final position, the two points are now at A´ and B´. Connect a line from A to A´ and from B to B´. Draw a perpendicular bisector on line AA´, that is, at the halfway point of line AA´ draw a line perpendicular to AA´. Draw a perpendicular bisector for BB´. Where the two perpendicular bisectors intersect is the COR. (b) The ICR can be calculated for each instant in time if the velocity and angular velocity of a rigid body are known. The ICR follows a path but the path of the ICR does not have to include the point where the COR is.*

(Figure 5.3a). The COR can be in the body or on a point outside the body. Figure 5.3a shows a method for locating the centre of rotation, given two positions for a rigid body.

The further the COR is from the centre of a joint, the greater the translation of that joint. A large joint translation can be indicative of injury, thus, the location of the COR could be used to distinguish normal from abnormal joint motion. Attempts have been made to establish normal ranges for the location of the

COR for most body joints. For example, Figure 5.4 illustrates the location of the COR for each cervical spine joint for a group of normal subjects [6]. The broken lines indicate 2 SD from the average COR. Note the COR is more inferior for the mid-cervical spine compared with the lower cervical joints where the COR is closer to the disc. This indicates that for normal subjects there is more translation at the C2/C3 through C4/C5 joints compared to the C5/C6 and C6/C7 joints.

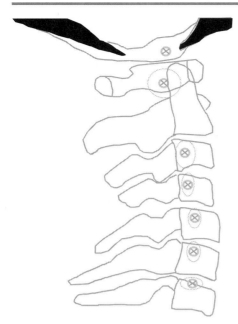

Figure 5.4 *COR for cervical spine joints in flexion and extension. The centre of rotation (COR) is illustrated for cervical spine joints for flexion/extension motion. The data are an average of normal subjects. The broken lines indicate ± 2 standard deviations. (Modified from Dvorak* et al. *[6].)*

Instantaneous centre of rotation

The instantaneous centre of rotation (ICR) is similar to the COR, but is used to describe continuous motion, where the velocity and angular velocity of the body are known. For example, with a video-fluoroscope, the entire motion of a vertebral joint can be recorded from full flexion to full extension. The path the ICR follows may vary and need not be the same as the COR (Figure 5.3b).

Three-dimensional motion

Three-dimensional motion is more difficult to describe than the two-dimensional motion discussed above. Listed below are three methods that are commonly used for describing three-dimensional (3D) motion:

1. Measure the displacement of at least three non-linear points on a rigid body (Figure 5.5a). The 3D translation of the rigid body can be described using any of the points and the angle changes about three non-planar axes can be calculated (Figure 5.5a). This method is probably the most widely used to describe 3D motion. The familiar flexion-extension, lateral flexion and axial rotation are examples of describing 3D motion.
2. The helical axis of motion (HAM) (also called a screw axis) can be used to describe 3D movement. All motions can be reduced to a rotation about a line as well as a translation parallel to the line, similar to the motion of a screw. The HAM is a succinct means of describing motion between two end points; for example, the motion of a vertebral joint from a neutral posture to lateral flexion could be described using the HAM (Figure 5.5b).
3. The instantaneous helical axis (IHA) is the continuous equivalent to the HAM. Given the full 3D velocity and angular velocity of a rigid body, the IHA can be determined. Recent work on head/chest motion indicates that the path of the IHA is more erratic in subjects with neck injury than the IHA path reported for normal subjects (Figure 5.6) [7–9].

Active and passive range of motion

Active range of motion (AROM) is the maximum motion that a person can obtain by moving a joint using his/her own muscles. After the AROM is achieved, a trained examiner can obtain a few more degrees of motion by gently moving the joint in the proper direction so that the joint is at its most extreme position. This is termed the passive range of motion (PROM). In general, most joints have slightly more motion with PROM. The PROM is more repeatable than AROM. AROM has been shown to have more variability than PROM by as much as 5–10 degrees [10]. As a result, it is preferable to use passive motion when measuring the range of motion of a joint. Unfortunately, many research papers overlook this important point and often do not indicate the type of motion measured.

Neutral zone

Figure 5.7 illustrates a typical load-displacement curve for a spinal joint. Note that there is a region on the graph, termed the neutral zone (NZ) [5] where there is a large amount

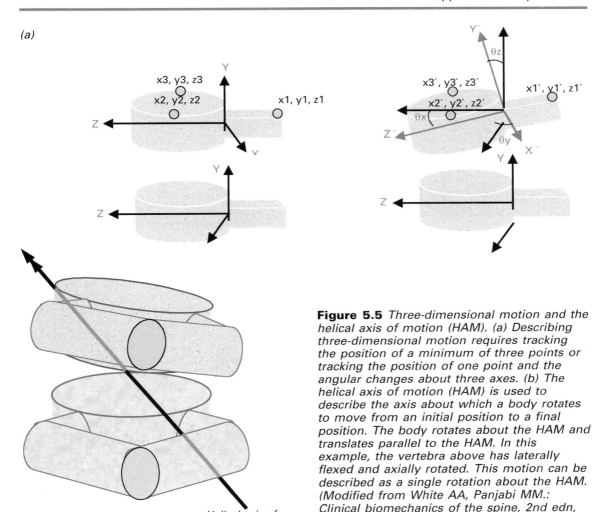

(a)

(b)

Helical axis of motion (HAM)

Figure 5.5 *Three-dimensional motion and the helical axis of motion (HAM). (a) Describing three-dimensional motion requires tracking the position of a minimum of three points or tracking the position of one point and the angular changes about three axes. (b) The helical axis of motion (HAM) is used to describe the axis about which a body rotates to move from an initial position to a final position. The body rotates about the HAM and translates parallel to the HAM. In this example, the vertebra above has laterally flexed and axially rotated. This motion can be described as a single rotation about the HAM. (Modified from White AA, Panjabi MM.: Clinical biomechanics of the spine, 2nd edn, Philadelphia: JB Lippincott Co., 1990.)*

Table 5.2 Neutral zones for spinal joints. Neutral zones are defined for each region of the spine for flexion-extension, lateral flexion and axial rotation

Region	Flexion-extension	Lateral bend	Axial rotation
C0–C1	1.1°	1.6°	1.5°
C1–C2	3.2°	1.2°	29.6°
C3–C6	4.9°	4.0°	3.8°
C7–T11	1.5°	2.2°	1.2°
L1–L4	1.5°	1.6°	0.7°
L5–S1	3.0°	1.8°	0.4°

of motion resulting from very small forces. In general, the NZ is the normal physiological range of motion for the joint. The elastic zone (EZ) is near the ends of the ROM where the joint capsules and ligaments begin to tighten. In the plastic zone (PZ) there is irreversible stretching of the ligaments (ligamentous damage). Table 5.2 lists the range of NZ for

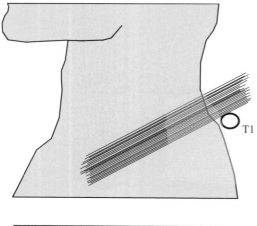

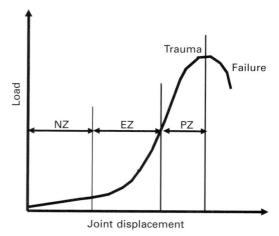

Figure 5.7 *Neutral zone (NZ) for spinal joints. In the graph the force acting on a joint is plotted against the displacement of the joint. The neutral zone (NZ) is the region of the graph where small forces can cause a large displacement in joint position. The elastic zone (EZ) is the region where the force causes a proportional change in joint position and the plastic zone (PZ) is the region of the graph where the force applied to the joint is causing damage to the tissue.*

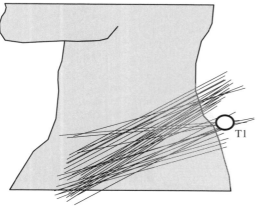

Figure 5.6 *The instantaeous helical axis (IHA). The instantaneous helical axis (IHA) describes the axis about which a body is rotating and translating for any given instant in time. The 3D velocity and angular velocity must be known to calculate the IHA. The series of IHAs generated from a motion generate a ruled surface (a surface generated by the motion of a line in space). The IHA has been used to describe normal head motion as well as head motion as a result of cervical spine injury. The ruled surface of the IHA is smooth, continuous with very little change in the direction of the IHAs for subjects with normal head motion (top). For subjects with whiplash trauma, the ruled surface is discontinuous, fluctuates and has greater oblique variability (bottom).*

KINEMATICS OF THE UPPER CERVICAL SPINE

The range of motion (ROM) for all cervical vertebrae are summarized in Figure 5.8 for flexion/extension, lateral flexion and axial rotation. In flexion/extension, C0–C1 (atlanto-occipital joint) has the largest ROM. In axial rotation, the C1–C2 joint dominates the cervical spine. However, on lateral flexion the upper cervical spine motion is more limited than the remainder of the cervical joints. In the following paragraphs the motions of the upper cervical spine will be examined in more detail.

Kinematics of the atlanto-occipital joint (C0–C1)

Flexion-extension $(+\theta_x$ and $-\theta_x)$

Using the coordinate system illustrated in Figure 5.1, flexion-extension occurs about the

the cervical vertebrae. The C1/C2 (atlas/axis) joint dominates the NZ in rotation, while the lower cervical vertebrae dominate the NZ for flexion/extension as well as lateral flexion.

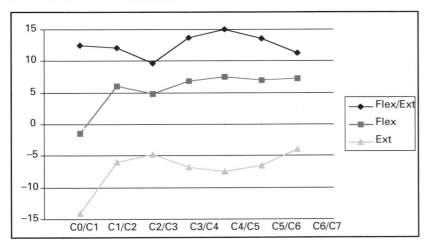

(a)

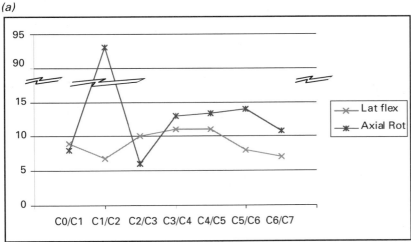

(b)

Figure 5.8 *Cervical spine range of motion (ROM). Range of motion for cervical spine joints. (a) Flexion, extension and full flexion-extension ROM for each cervical vertebra. (b) Lateral flexion and axial rotation ROM for each cervical vertebra.*

X-axis, with a positive rotation $(+\theta_x)$ causing flexion and a negative rotation $(-\theta_x)$ causing extension. The primary motion of the C0–C1 (occipital-atlantal) joint is flexion/extension. Although it can also laterally flex and rotate, these motions are small compared to flexion/extension. The limitations of motion at this joint are primarily determined by osseous structure. The joint is long posterior to anterior and narrower left to right (Figure 5.9). The occipital portion is convex and the atlas portion of the joint is concave. This arrangement allows for extensive flexion/extension but limits lateral flexion and axial rotation.

Flexion is limited by contact between the anterior margin of the foramen magnum and the odontoid process as well as tightness of the articular capsules and tightness of the nuchal ligament. Extension is limited by contact between the arch of atlas and the occiput, contact between the arch of atlas and C2 spinous and tightness of the tectorial membrane (posterior longitudinal ligament).

Clinically, flexion and extension at the C0–C1 joint reach their maximum during retraction and protrusion, respectively. Protrusion occurs when the entire head is translated forward, jutting the chin outward. This causes upper cervical extension and lower cervical flexion, generating an S-shaped cervical spine. Retraction occurs when the head is translated rearward, flexing the upper cervical spine and

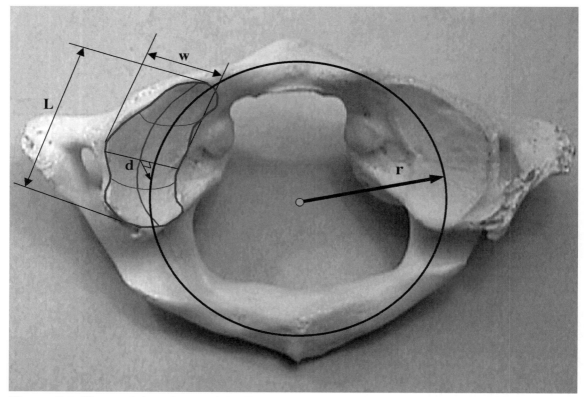

Figure 5.9 *Shape of the atlas condyle. The shape of the atlas articular surface and the corresponding mating shape of the occipital condyle limit the motion of the C0–C1 (occiput-atlas) joint. The length, L, is greater than the width, w, of the articular surface, allowing more flexion-extension motion than lateral flexion. The depth, d, of the articular surface is shallow compared to L and w, and the overal shape of the two articular surfaces combined is roughly spherical with a radius, r.*

extending the lower cervical spine. During protrusion and retraction, the upper cervical spine reaches its limit in both extension and flexion. During active flexion of the head, the C0–C1 joint only flexes about half the extent that can be achieved with retraction. Similarly, active extension of the head results with C0–C1 extending only about half of what can be achieved with protrusion [11].

Paradoxical motion of occiput/atlas on flexion

During full cervical spine flexion the C0–C1 joint extends a few degrees (Figure 5.8a), when motion is measured relative to McGregor's line. This is termed the paradoxical motion of the occiput-atlas joint. Data from Kraemer and Patris [12] are summarized in Table 5.3 and

Figure 5.10. The paradoxical motion of the atlas appears to be a normal condition, especially in younger people. The shape of the occiput/atlas condyles is probably the most important factor. Changes in the condyle with age is speculated to cause the progressive tendency toward flexion in this joint as a person ages [12].

Lateral flexion and axial rotation

Lateral flexion and axial rotation at C0–C1 are both limited, primarily due to the fit between the occipital condyles and the lateral mass of atlas. Being relatively narrow side-to-side limits the axial rotation of the joint (Table 5.4). The role of the condyle in restricting motion has been studied by the progressive unilateral removal of a condyle from intact C0–C1 joints. Vishteh, *et al.* [13] reported that a 50%

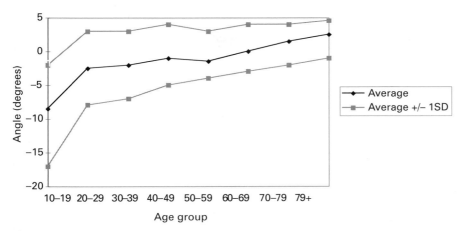

Figure 5.10 *Paradoxical motion of the occiput-atlas (C0–C1) joint on flexion. On average, the C0–C1 joint actually extends when the cervical spine is in full flexion. This extension changes with age; the younger the individual the greater the extension.*

Table 5.3 Changes in C0–C1 flexion paradoxical motion with age. The paradoxical motion which occurs at the C0–C1 joint during global head flexion is described as a function of age. Over 90% of those younger than 20 years will have a slight extension of the C0–C1 joint when the head is at full flexion. This drops to less than 30% for those over age 80 years

Age range	% of subjects with paradoxical motion
10–19	94%
20–29	70%
30–39	61%
40–49	50%
50–59	49%
60–69	46%
70–79	35%
>80	28%

condylectomy results in an increase of 15.3% in flexion-extension, 40.8% increase in lateral bending and a 28.1% increase in axial rotation. Thus, the occipital condyles play an important part in limiting all C0–C1 motions. Successive removal of the condyle increases the NZ, indicating that the condylar portion of the joint restricts the NZ.

The alar ligaments also play an important role in limiting C0–C1 motion. The anatomical locations of these ligaments are illustrated in Figure 5.11. The alar ligament originates in the upper portion of the dens and inserts into the occiput and has a portion insert on the lateral masses of atlas. There is some disagreement over the role of the alar ligaments in restricting C0–C1 motion. Early evidence indicated that lateral flexion is limited by the contralateral upper alar ligament so that right lateral flexion is opposed by the left upper alar ligament [14]. However, in more recent work, it has been shown that sectioning the left alar ligament does NOT increase lateral bending, although it does increase the neutral zone for right lateral bending [14]. Increasing the neutral zone probably increases the stresses on other ligaments and may initiate osteoarthritic changes in the C0–C1 articulations.

Axial rotation is limited by the contralateral upper alar ligament (right rotation is limited

Table 5.4 Role of osseous and ligamentous structures in motion restriction and stabilization of the upper cervical spine. The stabilization of the upper cervical spine is dependent on both osseous and ligamentous structures. The major sources of joint stabilization (and therefore motion restriction) are listed in this table

Ligament/structure	Major motion restriction	Axis
C0–C1 joint:		
C0–C1 facet joint shape	C0–C1 axial rotation	θ_Y
	C0–C1 lateral flexion	θ_Z
C0–C1 capsular ligaments	C0–C1 lateral flexion	θ_Z
Unilateral alar ligament	C0–C1 contralateral lateral flexion	θ_Z
	C0–C1 contralateral rotation	θ_Y
Unilateral alar ligaments	C0–C1 flexion	θ_X
C1–C2 joint:		
C1–C2 facet joint shape	None	
Transverse ligament	C1–C2 flexion	θ_X
	C1 anterior translation	Z
Unilateral alar ligament	C1–C2 contra- and ipsilateral rotation	ϑ_Y
	C1–C2 contralateral lateral flexion	ϑ_Z
	C1–C2 flexion	$+\vartheta_X$
	C1–C2 extension	$-\vartheta_X$
Bilateral alar ligament	C1–C2 bilateral axial rotation	ϑ_Y
	C1–C2 bilateral lateral flexion	ϑ_Z
	C1–C2 flexion	$+\vartheta_X$
	C1–C2 extension	$-\vartheta_X$
Unilateral capsular ligament	Contralateral axial rotation	ϑ_Y
Bilateral capsular ligament	Bilateral axial rotation	ϑ_Z
	Bilateral lateral flexion	ϑ_Z

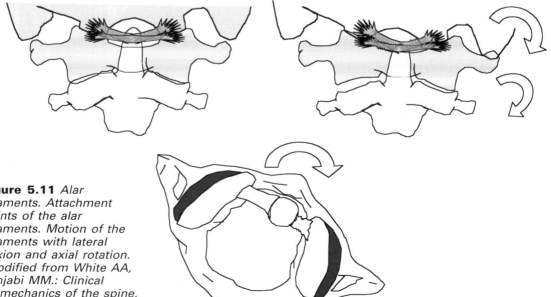

Figure 5.11 *Alar ligaments. Attachment points of the alar ligaments. Motion of the ligaments with lateral flexion and axial rotation. (Modified from White AA, Panjabi MM.: Clinical biomechanics of the spine, 2nd edn, Philadelphia: JB Lippincott Co., 1990.)*

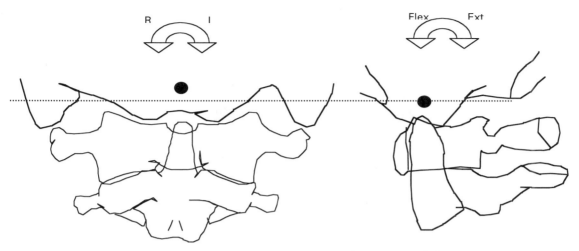

Figure 5.12 *COR for C0–C1 flexion-extension and lateral flexion. The COR for flexion-extension of C0–C1 occurs slightly above the dens of C2 approximately on a line that passes through the centres of the mastoid processes. On lateral flexion, the COR is about 2–3 cm above the dens, slightly more superior than for flexion-extension. (Modified from White AA, Panjabi MM.: Clinical biomechanics of the spine, 2nd edn, Philadelphia: JB Lippincott Co., 1990.)*

by the left upper alar ligament) [5]. Sectioning the alar ligaments bilaterally results in an increase in flexion at C0–C1, but no change in extension [14]. C0–C1 lateral flexion is also limited by both articular capsules (Table 5.4).

Centres of rotation

The COR between C0–C1 has been poorly studied. Over a century ago, Henke [15] measured the COR in flexion/extension and lateral flexion. The COR for both flexion/extension and lateral flexion is just slightly superior to the dens (Figure 5.12). The COR in axial rotation (θ_Y rotation) has been reported in only one study. The average location of the COR during axial rotation is slightly anterior to the foramen magnum [16].

Coupled motions

When the motion of the head is axial rotation, the occiput also axially rotates but it also has two coupled motions: extension and lateral flexion to the opposite side. There is between 4° and 8° of axial rotation at C0–C1. The amount of coupled extension ranges from 1:4 to 1:1, that is, the joint has been reported to extend 1° for every 4° of axial rotation, up to 1° of extension for every 1° of axial rotation.

The coupled lateral flexion is to the opposite side of the axial rotation with a ratio of nearly 1:1. That is, for every degree of right axial rotation, the occiput laterally flexes to the left approximately 1°.[17].

When the head laterally flexes, the occiput laterally flexes on C1, but it also extends and axial rotates to the opposite side. The degree of the coupling motion is less. For every degree of left lateral flexion, there is less than 0.5° of right axial rotation and about 0.5° of extension [17].

Posture does not appear to affect the axial to lateral rotation-coupling pattern at the C0–C1 joint. Whether the occiput is flexed, neutral or extended, the coupling between axial rotation and lateral bending is the same. However, when the head is extended, the C0–C1 joint remains extended during axial rotation and when the head is flexed, the C0–C1 joint remains flexed during axial rotation.

As mentioned earlier, most research into spinal joint motion is performed on cadaver spines. Owing to the complexity of measuring such small motions, very little research is available on the in-vivo motions of the spine. Iai *et al.* [16] found that the C0–C1 joint behaves very differently in vivo from in vitro. They reported that during axial rotation of the head, the C0–C1 joint rotates in the opposite direction of the head. The coupled lateral flexion is to the same side as the rotation. Thus, during right axial rotation of the head, the C0–C1 joint axially rotates to the left and laterally flexes to the right. The coupling characteristics agree with those described above, that is, C0 laterally flexes to the opposite side of the local (C0–C1) axial rotation. In addition, Iai reported that C0–C1 extends during axial rotation of the head, which agrees with in-vitro studies, but with the extension averaging 10°, which is two to three times the extension reported by others [17].

The paradoxical counter-rotation at C0–C1 has not been reported by any others. Iai [16] argues that the counter-rotation is a required 'buffer function'. In a CT study of axial rotation, Dvorak [18] did not report any paradoxical motion at C0–C1. However, there were differences between the procedures used by these two studies that may explain the conflicting results. Iai [16] had subjects sitting and required active muscle contraction during the data collection, while Dvorak [18] measured subjects supine, allowing subjects to relax the muscles required to maintain the posture. Thus, it is highly likely that muscle activity plays a part in this paradoxical motion.

The bony structure is the primary source of motion limitation for C0–C1 as described above; however, it is also a primary cause of the coupled motion at this joint. The progressive removal of the condyle from medial to lateral progressively increases the ROM in all directions and also decreases the coupled motions. For example, during axial rotation, the coupled lateral flexion decreases as the condyle is removed [13].

Atlanto-axial joint (C1–C2)

The primary motion of the C1–C2 (atlanto-axial) joint is axial rotation. However, this joint also allows flexion-extension as well as lateral flexion. Studying in-vivo axial rotation is a difficult task and thus most data is from in-vitro studies. The advent of CT scans and stereo-radiography have helped tremendously in the in-vivo analysis of the upper cervical spine [18,19,26]. Stereo-radiography has aided in understanding the complex coupling motions that occur during both axial rotation and lateral flexion.

Flexion-extension ($+\theta_X$ and $-\theta_X$)

The combined flexion-extension of the C1–C2 is 20° [5], however; the data from this reference is mostly from in-vitro work. More recent, in-vivo work indicates that there is about 7° in flexion and about 3° in active extension, for a total range of about 10° [11]. However, during extension of the head (i.e., extension of the whole cervical spine), the C1–C2 joint does not extend as far as it does during protrusion of the head [11]. During whole cervical spine extension, the C1–C2 joint extends only about half the extent achievable with protrusion. However, with whole cervical spine flexion, the maximum C1–C2 flexion reaches the same degree of flexion as that which occurs during retraction.

Cineradiography has been used to study cervical spine motion for flexion and extension. Moving from extension to flexion, the motion begins at the upper cervical spine. In a 2-second-long motion from full extension to full flexion, the time lag between the initiation of motion at each motion segment is about 0.4 seconds. For example, after C1–C2 begins to flex, C2–C3 does not begin to flex for another 0.4 seconds [20]. This pattern of delay in the initiation of motion continues, with C3–C4 flexing 0.6 seconds after C2–C3 begins to flex, followed by an additional 0.4 seconds before C4–C5 starts flexing and another 0.4 seconds before C5/C6 flexes.

Axial rotation ($+\theta_Y$)

The C1–C2 joint dominates the spine in axial rotation. Over 50% of cervical spine axial rotation ($+\theta_Y$) comes from the atlas-axis joint [21]. The first 40–50° of rotation come from C1/C2. Only after this point do the lower cervical vertebrae begin to rotate. C0/C1 is speculated to rotate axially only after all other vertebrae have reached full rotation. On axial rotation, C1/C2 has about 2° of lateral flexion to the opposite side as well as about 14° of extension.

C1–C2 stability

The osseous structure of the C1–C2 facet joints plays only a small part in constraining the overall C1–C2 motion. The biconvex shape of atlas-axis facet joints allows for a large range of motion. It is primarily the ligamentous structures that constrain this joint, with the stability of the atlanto-axial joint complex dependent on three major ligaments. The most important is the transverse ligament for restricting flexion and anterior translation of the atlas [22]. Second to the transverse ligament are the alar ligaments (Figure 5.11), which limit both axial rotation and lateral flexion, as well as flexion and extension (Table 5.4). The capsular ligaments also limit axial rotation and lateral flexion. Although there are many other ligaments, these three (transverse, alar and capsular ligaments) are the most important for joint stability. Damage to either the transverse or alar ligaments can lead to severe neurological problems, requiring joint stabilization.

Both alar ligaments must be intact to adequately constrain atlas rotation on axis [21,23]. The unilateral sectioning of an alar ligament results in an increase in both left and right axial rotation, although contralateral rotation increases more than ipsilateral rotation. Previously, it was thought that unilateral injury to the alar ligament resulted in an increase in only the contralateral rotation [5]. In addition to instability, injury to the alar ligaments also causes an increase in the range of the neutral zone so that the normal day-to-day range of motion of the joint increases.

The alar ligaments also restrict C1–C2 flexion and extension (Table 5.4). Both left and right ligaments are required to adequately constrain flexion and extension motions. The unilateral sectioning of one alar ligament causes an increase in both flexion and extension ROM, while the subsequent sectioning of the opposite ligament results in further increasing flexion ROM [14].

Lateral flexion at C1–C2 is constrained by the contralateral alar ligament. Sectioning of the left alar ligament increases the ROM for C1–C2 on right lateral bending but does not change left lateral bending. Sectioning of both alar ligaments leads to a significant increase in both right and left lateral flexion [14].

The atlas-axis facet joint capsule also plays an important part in limiting rotation and lateral flexion (Table 5.4). Sectioning of one facet capsule results in an increase in contralateral rotation. That is, sectioning of the left C1–C2 facet capsule increases axial rotation to the right. Lateral flexion increases only on the transection of both joint capsules [24]. Computer models of the atlas-axis facet joints predict that the capsular ligaments undergo significant strains in all motions, with the capsular ligaments experiencing larger strains than the alar and transverse ligaments [25]. It must be pointed out that large strains do not necessarily mean the ligaments are resisting with the same forces carried by the alar and transverse ligaments. The ligamentum flavum is an excellent example of a ligament that undergoes a large strain but carries a very small load compared to other ligaments such as the posterior and anterior longitudinal ligaments.

Centre of rotation

In flexion/extension, the COR is located just posterior to the dens, indicating that the atlas pivots at or near the transverse ligament during flexion and extension (Figure 5.12). In axial rotation, the COR passes through the dens, as would be expected given the architecture of the joint [5]. In lateral flexion, the motion is too complex and cannot be described in the simple planar terms required for calculating the COR.

Coupled motions

During axial rotation the C1–C2 joint displays a unique coupled motion: the joint vertically translates during axial rotation [26]. The biconvex shape of the condyles cause the atlas to drop 2–3 mm along the Y-axis (-Y translation) as the atlas rotates. In the neutral position, the biconvex surfaces of each joint are contacting at the mid-point of the joint, so that the atlas is as high as possible on the axis. During axial rotation, the atlas condyles slide down the axis facets, thus the atlas drops vertically.

Axial rotation (θ_Y) of the atlas on the axis is coupled with flexion and lateral bending to the opposite side. Thus, right axial rotation ($-\vartheta_Y$ rotation) is coupled with left lateral flexion ($-\vartheta_Z$) and flexion of atlas with respect to axis ($+\vartheta_X$) [17]. An in-vivo study found the same-coupled motions, with the exception that there is extension as a coupled motion during axial rotation. This discrepancy may be due to a postural dependency for the coupled motion [16]. Panjabi, *et al.* [17] have shown that the flexion/extension-coupled motion depends on posture. If the C0–C2 complex is in extension, the coupled motion on axial rotation is extension, and if the C0–C2 complex is neutral or in flexion, the coupled motion on axial rotation is flexion. Thus, it is likely that the subjects in the in-vivo study had a slight degree of extension.

Lateral flexion (θ_Z) of atlas on axis is coupled with flexion and axial rotation to the opposite side. Thus, in the neutral posture, right lateral flexion $(+(_Z)$ has coupled flexion $(+\vartheta_X)$ and left axial rotation $(+\vartheta_Y)$. The degree to which the atlas axially rotates is very large, with the axial rotation exceeding the primary motion by 3:1, so that for every 1° of right lateral flexion there is about 3° of left axial rotation [17]. There is a postural dependency to the coupling motion on lateral flexion. If the C0–C2 complex is in extension, then during lateral flexion, the coupled motion is extension and axial rotation to the opposite side.

If the C0–C2 complex is in flexion, then the coupled motion during lateral flexion is flexion and axial rotation to the opposite side. However, when the C0–C2 complex is flexed, the amount of lateral flexion that can be achieved is decreased by a factor of 6. In the neutral posture, there is 8°–10° of lateral flexion, coupled with about 24° of axial rotation and 2° of flexion. When the C0–C2 complex is flexed, the lateral flexion is decreased to 1°–2°, but the coupled axial rotation is 10°–12° [17].

BIOMECHANICAL FUNCTION OF CERVICAL MUSCLES

Muscle is the most complex tissue in the body. Other tissues, such as ligaments, have a distinct relation between force and length; that is, one can generate an equation that predicts the force acting on the tissue as a function of the length. However, muscle is able to generate an internal force independent of length. As a result, mathematical models for predicting the forces generated by muscles are far more complex but less robust than those for passive tissue. In addition to the biomechanical role of generating force, muscle also acts as a joint position sensor. The importance of the propri-

oceptive role of muscle is growing as more research becomes available. Finally, the role of injury in the changes of muscle function is an area of intense research. In this section, a biomechanical model for muscle will be briefly described and the role of muscle will be reviewed as a force generator, a position sensor and as a source of pain.

Hill's model

The standard biomechanical model of muscle is based on the work of Hill [27]. Muscle is modelled as having three elements (Figure 5.13). The most important is the contractile element, which models the actions of the myosin and actin filaments. The other two elements are springs; one in series and the other in parallel with the contractile element. The series and parallel springs are not intended to model any specific tissue, however, one could argue that the series spring models the elastic nature of the tissue associated with the contractile element, while the parallel spring models the tissue surrounding the muscle such as the epimysium, perimysium and endomysium.

The total force a muscle generates is the sum of the active force and passive force. The active force is generated by the contractile component of muscle (actin-myosin bond) while the passive force is the reaction of the surrounding tissue (epimysium, perimysium and endomysium) and the muscle fibres to the

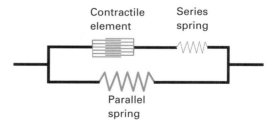

Figure 5.13 *Hill's muscle model. The model consists of two components in parallel. The contractile element and series spring make up one component and the parallel spring makes up the second component. The contractile element represents the ability of muscle to change length and/or generate force. The series and parallel springs model the behaviour of tissues such as the epimysium, perimysium and endomysium.*

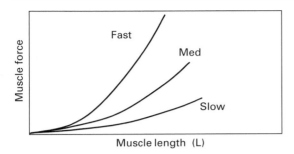

Figure 5.14 *Force-length curve for passive muscle tissue. Because of the viscoelastic nature of passive muscle tissue, the force generated by stretching the tissue is dependent on the velocity of the stretch. The faster the stretch of the tissue, the greater the resistance force to stretch.*

internal and external forces acting on the muscle. Thus, the series and parallel springs in Figure 5.13 represent the passive force that can be generated by muscle, while the contractile element represents the active force.

When a muscle is passive, the behaviour is very similar to that of a ligament or a tendon. The force generated by the passive tissue is dependent on the velocity the muscle is stretched, as shown in Figure 5.14. In Figure 5.14, the load on a muscle is measured while it is being stretched. The faster the muscle is stretched, the greater the force required to cause the stretch. Muscle requires an external force to cause the stretch, hence the need for antagonistic muscles. The passive force plays a significant part in cyclic motions (i.e., running). The muscle stretch acts as a means of storing energy. If the muscle contracts within a short time of stretching, the energy in the passive tissue can be used to assist in the contraction of the muscle.

The active contraction of muscle causes shortening of the whole muscle, or the resistance of the muscle to stretch. The amount of force that can be generated by the contraction of a muscle is dependent on the length of the muscle relative to its resting length. As illustrated in Figure 5.15, the maximum force generated by a muscle is near the resting length, while the force decreases when the muscle is fully stretched or fully contracted. On a microscopic level this behaviour is caused by the number of actin-myosin bonds available. At the resting length, the number of contractile bonds that can be achieved is highest, with the number decreasing at both full contraction and full stretch.

Also illustrated in Figure 5.15 is the increase in force that can be generated when active and

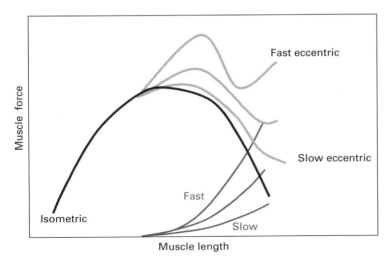

Figure 5.15 *Maximum isometric muscle force versus muscle length and maximum eccentric muscle force versus muscle length. The maximum isometric contraction (i.e., length of the muscle is held constant for each contraction measured) force is dependent on the length at which the muscle is fixed. The maximum force is generated when the muscle is near its resting length and the force decreases as the muscle is set at longer or shorter lengths. The maximum eccentric contraction (i.e., lengthening contraction) force is dependent on the speed of the eccentric contraction and is the sum total of the force-length curve for passive muscle plus the maximum isometric force at a given length.*

passive forces are combined. During a muscle lengthening (eccentric) contraction, the passive resistance in the muscle is added to the force generated by the active contraction. The faster the stretch, the greater the force that can be generated. This is why it is easier to lower a weight than to lift a weight. More force can be generated by a muscle when it stretches than when it contracts. The passive stretch during an eccentric contraction can also be reused by a muscle if there is an immediate concentric contraction. If followed by an immediate muscle contraction, the energy in the passive tissue can be used to accelerate the contraction and generate more force. If too much time elapses between stretch and contraction, the energy stored in the tissue is dissipated as heat. The stretch in the passive tissue acts like a stretched spring; this is why it is easier to lift weights if done in a quick cycle. It is also why you are able to jump higher if you first squat slightly before jumping. By going into a slight squat, the quadriceps muscles are stretched, the energy in the stretch can be added to the energy of a forceful contraction if the contraction immediately follows the stretch. The stretching energy in the passive tissue generated during the squat phase is added to the contraction force, increasing the overall force and therefore allowing you to jump higher.

Muscle damage and eccentric contractions

There is a price to pay for the added force generated by eccentric contractions: there is greater chance of injury to the muscle during eccentric contractions. In untrained muscle, microscopic tears occur after only a single eccentric contraction, even when the eccentric contraction resists only a minor load [28]. The damage to muscle tissue is a function of both training as well as the magnitude of the load being resisted by the eccentric contraction. Repeated eccentric contractions lead to inflammation and muscle tenderness in untrained muscles [29], while repeated concentric contractions with the same force do not cause injury [30]. However, eccentric contraction injuries repair with time and similar eccentric exercises do not generate damage after training. Unfortunately, the training of muscle will reverse with disuse.

In the cervical spine, whiplash could be considered to be a very large force eccentric contraction. Given that a single eccentric contraction resisting a small load can injure the biceps muscle [28] then minor whiplash could be expected to cause damage to the cervical muscles, even if the passive tissue remains uninjured. The larger the force of the whiplash, the greater the eccentric load resistance and the greater the injury to the muscle. Above a certain level, passive tissue injury would exist along with the muscle injury.

Muscle actions

Very little work has been done to accurately describe the mechanical actions and interactions of cervical spine muscles. Most muscle actions described in anatomical texts have been determined from in-vitro examinations of origins and insertions. In-vivo investigations of muscle function are scarce primarily because of the limited tools for such research. Until recently, only EMG (electromyography) has been available to measure muscle function during specific motions. However, EMG can only be applied to measure surface muscles or the activity at specific needle insertion sites. Thus, relatively few studies have been done to document the function of cervical spine musculature [31,32]. MRI has been shown to be a useful tool for documenting muscle function. The T2 contrast shifts from MRI images are highly correlated with EMG activity [2] with the half-life of exercise-induced changes lasting approximately 7 minutes [1]. In addition, there is strong evidence that changes in the T2 images after exercise are related to glycogenolysis and lactate production [33].

A study of cervical spine muscle function using MRI has been shown to agree with similar EMG studies [33]. The muscles most active with specific motions are summarized in Table 5.5. Missing from the table are the actions of smaller muscles such as the rectus capitis posterior major and minor (RCPMaj, RCPMin). The small size of these muscles makes them difficult to locate and measure using MRI.

In general, head rotation involves a broader use of neck muscle activity than other motions. That is, more muscles are active during rotation than during extension, flexion or

Table 5.5 Muscle actions for cervical spine motion. Listed in this table are the major and minor muscles for each motion of the cervical spine

Action	Major muscle	Minor muscles
Extension ($-\theta_X$)	Semispinalis capitis	Splenius capitis Longissimus capitis Longissimus cervicis Semispinalis cervicis Multifidus muscles
Flexion ($+\theta_X$)	Sternocleidomastoid	Longus capitis Longus colli
Latera flexion ($\pm\theta_Z$)	Sternocleidomastoid	Levator scapulae Longissimus capitits and cervicis Scalenus medius and anterior Longus capitis and colli
Axial rotation ($\pm\theta_Y$)	Splenius capitis (ipsilateral)	Sternocleidomastoid (contralateral) Semispinalis capitis Contralateral for moderate action Bilateral for intensive action

lateral flexion. However, the most force that can be generated by the cervical spine is in extension, followed by flexion (~60% of extension), then lateral flexion (~60% of extension) and finally rotation (~40% of extension) [33,34]. Although more muscles are active during rotation, the mechanical advantage of these muscles is less effective for rotation than it is for extension. Given the structure and function of the cervical muscles, the finding that muscles are strongest in extension is expected owing to the need to counteract gravity and hold the head upright.

The postural muscles have also been examined using MRI [33]. The semispinalis cervicis and multifidus muscles show considerable activity with the head in a normal upright posture. However, the semispinalis capitis and splenius capitis muscles are only active during moderate and intense head extension; they are not active during normal postural activity.

Muscle as a sensory organ

Muscle tissue has two important roles: it generates force and therefore motion, but in addition, muscle tissue is extensively endowed with proprioceptors and thus acts as a sensory organ. In general, smaller muscles have a greater number of muscle spindles per gram than larger muscles. For example, small muscles, such as the RCPMin have an average of 36 spindles/g while larger muscles such as the splenius capitis average 7.6 spindles/g and larger muscles such as the gluteus maximus have only 0.8 spindles/g.

There is a biomechanical advantage to having more muscle spindles in smaller muscles than in larger muscle. An example can be illustrated by the gastrocnemius versus the plantaris muscles. Both have similar origins and insertions; however, the actual muscle tissue length of the gastrocnemius is about three times longer than that of the plantaris, with significantly more bulk (Figure 5.16). In Figure 5.16, an example of the change in length as a function of the resting length of the muscle is given. Expressed as a percentage change (strain) the smaller muscle has a much larger strain for the same change in length. Thus, a muscle spindle buried within the smaller muscle will 'see' a larger change than if it were within the larger muscle. As a result, it is mechanically advantageous to have more muscle spindles in smaller muscles than in larger muscles. This also helps explain why the body has so many redundant small muscles.

Muscle pain

Within the past decade our understanding of the role of muscle in pain and pain referral has

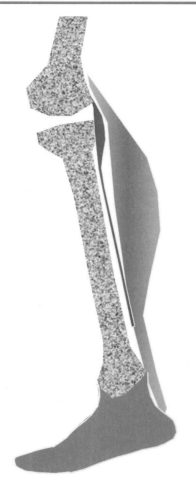

Figure 5.16 *Sensory role of small muscles. Muscle tissue of all sizes can change length and generate force via the contraction generated by the actin-myosin bond. However, small muscles are more sensitive to changes in joint position as illustrated in this figure. In this example, the gastrocnemius has an estimated resting length of ~20 cm and the plantaris has a resting length of ~6 cm. Assume the ankle moves so that both shorten by 3 cm. Then the strain (change in length divided by original length) is: Gastroc 3/20 = 0.15 (15% strain); Plantaris 3/6 = 0.50 (50% strain). Thus, the spindles in the plantaris would see a change in length of 50% while the spindles in the gastrocnemius see a change in length of only 15%. This provides insight as to why the plantaris has nine times the spindle density as the gastrocnemius. In general, smaller muscles are configured so that a large strain results on the muscle spindle, making the muscle more sensitive to joint position changes.*

grown dramatically [35–37]. Muscle pain is diffuse while cutaneous pain is well localized. In fact it is more difficult to localize the source of pain as the muscle pain increases. In addition, as muscle pain increases it is referred to other regions such as other muscles, fascia, tendons, joints and ligaments while a similar increase in cutaneous pain does not change the perceived location of the receptive field [35,38,39].

Not only does injured muscle refer pain to surrounding joints and ligaments, but it can also increase the sensitivity of the tissue at the site of referral. In studies of experimentally induced referred muscle pain, touch and other stimuli applied to the area of pain referral can increase the pain at the referred site even though there is no damage at that site [40].

Special role of the rectus capitis posterior minor (RCPMin)

In the cervical spine, the RCPMin has been found to be a very important muscle with respect to its anatomical insertions into the dura, loss of muscle mass with trauma and an important source of pain radiation [41]. Irritation of the RCPM initiates reflex EMG activity in other head and neck muscles such as the trapezius and surrounding cervical muscles and extending as far as the masseter muscles in the head [36]. The reflexive EMG activity of the neck and jaw muscles caused by RCPM irritation mimic the pattern of that initiated by irritation of the meningeal/dural vasculature in the upper cervical region [42]. However, direct irritation of the RCPM causes only a temporary reflexive reaction that typically resolves within 30 minutes [37].

There is a mechanical link between the RCPM and the dura matter whereby the chronic dysfunction of the RCPM may lead to repeated mechanical irritation to the dura. The RCPM has partial attachments to the posterior atlanto-occipital membrane that in turn is directly attached to the dura mater by fine connective tissue [43]. Thus, chronic dysfunction of the RCPM may cause persistent mechanical irritation to the dura, resulting in reflexive activity of cervical and jaw musculature [41].

Hallgren *et al.* [44] used MRI of the upper cervical spines to compare chronic neck pain subjects with normal subjects. They reported severe degeneration of the RCPMin with fatty infiltration and atrophy of the muscle while surrounding cervical muscles had no signs of degeneration. They speculated that the cause of the degeneration is from the loss of innervation to the muscle due to a hyperflexion injury of the cervical spine. The muscle degeneration would cause the loss of the proprioceptive input to the dorsal horn of the spinal cord, removing the proprioceptive signals and thus opening the 'gate' that normally blocks nociceptor transmissions to higher centres [45].

A loss of proprioceptive input should also have an effect on tasks such as standing balance. McPartland and Brodeur [46] found that patients with chronic neck pain with atrophy of the RCPMin also had a decrease in standing balance parameters compared to asymptomatic subjects having no muscle atrophy. In addition, they reported that patients with chronic neck pain had twice as many palpable dysfunctions of the upper cervical spine.

Loss of muscle mass due to trauma will increase the likelihood of muscle fatigue. Fatigue of muscle has been shown to be related to muscle spasm [47]. Fatigued muscles have an increase in output from the muscle spindle. During a stretch, a normal muscle has an increase in spindle output that is proportional to the rate of stretch; however, a fatigued muscle has an immediate increase in output as well as higher frequency of output. There is also an effect of fatigue on the Golgi organ output [47]. During stretch a normal muscle has an immediate increase in Golgi output with the output proportional to load; however, when a muscle is fatigued, the Golgi organ has almost no output. During a constant tension load the Golgi organ of a fatigued muscle has almost no output whereas the Golgi organ of a normal muscle has relatively constant output.

The hypersensitivity of the muscle spindle and the hypoactivity of the Golgi organ in a fatigued muscle set the stage for the initiation of a muscle spasm. If the muscle is contracted when in a shortened position a positive feedback loop will be initiated where the rate of spindle output increases, further causing a muscle spasm. In normal muscle the Golgi organ would fire to inhibit the muscle contraction, but in a fatigued muscle, the Golgi output is reduced or silent, and thus the muscle contraction continues unchecked.

The increased frequency of palpable joint dysfunctions in chronic neck pain subjects [46] is probably initiated by overworked cervical muscles. The loss of muscle mass from past trauma increases the load on the remaining muscle tissue. This in turn increases the frequency of muscle fatigue, and therefore muscle spasm. These muscle spasms are palpable; they generate pain, and sustain the muscle in the fatigued state.

Fatigue of muscle tissue also decreases the ability to sense a change in joint position. Traditionally, joint position has been viewed to be a function of ligaments and joint capsules; however muscle is now considered to be the primary sensor. Fatigue back muscles [48,49] and leg muscles [50] have been shown to cause a decrease in the ability of a subject to determine a change in joint position.

Clinical significance

Damage to any of the ligaments that maintain joint integrity will have the effect of increasing the neutral zone of the joint. Muscle tissue can easily compensate for damaged ligaments by controlling motion within the neutral zone [51,52]. However, any trauma to joint ligaments is likely to also damage surrounding muscle. The need for excessive muscle activity to maintain stability in a region that also has damaged muscle is likely to increase the frequency of fatigue and increase the possibility of muscle spasm. In addition, fatigue decreases the ability to accurately determine joint position, which increases the chances of further injury by overstretching a joint or underestimating the force needed to respond to a sudden change in position.

REFERENCES

1. Fisher MJ, Meyer RA, Adams GR, Foley JM, *et al*. Direct relationship between proton T2 and exercise intensity in skeletal muscle MR images. *Invest Radiol* 1990;**25**:480–485.
2. Adams GR, Duvoisin MR, Dudley GA. Magnetic resonance imaging and electromyography as indexes of muscle function. *J Appl Physiol* 1992;**73**:1578–1583.
3. Adams GR, Harris RT, Woodard D, Dudley GA. Mapping of electrical muscle stimulation using MRI. *J Appl Physiol* 1993;**74**:532–533.

4. Muhle C, Bischoff L, Weinert D, Lindner V, *et al.* Exacerbated pain in cervical radiculopathy at axial rotation, flexion, extension, and coupled motions of the cervical spine: evaluation by kinematic magnetic resonance imaging. *Invest Radiol* 1998;**33**(5):279–288

5. White AA, Panjabi MM. *Clinical biomechanics of the spine*, 2nd edn, Philadelphia: JB Lippincott Co., 1990.

6. Dvorak J, Panjabi MM, Novotny JE, Antinnes JA. In vivo flexion/extension of the normal cervical spine. *J Orthop Res* 1991;**9**(6):828–834

7. Woltring HJ, Long K, Osterbauer PJ, Fuhr AW. Instantaneous helical axis estimation from 3-D video data in neck kinematics for whiplash diagnostics. *J Biomech* 1994;**27**(12):1415–1432

8. Osterbauer PJ, Long K, Ribaudo TA, Petermann EA, *et al.* Three-dimensional head kinematics and cervical range of motion in the diagnosis of patients with neck trauma. *J Manipulative Physiol Ther* 1996;**19**(4):231–237

9. Winters JM, Peles JD, Osterbauer PJ, Derickson K, *et al.* Three-dimensional head axis of rotation during tracking movements. A tool for assessing neck neuromechanical function. *Spine* 1993;**18**(9):1178–1185

10. Dvorak J, Antinnes JA, Panjabi M, Loustalot D, *et al.* Age and gender related normal motion of the cervical spine. *Spine* 1992;**17**(10 Suppl):S393–S398

11. Ordway NR, Seymour RJ, Donelson RG, Hojnowski LS, *et al.* Cervical flexion, extension, protrusion and retraction. A radiographic segmental analysis. *Spine* 1999;**24**(3):240–247.

12. Kraemer M, Patris A. Radio-functional analysis of the cervical spine using the Arlen method. A study of 699 subjects. Part Two: Paradoxical tilting of the atlas. *J Neuroradiol* 1989;**16**(1):65–74

13. Vishteh AG, Crawford NR, Melton MS, Spetzler RF, *et al.* Stability of the craniovertebral junction after unilateral occipital condyle resection: a biomechanical study. *J Neurosurg* 1999;**90**(1 Suppl):91–98

14. Panjabi M, Dvorak J, Crisco J, Oda T, *et al.* Flexion, extension, and lateral bending of the upper cervical spine in response to alar ligament transections. *J spinal Disord* 1991;**4**(2):157–167.

15. Henke, as reported by White AA, Panjabi MM. *Clinical biomechanics of the spine*, 2nd edn, Philadelphia: JB Lippincott Co., p 95, 1990.

16. Iai H, Moriya HH, Goto S, Takahashi K, *et al.* Three-dimensional motion analysis of the upper cervical spine during axial rotation. *Spine* 1993;**18**(16):2388–2392

17. Panjabi MM, Oda T, Crisco JJ, Dvorak J, *et al.* Posture affects motion coupling patterns of the upper cervical spine. *J Orthop Res* 1993;**11**(4):525–536.

18. Dvorak J, Hayek J, Zehnder R. CT-functional diagnostics of the rotatory instability of the upper cervical spine: part 2: an evaluation on healthy adults and patients with suspected instabilities. *Spine* 1987;**12**:726–731.

19. Panjabi M, Dvorak J, Duranceau J, Yamamoto I, *et al.* Three-dimensional movements of the upper cervical spine. *Spine* 1988;**13**(7):726–730

20. Hino H, Abumi K, Kanayama M, Kaneda K. Dynamic motion analysis of normal and unstable cervical spinew using cineradiography. *Spine* 1999;**24**(2):163–168.

21. Crisco JJ, Pahjabi MM, Dvorak J. A model of the alar ligaments of the upper cervical spine in axial rotation. *J Biomech* 1991;**24**(7):607–614.

22. Dvorak J, Schneider E, Saldinger P, Rahn B. Biomechanics of the craniocervical region: the alar and transverse ligaments. *J Orthop Res* 1988;**6**(3):452–461.

23. Panjabi M, Dvorak J, Crisco JJ, Oda T, *et al.* Effects of alar ligament transection on upper cervical spine rotation. *J Orthop Res* 1991;**9**(4):584–593.

24. Crisco JJ, Oda T, Panjabi MM, Bueff HU, *et al.* Transections of the C1–C2 joint capsular ligaments in the cadaveric spine. *Spine* 1991;**16**(10 Suppl):S474–S479.

25. Godel VK, Yamanishi TM, Chang H. Development of a computer model to predict strains in the individual fibers of a ligament across the liagamentous occipito-atlanto-axis (C0–C1–C2) complex. *Ann Biomed Eng* 1992;**20**(6):667–686.

26. Mimura M, Moriya H, Watanabe T, Takahashi K, *et al.* Three-dimensional motion analysis of the cervical spine with special reference to the axial rotation. *Spine* 1989;**14**(11):1135–1139

27. Hill AV. Heat of shortening and dynamic constants of muscle. *Proc R Soc Lond* B126:**136**, 1939.

28. Warren GL, Hayes DA, Lowe DA, Armstrong RB. Mechanical factors in the initiation of eccentric contraction-induced injury in rat soleus muscle. *J Physiol (Lond)* 1993;**464**:457–475

29. Nosaka K, Clarkson PM. Changes in indicators of inflammation after eccentric exercise of the elbow flexors. *Med Sci Sports Exerc* 1996;**28**(8):953–961

30. Shellock FG, Fukunaga T, Mink JH, Edgerton VR. Exertional muscle injury: evaluation of concentric versus eccentric actions with serial MR imaging. *Radiology* 1991;**179**(3):659–664

31. Takebe K, Vitti M, Basmajian JV. The functions of semispinalis capitis and splenius capitis muscles: an electromyographic study. *Anat Rec* 1974;**179**:477–480.

32. Vitti M, Fujiwara M, Basmajian JV, Iida M. The integrated roles of longus colli and sternocleidomastoid muscles: an electromyographic study. *Anat Rec* 1974;**177**:471–484.

33. Conley MS, Meyer RA, Bloomberg JJ, Feeback DL, *et al.* Noninvasive analysis of human neck muscle function *Spine* 1995; **20**(23):2505–2512.

34. Berg HE, Berggren G, Tesch PA. Dynamic neck strength training effect of pain and function. *Arch Phys Med Rehabil* 1994; **75**:661–665.

35. Mense S, Skeppar P. Discharge behavior of feline gamma-motoneurones following induction of an artificial myositis. *Pain* 1991; **46**:201–210.

36. Hu JW, Yu XM, Vernon H, Sessle BJ. Excitatory effects on neck and jaw muscle activity of inflammatory irritant applied to cervical paraspinal tissues. *Pain* 1993;**55**:243–250

37. Hu JW, Tatourian I, Vernonr H. Opioid involvement in electromyographic (EMG) responses induced by injection of inflammatory irritant into deep neck tissues. *Somatosens Motor Res* 1996;**13**:139–146.

38. Mense S, Stahnke M. Responses in muscle afferent fibres of slow conduction velocity to contractions and ischaemia in the cat. *J Physiol* 1983;**342**:383–397.

39. Mense S, Meyer H. Different types of slowly conducting afferent units in cat skeletal muscle and tendon. *J Physiol* 1985;**363**:403–417.

40. Graven-Nielsen T, Arendt-Nielsen, Svensson P, Jensen TS. Stimulus-response functions in areas with experimentally induced referred muscle pain – a psychophysical study. *Brain Res* 1997;**744**(1):121–128

41. McPartland JM, Brodeur RR. Rectus capitis posterior minor: a small but important suboccipital muscle. *Journal of Bodywork and Movement Therapies* 1999;**3**(1):30–35.

42. Hu JW, Vernon H, Tatourian I. Changes in neck electromyography associated with meningeal noxious stimulation. *J Manipulative Physiol Ther* 1995;**18**(9):577–581

43. Hack GD, Koritzer RT, Robinson WL, *et al.* Anatomic relation between the rectus capitis posterior minor muscle and the dura mater. *Spine* 1995;**20**:2484–2486.

44. Hallgren RC, Greenman PE, Rechtien JJ. Atrophy of suboccipital muscles in patients with chronic pain: a pilot study. *JAOA* 1994; **94**:1032–1038.

45. Wall PD. The dorsal horn. In *Textbook of pain* (eds. PD Wall, R. Melzack), 2nd edn, Edinburgh: Churchill Livingstone, pp 102–111, 1989.

46. McPartland JM, Brodeur RR, Hallgren RC. Chronic neck pain, standing balance, and suboccipital muscle atrophy-a pilot study. *J Manipulative Physiol Ther* 1997;**20**(1):24–29

47. Schwellnus MP, Derman EW, Noakes TD. Aetiology of skeletal muscle 'cramps' during exercise: A novel hypothesis. *J Sports Sci* 1997;**15**:277–285

48. Taimela S, Kankaanpaa M, Luoto S. The effect of lumbar fatigue on the ability to sense a change in lumbar position. *Spine* 1999;**24**:1322–1327.

49. Parnianpour M, Nordin M, Kahanovitz N, Frankel V. Volvo award in biomechanics. The triaxial coupling of torque generation of trunk muscles during isometric exertions and the effect of fatiguing isoinertial movements on the motor output and movement patterns. *Spine* 1988;**13**(9):982–992

50. Skinner HB, Wyatt MP, Hodgdon JA, Conard DW, *et al.* Effect of fatigue on joint position sense of the knee. *J Orthop Res* 1986;**4**:112–118.

51. Panjabi M, Abumi K, Duranceau J, Oxland T. Spinal stability and intersegmental muscle forces: A biomechanical model. *Spine* 1989; **14**:194–200.

52. Wilke HJ, Wolf S, Claes LE, Arand M, *et al.* Stability increase of the lumbar spine with different muscle groups: A biomechanical in-vitro study. *Spine* 1995;**20**:192–198.

Chapter 6

Mechanisms and pain patterns of the upper cervical spine

Nikolai Bogduk

INTRODUCTION

As a class, neurologists and other headache specialists seem to have been reluctant to embrace the notion that headaches can arise from the cervical spine. Part of the difficulty lies in the lack of valid criteria whereby cervicogenic headaches can be diagnosed clinically. Clinicians accustomed to diagnosing headache on the basis of history and clinical examination find that the features of so-called cervicogenic headache are not unique, and overlap greatly with those of migraine and tension-type headache [1,2].

In contrast, the notion of cervicogenic headache rests comfortably with pain specialists and practitioners of spinal medicine. They are accustomed to the phenomenon of somatic referred pain. It is well established, for example, that pain from the lumbar zygapophysial joints [3–5], the lumbar back muscles [6], and the lumbar dura mater [7] can be referred to the buttocks and thighs. In a reciprocal manner, cervicogenic headache is pain referred into the head from the upper cervical spine.

Ironically, although cervicogenic headache remains controversial with respect to clinical diagnosis, with respect to mechanism it is one of the best-understood forms of headache. Numerous studies have established how pain from various structures in the upper cervical spine can be referred to different parts of the head and, thereby, present as headache.

NEUROANATOMY

The fundamental basis of somatic referred pain is convergence. It occurs when afferents from one particular somatic structure or region converge on second-order neurons in the spinal cord that happen also to receive afferents from another somatic region. As a result, pain stemming from the first region may be perceived, or misinterpreted, as arising also in the second region.

The structure that mediates pain from the head and upper neck is the trigeminocervical nucleus. This is not a discrete nucleus in the sense that it has distinct rostral and caudal, morphological boundaries. Rather, it is a continuous column of grey matter consisting of the pars caudalis of the spinal nucleus of the trigeminal nerve and the apical grey matter of the dorsal horns of the upper three segments of the spinal cord. What defines the nucleus as an entity is not any intrinsic feature, but the afferents that relay to it.

The trigeminocervical nucleus receives afferents from the spinal tract of the trigeminal nerve and from the upper three cervical spinal nerves. Within the nucleus, there is considerable overlap of the terminal fields of the afferents. Trigeminal afferents relay to the grey matter of at least the first three cervical segments; some reach as far as C4, but the majority terminate above the middle of the C3 segment [8,9]. Afferents from the second cervical segment ramify not only at their level of entry into the spinal cord, but also ascend to the C1 level, and descend to the C3 level [10,11]. Afferents from C3 ascend to the C2 level and sparsely to the C1 level. Afferents from C1 are largely restricted to their level of entry, but few enter the substantia gelatinosa of the dorsal horn.

Conspicuously, cervical afferents do not ascend to ramify in the spinal nucleus of the trigeminal nerve. Rather, the pattern of overlap is converse: trigeminal afferents end in the spinal nucleus but also extend into the cervical spinal cord, with the overlap between trigeminal and cervical afferents densest at the C2 and C1 levels [10,11].

As a result of these connections, pain may be referred between cervical and trigeminal fields, and between different cervical fields. Noxious stimuli mediated by cervical nerves may evoke pain in the forehead, constituting cervical-trigeminal referral; or noxious stimuli from deep cervical afferents may evoke pain in the occiput, constituting cervical-cervical referral. The exact circuitry for these patterns of referral has not been corroborated by explicit anatomical studies, but they have been clearly demonstrated in clinical experiments.

PERIPHERAL ANATOMY

The catchment area for potential cervical-trigeminal referral of pain is dictated by the peripheral distribution of the upper three cervical spinal nerves. This is illustrated systematically in Figure 6.1.

At the deepest level of the cervical spine, the sinuvertebral branches of the C1–C3 ventral rami run along the floor of the vertebral canal (Figure 6.1a). There they supply the atlanto-axial ligaments and spinal dura mater before entering the foramen magnum to innervate the dura mater over the clivus [12]. The remainder of the dura mater in the posterior cranial fossa, including the inferior surface of the tentorium cerebelli, is innervated by cervical nerves that leave the cervical plexus and follow the vagus and hypoglossal nerves in a retrograde fashion in order to enter the skull through the jugular foramen and hypoglossal canal.

The atlanto-occipital and lateral atlanto-axial joints lie ventral to the neuraxis, and receive their innervation from the ventral rami of the C1 and C2 spinal nerves, respectively

[13] (Figure 6.1b). The C2–3 zygapophysial joint lies behind the neuraxis and is innervated by the dorsal ramus of C3, specifically by the third occipital nerve as it winds around the lateral and posterior aspects of this joint [14] (Figure 6.1b).

Anteriorly, the ventral rami of the upper three cervical spinal nerves join the cervical plexus, from which they contribute to the innervation of the prevertebral muscles – longus cervicis and longus capitis, and the scalenus medius, levator scapulae, sternocleidomastoid and trapezius. In this context, although the motor innervation of sternocleidomastoid and trapezius is from the spinal accessory nerve, their sensory innervation is mediated by the upper three cervical spinal nerves, whose fibres join the spinal accessory deep to the sternocleidomastoid.

Posteriorly, the dorsal rami of the upper three cervical spinal nerves innervate the posterior neck muscles [14]. The C1 dorsal ramus supplies the suboccipital muscles (Figure 6.1c). The deep medial branch of the C3 dorsal ramus supplies those fibres of multifidus and semispinalis cervicis that arise from the C2 spinous process, and the interspinalis at that level. The medial branch of the C2 dorsal ramus – the greater occipital nerve, and the superficial medial branch of C3 – the third occipital nerve, supply the overlying semispinalis capitis. The lateral branches of the C2 and C3 dorsal rami supply the longissimus capitis and splenius capitis.

The greater occipital nerve pierces the semispinalis capitis and ascends onto the scalp of the occiput between the trapezius and sternocleidomastoid where they insert into the superior nuchal line (Fig. 6.1d). This nerve supplies the skin of the scalp as far forwards as the coronal suture. The third occipital nerve winds around the medial border of the semispinalis capitis to supply the skin over the suboccipital region. The lesser occipital nerve is derived from the cervical plexus and reaches the occiput by following the posterior border of sternocleidomastoid. The greater auricular nerve also arises from the cervical plexus and innervates the skin of the pinna and adjacent parts of the occiput.

Classical anatomy teaching attributes root values of C2 and C3 to the lesser occipital and greater auricular nerves. Accordingly, the C2 dermatome has classically been depicted as

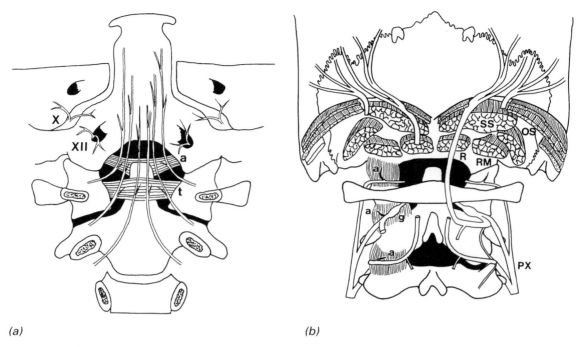

(a)   *(b)*

Figure 6.1 *The anatomy of the suboccipital region, by layers. (a) A sketch of the floor of the upper cervical vertebral canal. The occiput, the posterior arch of the atlas and the lamina of C3 have been removed. The C1–C3 sinuvertebral nerves supply the transverse (t) and alar (a) ligaments before passing through the foramen magnum to innervate the dura mater over the clivus. The meningeal branches of the vagus (X) nerve and hypoglossal nerve (XII) emerge from the jugular foramen and hypoglossal canal respectively to supply the remaining dura mater of the posterior cranial fossa. (b) A sketch of the dorsal aspect of the upper cervical vertebral column. All posterior muscles have been resected, leaving only their occipital attachments, to show the entire course of the greater occipital nerve, and the course of the third occipital nerve across the C2–C3 zygapophysial joint. The ganglion of the C2 spinal nerve (g) lies behind the lateral atlanto-axial joint. Articular branches (a) arise from the C1 ventral ramus to the atlanto-occipital joint, from the C2 ventral ramus to the lateral atlanto-axial joint, and from the third occipital nerve to the C2–C3 zygapophysial joint. The C1–C3 ventral rami enter the cervical plexus.*

covering the ear and lower lateral jaw. However, clinical studies, in which the C2 spinal nerve has been anaesthetized or transected, have revealed that C2 is expressed only in the greater occipital nerve [15,16]. Consequently, the C2 dermatome lies over the occiput but not over the face. The lower lateral aspect of the jaw belongs to the C3 dermatome.

Other structures innervated by the upper cervical nerves are the vertebral artery and the C2–3 intervertebral disc. Sensory fibres from the vertebral artery can be traced to the C1 dorsal root ganglion [17] and branches of the

C3 sinuvertebral nerve supply the back of the C2–3 intervertebral disc [18].

PAIN PATTERNS

The earliest demonstration in normal volunteers of referred pain from the neck to the head can be ascribed to Cyriax [19]. He showed injection of hypertonic saline into the suboccipital muscles caused referred pain to the forehead. If injections were made progressively more caudally into the back of the neck, the referred pain receded from the forehead to the occiput.

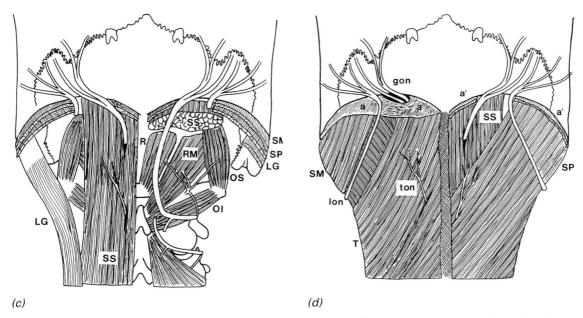

(c)

(d)

Figure 6.1 (cont) *(c) A sketch of the deep muscle layers of the upper cervical spine. On the left, the splenius has been resected to reveal the longissimus capitis (LG) and the extent of semispinalis capitis. On the right, the semispinalis capitis (SS) has been resected to reveal the course of the greater occipital nerve across the suboccipital muscles: rectus capitis posterior minor (R), rectus capitis posterior major (RM), obliquus inferior (OI) and obliquus superior (OS). The attachments of sternocleidomastoid (SM), splenius (SP) and longissimus capitis (LG) to the mastoid process remain in situ. (d) A sketch of the superficial muscle layers of the upper cervical spine. On the left, the most superficial muscle layer is shown, in which the sternocleidomastoid (SM) and trapezius (T) attach to the superior nuchal line by way of an aponeurosis (a) which connects the two muscles. The greater occipital nerve (gon) emerges through an aperture above the aponeurotic sling between these two muscles to become cutaneous. The lesser occipital nerve (lon) ascends parallel to sternocleidomastoid to reach the occiput. The third occipital nerve (ton) penetrates the trapezius to become cutaneous. On the right, the trapezius and sternocleidomastoid have been resected, leaving their aponeuroses (a') attached to the superior nuchal line, to reveal the splenius (SP) and the semispinalis capitis (SS) through which the greater occipital nerve passes. (Reproduced with permission of the publishers from Bogduk N. Anatomy and physiology. In The Headaches (eds. J Olesen, P Tfelt-Hansen and KMA Welch), New York: Raven Press, 1993.)*

The first and most detailed quantitative data were provided by Campbell and Parsons [20]. They defined certain regions of the head (Figure 6.2), and reported the frequency with which pain was perceived in these regions when selected sites in the neck were stimulated. The stimuli used were probing the periosteum of the occipital condyles with a needle, and injections of hypertonic saline into the midline structures of the neck at the levels of occiput-C1, C1–C2, C2–C3, C3–C4 and C4–C5. As the stimulus was advanced further caudally into the neck, the frequency of refer-

ral of pain to the head decreased, and the areas in which pain was felt withdrew caudally from the frontal and orbital regions (Figure 6.2).

Since the suboccipital structures are innervated by C1, and those in the C1–C2 space are innervated by C1 and C2, and since the interspinous muscles at each lower segmental level are innervated by the ipsisegmental nerve [14], the sites of stimulation used by Campbell and Parsons can be assigned a neural segmental value (Figure 6.2). Subsequently, it can be inferred that segments C1 and C2 are the more

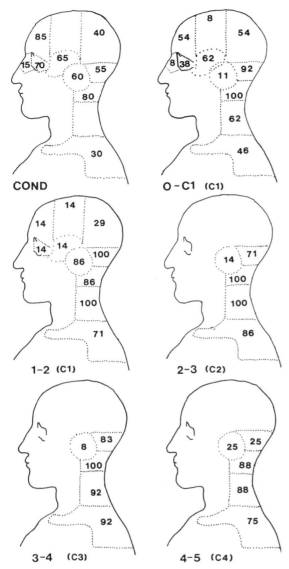

Figure 6.2 *The proportion (%) of subjects who experienced pain in the regions illustrated, following noxious stimulation of the occipital condyles (COND), or the interspinous muscles at the segmental level from occipito-C1 (O-C1) to C4–5, as labelled. In parentheses are shown the neural segment most likely to mediate the noxious stimulus. Based on Campbell and Parson [20].*

Similar patterns of referred pain were reported by Feinstein *et al.* [21] who used injections of hypertonic saline into the midline structures of the spine. Pain to the forehead was evoked when the occiput-C1 level was stimulated, and to the occiput when C1–C2 was stimulated.

These early studies demonstrated the patterns of referral of pain to the head largely from muscle tissues in the upper cervical spine. Interpreted in isolation, these studies could be misconstrued as indicating that cervicogenic headaches should have a muscular basis, which is what Campbell and Parsons [20], indeed, suggested. However, a more generic interpretation is that the studies established the principle that any structure, not just the muscles, innervated by the upper three or four cervical nerves might have the capacity to evoke referred pain to the head.

In modern times, investigators have targeted particular joints rather than the posterior midline muscles of the neck. Dwyer *et al.* [22] showed that, in normal volunteers, stimulation of the C2–3 zygapophysial joint with an injection of contrast medium evoked referred pain in the occiput. Dreyfuss *et al.* [23], using similar injections, showed that pain from the atlanto-occipital and lateral atlanto-axial joints was referred to the suboccipital regions; in some cases, from the atlanto-occipital joint, the pain extended caudally along the neck towards the shoulder girdle (Figure 6.3).

These observations in normal volunteers complement reports from clinical studies in which headache has been relieved by selectively anaesthetizing either the atlanto-occipital [24], lateral atlanto-axial joints [25,26], or the C2–3 zygapophysial joints [27–30]. They are also consistent with descriptions of headache in patients with upper cervical rheumatoid arthritis [31–34], and with median atlanto-axial osteoarthritis [35]. From extensive studies of patients, Lord and Bogduk [36] found that in patients presenting with headache after whiplash injury, the most common source of pain was the C2–3 zygapophysial joint, followed by the C3–4 joint; referral to the head from joints below C4–5 was distinctly uncommon.

Collectively, these studies in normal volunteers and in patients demonstrate that any of the joints or muscles innervated by the upper

likely to mediate referred pain to the frontal region of the head; while referral to the occiput occurs from segments C2 and C3, and to a lesser extent from C1 and C4.

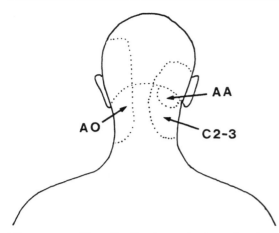

Figure 6.3 *The distribution of referred pain following stimulation of the atlanto-occipital (AO), lateral atlanto-axial (AA) and C2–3 zygapophysial (C2–3) joints in normal volunteers, using intra-articular injections of contrast medium to distend the joint.*

three or four cervical nerves are potential sources of pain in the head. However, although the studies in normal volunteers have focused on the muscles as a source, the clinical studies have implicated the upper cervical joints as the more common source of referred pain.

CHALLENGES

Experimental and clinical studies clearly demonstrate the capacity of upper cervical structures to cause referred pain to the head. The challenge that applies is how to distinguish in clinical practice these sources of headache from non-cervical sources. To date, no clinical features of cervicogenic head pain have been validated. The best statistical data stem from the studies of Lord *et al.* [36] who showed that the combination of headache as the dominant complaint and tenderness over the C2–3 zygapophysial joint had a positive likelihood ratio of 2:1 for the joint being the source of pain. This modest likelihood ratio, however, provides for a diagnostic confidence of only about 60%.

The lack of valid, clinical diagnostic features means that other criteria must be satisfied. To date, controlled diagnostic blocks have been the only means by which cervical sources of

head pain can be diagnosed. Techniques have been described by which any of the upper cervical joints, or the nerves that innervate them can be blocked, under fluoroscopic control [23,25,30]. Similar studies of blocks of upper cervical muscles have not been reported. Although cervical muscles are theoretically possible sources of cervicogenic head pain, no controlled studies have yet documented just how often muscles rather than joints are the source of pain.

Clinicians intent upon proving that the headaches of their patients arise from the cervical joints will need to implement the techniques available to anaesthetize these joints. Against the results of such diagnostic blocks, the validity of any putatively diagnostic clinical signs can be evaluated. Those intent on proving that the headaches arise from muscle will need to develop valid, objective tests that prove a muscle origin for the pain.

REFERENCES

1. Leone M, D'Amico D, Moschiano F, Farinotti M, *et al.* Possible identification of cervicogenic headache among patients with migraine: an analysis of 374 headaches. *Headache* 1995;**35**:461–464.
2. Leone M, D'Amico D, Grazzi L, Attanasia A, *et al.* Cervicogenic headache: a critical review of the current diagnostic criteria. *Pain* 1998;**78**:1–5.
3. Mooney V, Robertson J. The facet syndrome. *Clin Orthop* 1976;**115**:149–156.
4. McCall IW, Park WM, O'Brien JP. Induced pain referred from posterior lumbar elements in normal subjects. *Spine* 1979;**4**:441–446.
5. Fukui S, Ohseto K, Shiotani M, Ohno K, *et al.* Distribution of referred pain from the lumbar zygapophyseal joints and dorsal rami. *Clin J Pain* 1997;**13**:303–307.
6. Kellgren JH. On the distribution of pain arising from deep somatic structures with charts of segmental pain areas. *Clin Sci* 1939;**4**:35–46.
7. Smyth M J, Wright V. Sciatica and the intervertebral disc. An experimental study. *J Bone Joint Surg* 1959;**40A**:1401–1418.
8. Humphrey T. The spinal tract of the trigeminal nerve in human embryos between 71/2 and 81/2 weeks of menstrual age and its relation to early fetal behaviour. *J Comp Neurol* 1952;**97**:143–209.
9. Torvik A. Afferent connections to the sensory trigeminal nuclei, the nucleus of the solitary tract and adjacent structures. *J Comp Neurol* 1956;**106**:51–141.

10. Escolar J. The afferent connections of the 1st, 2nd, and 3rd cervical nerves in the cat: an analysis by Marchi and Rasdolsky methods. *J Comp Neurol* 1948;**89**:79–92.

11. Kerr FWL. Structural relation of the trigeminal spinal tract to upper cervical roots and the solitary nucleus in the cat. *Exp Neurol* 1961;**4**:134–148.

12. Kimmel DL. Innervation of the spinal dura mater and dura mater of the posterior cranial fossa. *Neurol* 1960;**10**:800–809.

13. Lazorthes G, Gaubert J. L'innervation des articulations interapophysaire vertebrales. *Comptes Rendues de l'Association des Anatomistes*, pp 488–494, 1956.

14. Bogduk N. The clinical anatomy of the cervical dorsal rami. *Spine* 1982;**7**:319–330.

15. Poletti CE. C2 and C3 radiculopathies. Anatomy, patterns of cephalic pain, and pathology. *Am Pain Soc J* 1992;**1**:272–275.

16. Poletti CE. C2 and C3 pain dermatomes in man. *Cephalalgia* 1991;**11**:155–159.

17. Kimmel DL. The cervical sympathetic rami and the vertebral plexus in the human foetus. *J Comp Neurol* 1959;**112**:141–161.

18. Bogduk N, Windsor M, Inglis A. The innervation of the cervical intervertebral discs. *Spine* 1988;**13**:2–8.

19. Cyriax J. Rheumatic headache. *BMJ* 1938; **2**:1367–1368.

20. Campbell DG, Parsons CM. Referred head pain and its concomitants. *J Nerv Ment Dis* 1944;**99**:544–551.

21. Feinstein B, Langton JBK, Jameson RM, Schiller F. Experiments on referred pain from deep somatic tissues. *J Bone Joint Surg* 1954;**36A**:981–997.

22. Dwyer A, Aprill C, Bogduk N. Cervical zygapophysial joint pain patterns I: a study in normal volunteers. *Spine* 1990;**15**:453–457.

23. Dreyfuss P, Michaelsen M, Fletcher D. Atlanto-occipital and lateral atlanto-axial joint pain patterns. *Spine* 1994;**19**:1125–1131.

24. Busch E, Wilson PR. Atlanto-occipital and atlanto-axial injections in the treatment of headache and neck pain. *Reg Anesth* 1989;**14**(Supp 2):45

25. McCormick CC. Arthrography of the atlanto-axial (C1–C2) joints: technique and results. *J Intervent Radiol* 1987;**2**:9–13.

26. Ehni G, Benner B. Occipital neuralgia and the C1–2 arthrosis syndrome. *J Neurosurg* 1984;**61**:961–965.

27. Bogduk N, Marsland A. On the concept of third occipital headache. *J Neurol Neurosurg Psychiatr* 1986;**49**:775–780.

28. Bogduk N, Marsland A. The cervical zygapophysial joints as a source of neck pain. *Spine* 1988;**13**:610–617.

29. Editorial. Third-nerve headache. *Lancet* 1986;**2**:374.

30. Lord S, Barnsley L, Wallis B, Bogduk N. Third occipital headache: a prevalence study. *J Neurol Neurosurg Psychiatr* 1994;**57**:1187–1190.

31. Cabot A, Becker A. The cervical spine in rheumatoid arthritis. *Clin Orthop* 1978;**131**:130–140.

32. Robinson, HS. Rheumatoid arthritis: atlanto-axial subluxation and its clinical presentation. *Can Med Assoc J* 1966;**94**:470–477.

33. Sharp J, Purser DW. Spontaneous atlanto-axial dislocation in ankylosing spondylitis and rheumatoid arthritis. *Ann Rheum Dis* 1961;**20**:47–77.

34. Stevens JS, Cartlidge NEF, Saunders M, Appleby A, *et al*. Atlanto-axial subluxation and cervical myelopathy in rheumatoid arthritis. *Quart J Med* 1971;**159**:391–408.

35. Zapletal J, Hekster REM, Straver JS, Wilmink JT, *et al*. Relationship between atlanto-odontoid osteoarthritis and idiopathic suboccipital neck pain. *Neuroradiol* 1996;**38**:62–65.

36. Lord SM, Bogduk N. The cervical synovial joints as sources of post-traumatic headache. *J Musculoskel Pain* 1996;**4**:81–94.

Chapter 7

Tension-type and cervicogenic headaches: Part 1 Clinical descriptions and methods of assessment

Howard T. Vernon

TENSION-TYPE HEADACHE

Tension-type headache (TTH) is the most prevalent form of benign, primary headache [1–4]. The terminology of this category of headache has undergone an evolution from the earliest classification of the NIH Ad Hoc Committee [5]. This type of headache has been called 'tension headache' as well as 'muscle contraction headache'. The most recent definitions derive from the classification of the International Headache Society (IHS) [6], where the term 'tension-type headache' was proposed. TTH has been described as: a bilateral headache of mild-to-moderate intensity experienced with an aching, tightening or pressing quality of pain that may last from 30 minutes to 7 days; which is not accompanied by nausea or vomiting; and in which only one of photo- or phonophobia may be experienced.

The IHS introduced two forms of TTH – namely, 'episodic' and 'chronic'. The distinction between the two forms is based solely on the frequency of headache days; in 'episodic' TTH (ETTH), headaches are experienced in no more than 180 days a year, while in 'chronic' TTH (CTTH), headaches occur more than 180 days a year.

Epidemiology of TTH

Prevalence/incidence

A small body of population-based studies on TTH exists, the most recent of these reporting on Canadian [7], US [8], Danish [9], German [10] and Finnish [11] populations (Table 7.1). These studies have employed various survey methods, including telephone interviews [7,8], mail surveys [10,11] and subject interviews [9]. All but one of the most recent of these studies have employed the IHS criteria for TTH described above. With one exception [9], these studies have involved large, randomly selected samples with good response rates.

Several studies reported a slight predilection for TTH in females [7–9,11]; but Gobel *et al.* [10] failed to confirm this. Similarly, some studies reported an increased prevalence in people aged 25–45 [7], while others found no increasing trend with age [8–11]. Schwartz *et al.* reported higher prevalence rates in white people and in those with higher education.

In summary, the reported prevalence rates vary from approximately 10–65%, depending on the classification as well as the description and severity of headache features. In general,

Table 7.1 Prevalence of tension-type headache: recent studies

Authors	Locale	Survey method	Sample size	Prevalence rate
Pryse-Phillips *et al.*, 1992 [7]	Canada	telephone	2905	Lifetime prevalence for headache = 58%; for TTH = 21%
Honskaalo *et al.*, 1993 [11]	Finland	mail	22 809	Prevalence for once weekly TTH = 7–17%
Gobel *et al.*, 1994 [10]	Germany	mail	5000	Lifetime prev. for TTH = 38.3%
Rasmussen *et al.*, 1995 [9]	Denmark	interview	1000	Lifetime prevalence for all TTH = 66%; for once-weekly TTH = 20–30%
Schwartz *et al.*, 1997 [8]	America	telephone	13 345	Lifetime prevalence for TTH = 38.3%

these rates derive from large, randomly selected, well-represented samples. The consistency of findings, particularly among urban populations, is notable leading to the conclusion that slightly more than one-third of the adult population suffers from this problem.

Frequency of headaches

The findings of several studies [7,10,11] agree that only 3% of TTH sufferers experience headaches more than 180 times yearly (in other words, are classified as CTTH). Rasmussen [9] reports that the percentage that suffer TTH more than once weekly (over 52/year) is 20–30%. Gobel *et al.* [10] reported that only 28% suffer TTH more than 36 times yearly. Honskaalo *et al.* [11] reported an increasing yearly frequency with age, varying from 7.3 and 13.5 per year for males and females aged below 30 years to 27.7 per year for both sexes older than 65 years. This increase appears to be linear from one decade of adulthood to the next.

Severity of headaches

TTH is, by definition, a milder, less severely painful form of headache than migraine or other primary categories (cluster headache, cervicogenic headache). Gobel *et al.* [10] reported that headache severity varied from mild, moderate to severe in 22, 68 and 10% of TTH sufferers, respectively. Rasmussen [9] reported that 58% of their TTH sample has 'mild, infrequent conditions.' Adding these subjects to their study produced the highest

reported prevalence rate. Schwartz *et al.* [8] used a pain-rating scale and reported mean (SD) headache severalties as 4.98 (1.99)/10 for ETTH and 5.55 (2.10)/10 for CTTH. In their sample, 62% were classed as moderately severe, while 25% were mild and 13% severe, closely matching Gobel *et al.*'s figures.

In summary, it appears that at least 50% of TTH sufferers rate their headaches as moderately or severely painful.

Psychosocial impact

The range of psychosocial impacts of TTH includes disturbances of daily activities, disturbed quality of life, workdays lost or disturbed as well as the costs of these disruptions. In Pryse-Phillips *et al.*'s study [7] 44% of TTH sufferers reported a significant reduction in their activities of daily living due to headache (with a mean duration of 18 hours per year) while 8% reported taking at least one day off work from their last headache. In a follow-up study of the Canadian sample, Edmeads *et al.* [12] reported that a high proportion of TTH sufferers endured adverse effects on their relationships with 89% reporting adverse effects within the family, 71% with friends and colleagues and 80% with their physical activities.

According to Rasmussen [9] 60% of TTH sufferers reported an adverse effect on work capacities, with 12% missing one or more workdays per year; 9% of their subjects had missed work in the previous year, with an interval of 1–7 days lost. He estimated a work loss rate of 820 days/1000 people per year for a total of 2 300 000 annual workdays lost in Danish society.

In Schwartz *et al*.'s US sample [8], 8.3% of subjects reported lost workdays (with a mean of 9 days per year) while 43.6% reported 'reduced-effectiveness' days (mean 5 days).

Treatment of TTH

Treatment of TTH varies widely both within medical and non-medical circles. Also, the patterns of healthcare utilization by TTH sufferers are variable. According to Edmeads *et al*. [12] 45% of their sample of TTH sufferers had consulted a physician and, of these, 32% were subsequently referred to a specialist. These figures are lower than those for migraine sufferers.

In contrast, the Danish results reported by Rasmussen [9] are much lower, with only 14% attending a physician and 4% receiving specialist referrals.

Medical approaches

Medications remain the mainstay of the medical approach to managing TTH. Two basic medication approaches exist – namely, symptom relief or abortive therapy (given every time a headache occurs) and prophylactic therapy (given on a regular basis for headache prevention). Edmeads *et al*. [12] reported that 90% of their TTH sample used over-the-counter (OTC) medications that typically include analgesic or anti-inflammatory drugs. Twenty-four percent used prescription medications, which typically include stronger doses of the OTC drugs as well as muscle relaxants and combination drugs. Only 3% were taking prophylactic medications, which include low-level antidepressants and serotonin-enhancing agents.

Wober-Bingol *et al*. [13] reported on 210 headache sufferers referred to two Austrian specialist centres. Thirty-nine percent of subjects were on some form of prophylactic regimen; however, in only 9% was this a medication regimen. Of the 19 cases that were receiving antidepressants, 11 reported them to be effective.

Non-medical approaches

There is considerable variety in the non-medical approaches to the treatment of TTH.

Edmeads *et al*. [12] reported that 34% of their headache sample has used non-medical forms of treatment, although these may have included a broad spectrum from psychological-based to physical therapies to non-pharmacological medications.

Rasmussen [9] reported that 5–8% of his headache respondents had sought care from physiotherapists or chiropractors. Wober-Bingol *et al*.'s [13] study of specialist-level patients reported that 29% had received prophylactic physiotherapy with only a quarter reporting that it was effective.

In an earlier study, Graff-Radford *et al*. [14] reported that 35% of their specialist-level headache subjects (US sample) had previously received chiropractic treatment.

The question of the percentage of chiropractic patients who present with headache is uncertain. Unfortunately, no study to date has accurately determined this, nor has any study employed the IHS criteria to determine the percentage of TTH versus migraine sufferers. Several studies from chiropractic college clinics (see references in Waalen *et al*. [15]) estimate between 5–10% of patients present to chiropractors with a primary complaint of headache. According to Kelner and Wellman [16], 10% of the chiropractic patients in their small survey of alternative health practitioners reported that headache was their primary complaint. Interestingly, this figure was the largest among the five complementary/alternative medicine (CAM) practitioners surveyed and was considerably larger than the percentage reported for the family physicians who were also surveyed.

Most recently, Hurwitz *et al*. [17] reported that 2.3% of US chiropractors' patients present primarily with headache, although 13.5% presented with neck pain which may include headache.

CERVICOGENIC HEADACHE (CH)

Description and epidemiology

The role of the cervical spine in headache has become increasingly well accepted. Despite the wealth of writing in chiropractic, osteopathic, physiotherapy and manual medicine circles (see reviews in Vernon [18–22]), as recently as the late 1980s, cervicogenic headache was poorly recognized in orthodox circles. The diagnostic label 'cervicogenic headache' (CH) was coined in 1983 by Sjaastad and colleagues [23–25], although numerous other labels existed such as 'headache of cervical origin', 'cervical headache', 'vertebrogenic headache' and 'spondylitic headache'.

As Pollman *et al.* [26] and Vincent and Luna [27] have noted, reports dating from 1926 (with the cases of Barre) to those of Bartschi-Rochaix [28] and Hunter and Mayfield [29] in 1949 to Campell *et al.*'s [30] in 1954 probably involved cases of putative cervicogenic headache. From 1983 to 1987 Sjaastad and colleagues [23,25] as well as other European investigators [31,32] expanded on the topic and provided sufficient basis for the International Headache Society classification [6] to include 'cervicogenic headache' as a distinct entity (category number 11). The criteria for this category, shown in Table 7.2, were broader and more inclusive than Sjaastad's original description, as this was challenged by some (Vernon [18,19], Bogduk [33–35]) as being so restrictive as to relegate this headache type to a rare variant. Recognizing this situation, Bogduk, one of the most prominent writers in this field, has proposed a new definition of CH, which has been adopted by the North American Cervicogenic Headache Society:

> 'Referred pain perceived in any region of the head caused by a primary nociceptive source in the musculoskeletal tissues innervated by cervical nerves' (Bogduk, personal communication.)

Furthermore, a recent classification from the International Association for the Study of Pain (IASP) [36] adds the additional criterion of successful abolishment of headache by anaesthetic blockade of the various upper cervical nerves as a diagnostic factor. The confusion in applying these various classification or diagnostic schemes is exemplified in two recent studies. Persson and Carlsson [37] reported on 81 subjects with cervical and/or radicular arm pain, 67% of whom also reported experiencing headache. When they applied the IHS criteria, 81% of these cases were classified as having CH. When using Sjaastad's 1990 criteria [38], only 28% received the same diagnosis. They concluded that 'cervical headache has no unique features that differ from those of tension-type headache, and it would perhaps be appropriate that the diagnosis of CH is incorporated in the diagnosis of TTH' (p. 223).

Leone *et al.* [39] applied all of the differing classification schemes to 940 primary headache cases and found very few who manifested any unique features of CH which could not be subsumed in either TTH or migraine diagnoses. In fact, the boundaries between cervicogenic headache, tension-type and migraine headaches were and continue to be quite blurred, particularly on the issue of bilaterality. Another conundrum which confuses the diagnostic picture is that many of the features of CH cited in Table 7.2 are physical signs which the astute clinician must obtain from careful physical and radiological examinations.

If the headache pain pattern is not so distinct as to immediately point to the diagnosis (as in cluster headache or, perhaps, migraine with aura), and if the less astute clinician does not include examination of the neck in his or her assessment, then those features critical to the CH diagnosis will be absent in the clinical

---

Table 7.2 Features of cervicogenic headache

1. Unilateral pain without sideshift.
2. Reduced range of neck motion.
3. Provocation of pain by neck movements, awkward neck positions or suboccipital pressure.
4. Associated neck or non-radicular shoulder/arm pain.
5. Pain radiates from neck to anterior head (particularly frontal and ocular).
6. Moderate pain intensity (no throbbing pain).
7. Varying durations of pain including continuous fluctuating pain.
8. Minor associated symptoms and signs (non-obligatory) including:
   - nausea, vomiting, dizziness
   - photo- and phonophobia
   - difficulty swallowing
   - 'blurred vision' in ipsilateral eye.

(Modified from International Headache Society [6]).

equation. An erroneous diagnosis of tension-type or migraine without aura might then be imposed, and the opportunity to address the possible cervicogenic aetiology of the headache will be lost. In this way, the prevalence of CH is very likely to be underestimated.

Given the diagnostic confusion cited above, it is understandable that studies of the prevalence of CH (in either the general population or in headache samples) are fraught with difficulties and variations. A wide range of frequencies is reported in the literature. As cited above, Leone *et al.* [39] found CH in only 0.7% of their headache sample, while Pffafenrath and Kaube [40] found CH in 13.8% of their larger headache sample, with 6% suffering exclusively from CH. Using the IHS criteria along with careful questioning about cervical dysfunction, Nilsson [41] found an annual prevalence of CH to be approximately 15% in a Scandinavian population. This is roughly at the lower end of prevalence estimates for tension-type headache [8,9] and is identical to the prevalence of migraine headaches cited in these reports. This is far from the rare variant headache of the early 1980s.

Mechanisms of cervicogenic headache

According to Bogduk the cervical source of headache may lie in any of the structures innervated by the first three cervical nerves. As such, a thorough knowledge of upper cervical innervation patterns is required. Before considering these patterns, it is convenient to categorize these somatic tissues according to localization, as follows:

Extrasegmental

Long occipito-thoracic muscles lie relatively superficial in the neck and include trapezius, sternocleidomastoid and splenius cervicus. The occipito-frontalis muscle is also an important consideration related to cranial pain. Other important structures lying extrasegmentally include the vertebral artery (implicated in the Barre-Lieou syndrome [22,42,43] and vertebrobasilar ischaemic syndrome) as well as the ascending sympathetic chain and superior cervical ganglion. Older theories implicated compression or irritation of these sympathetic structures in generating cranial pain and cranial vasomotor dysregulation. These theories have fallen out of favour.

Intersegmental

These structures include the classic spinal joints and deep spinal muscles, i.e., the semispinalis occiput and cervicalis, multifidus and suboccipital muscles (posterior, lateral and anterior). Remember that there is no intervertebral disc between C0–1 and C1–C2. The suboccipital articulations include the bilateral atlanto-occipital joints, the bilateral atlanto-axial joints, the atlanto-dental joint, joints of Luschka and the C2–C3 intervertebral disc. The suboccipital region contains a large number of specialized ligamentous structures (see: Kapandji [44] for an excellent review).

Intrasegmental

This category involves the neural and vascular structures contained in the intervertebral environment of C1–C2 and the intervertebral foramina of C2–C3. Specifically, the anterior and posterior rami of C1 and C2, the C2 dorsal root ganglion as well as the C3 posterior nerve root. Bogduk's reviews of upper cervical anatomy [33,34,45] are particularly extensive.

Infrasegmental

This category includes the spinal cord and lower brainstem. Of particular importance is the spinal tract of the trigeminal nerve which contains descending afferents from the trigeminal sensory ganglion which terminate as far caudally as C3 in the spinal nucleus of the V nerve. The descending tract contains three components: the pars oralis (upper), pars intermedialis and the pars or subnucleus caudalis (lowest). These afferent fibres terminate on the same second order neurons as do the afferents from the upper three cervical roots. The second order neurons form a continuous column of cells called the 'trigemino-cervical nucleus' by Bogduk [33] and the 'medullary dorsal horn' by Gobel [46]) This 'neural anastomosis' of converging afferents is the fundamental neuroanatomical basis by which painful structures in the upper cervical region might generate referred pain to the cranium (see below).

Innervation patterns

C1 and C2 anterior ramus:

- deep anterior suboccipital muscles
- posterior dura
- posterior cranial vessels
- the C2 anterior ramus contains the sensory fibres of the hypoglossal nerve which run in the ansa hypoglossus

C1 posterior ramus:

The C1 posterior ramus is very small, but its existence was proven by Kerr [47] decades ago.

The C1 anterior ramus:

- superior oblique muscle

C2 posterior ramus:

- the C2 posterior ramus has two branches – the medial branch becomes the lesser occipital nerve and innervates rectus capitus posterior major and minor and the medial C1–C2 joint and ligaments.
- the lateral branch is the largest posterior ramus of the spine and is called the greater occipital nerve (GON). The GON gives off an articular branch to the lateral C1–C2 joint as well as a muscular branch to the inferior oblique. It then courses posteriorly and superiorly to pierce between the semispinalis capitus and trapezius muscle insertions where it becomes cutaneous and innervates the skin of the posterior skull till the midline.
- The C3 posterior ramus has been called the 'third occipital nerve' by Bogduk [33,35] and it innervates the C2–C3 Z-joint and deep muscles as well as providing a recurrent meningeal nerve which innervates the C2–C3 IVD.

Clinical mechanisms

Numerous mechanical and arthritic processes affect the region and may give rise to upper cervical pain (i.e., develop into a 'pain generator'). This discussion will omit mention of the many pathological processes which can afflict the region and give rise to pain.

Extrasegmental

Postural strain and micro- or macrotrauma can create myofascial dysfunction. Trigger points in the large regional muscles have been charted by Travell and Simons [48] and create typical referred pain patterns. Stress and occupational repetitive strain can produce static overload of these muscles predisposing to local and referred pain.

Intersegmental

Painful disorders of the C0–C3 joint structures are currently thought to be the most common disorder in cervical headaches. Pain patterns, both local and referred, have been mapped by provocation and anaesthetic procedures in humans for the C0–C1 joint by Dreyfuss *et al.* [49] and for C1–C2 and C2–C3 by Feinstein *et al* [50] (for both joints) and April and Bogduk [51–53]. Barnsley *et al.* [54,55] have used double-blind anaesthetic blockades to identify the C2–C3 2–joint as the primary pain generator in over 50% of a group of whiplash sufferers with headaches.

Trigger points have also been mapped in the deeper intersegmental and suboccipital muscles. Tenderness in the deep suboccipital muscles is the most commonly reported finding in the large number of clinical reports (see review by Vernon *et al.* [32]). In our 1992 study [56] at least one tender point was identified in at least 84% of a sample of tension-type and migraine sufferers with most having two or more. Sjaastad *et al.* [24] reported on the high prevalence of paraspinal tenderness at the C2–C3 level. This finding has eventually become a hallmark of CH. Bouquet *et al.* [57] reported on 24 cervicogenic headache sufferers, 21 of whom had an ipsilateral trigger point at C2–C3. They also commented on a frequently noted finding of what they called an 'enlarged C2 spinous process', which they proposed was due to rotational misalignment at that level. In Jaeger's report on 11 cervicogenic headache patients [58], tenderness and misalignment around the transverse process of C1 were the most frequently noted findings.

Several authors have reported on standardized methods of measuring tender points in the cranio-cervical region. In 1989, Langemark *et al.* [59] developed a method of rating manual palpation for muscular tenderness. Tender points are rated on a four-point scale to a standardized manual pressure. It was determined that the pressure sufficient to blanch the examiner's thumbnail was sufficient to elicit tenderness which is then rated as follows:

0 = no reaction
1 = slight reaction, no vocalization, no movement
2 = moderate reaction with vocalization
3 = severe reaction with vocalization and flinching or other movements

Scores for a variety of muscles are added up bilaterally for a 'total tenderness score' (TTS). TTS in 50 tension-type headache subjects were found to be highly reproducible on two examinations separated by 3 weeks. Comparison of findings in 24 healthy controls indicated significantly higher TTS in headache subjects. Numerous replications of this methodology have verified its reliability and validity [60,61]. While the manual palpation method has been employed in both neck pain and headache subjects and has been found to very reliable, no study has yet investigated the role of tenderness in cranial, suboccipital *and* neck/scapular muscles in TTH sufferers. In an unpublished study, the author used pressure algometry, another method frequently reported to measure tender points [62–70] in a comparison of 14 headache and 14 control subjects. There was a significant trend towards multiple tender points to be found in headache subjects (four or more). Overall values for each of eight tender points were lower in the headache compared with control subjects.

Intrasegmental mechanisms

Entrapment of the GON and its ganglion has long been purported to cause greater occipital neuralgia. Recent evidence by Bogduk [34,71] casts more doubt on this theory, as anaesthetizing the GON would reduce pain from any of the tissues it innervates. Irritation of the sensory fibres in the anterior ramus of C2 by inflammation or osteophytic outgrowths from the C1–C2 lateral joint has been implicated as a cause of the uncommon 'neck-tongue syndrome' [72].

Infrasegmental

Only two direct mechanisms related to mechanical disturbances have been identified for the upper cervical cord. The first concerns a controversial mechanism reported by Hack and Koritzer [73] involving a ligamentous connection between the rectus capitis posticus minor and the dural lining at the foramen magnum. In a small number of reported cases, surgical ligation of this ligament has resulted in improvement in headache.

The second mechanism involves a herniation of the C2–C3 IVD. This is relatively rare, and, up until recently, only Elvidge and Choh-Luh [74] had reported on it. Recently, the use of C2–C3 discograms and disc fusion surgery have resurrected this idea.

The most important role for the spinal cord in CH lies in the phenomenon of afferent convergence of the upper cervical and trigeminal systems, as described above [22,75]. This mechanism is undoubtedly the explanation for referred pain to the cranium resulting from upper cervical deep tissue pain. It should be remembered that the same convergence phenomenon explains why posterior intracranial pathologies result in referred upper cervical pain. This may be one of the mechanisms underlying the creation of upper cervical pain and myofascial dysfunction in migraine. Painful and inflamed posterior cranial vessels can refer pain to the suboccipital region – one more cause of diagnostic confusion!

CERVICAL ASSESSMENT OF TTH AND CH

Table 7.3 lists the procedures and their purported pathophysiological mechanisms associated with chiropractic assessment in CH. These procedures and their associated dysfunction targets are described in depth below.

Physical assessment

Regional considerations

General posture
Anterior head posture has been correlated with increased incidence of headache and neck pain [76–79]. Many sedentary occupational postures in our modern world predispose to anterior head posture. Watson and Trott [78] provide a theoretical explanation as follows: shortened anterior neck and shoulder muscles induce an anterior shift of the head and neck. In order to compensate for this and maintain

Table 7.3 Methods of clinical assessment in TTH and CH

Regional	*Mechanism*
1. Plumb line/postural observation	1. Anterior head carriage.
	2. Lateral and/or rotational craniocervical distortion.
2. Range of motion	1. Reduced regional ranges of motion.
3. Radiography - plain film	1. Visualization of neutral regional postural configuration.
Segmental	
1. Static palpation	1. Segmental alignment.
	2. Myofascial tender or trigger points.
2. Algometry	1. Quantification of myofascial tenderness.
3. Motion palpation	1. Detection of joint fixation or hypomobility.
	2. Appreciation of myofascial tissues during movement.
4. Dynamic x-rays	1. Detection of intersegmental motion abnormalities.

optimal horizontal alignment of the cranium, the suboccipital and long occipital extensors would tighten. This would induce suboccipital joint compression and pain, as well as create myofascially generated pain in the affected muscles.

In their study, 30 subjects with cervical headache were found to have significantly greater forward head posture than a similar number of control subjects. Treleaven *et al.* [79], however, failed to confirm this in a smaller group of post-traumatic headache sufferers.

Grimmer *et al.* [80] recently reported that CH sufferers have significantly longer anterior neck-length measurements than do non-headache sufferers, implying that anterior head shift may be present. Placzek *et al.* [81] found no difference in head posture between chronic headache sufferers and normal controls.

Two x-ray studies (Vernon *et al.* [56], Nagasawa *et al.* [82]) have demonstrated higher levels of straightened lordotic curves in headache subjects which is likely associated with forward head posture.

Anterior head carriage can be assessed using a plumb line and by photographic analysis [80,81].

Ranges of motion
Reduced active ranges of motion (AROM) in the neck have been reported frequently in subjects with neck pain and headaches. Several devices for measuring active and passive ranges of neck motion have been reported, including cap goniometers [83,84] and magnetic inclinometers [85–88], with findings of good test-retest and interexaminer reliability.

Several studies have reported on AROM in headache subjects. Stodolny and Chmielewski [89] used a goniometer to measure cervical AROM as an outcome of manipulation therapy in patients with 'cervical migraine'. After several treatments, AROM values were reported to be increased in these subjects. Kidd and Nelson [90] used a simplistic visual assessment of cervical AROM in benign headache subjects, reporting that two or more ranges were reduced in headache subjects more frequently than in controls.

Sandmark and Nisell [91] studied the degree to which active rotations and flexion/extension reproduced pain in neck pain subjects compared with healthy controls. No actual measure of the range of motion was taken. The sensitivity and specificity of rotations and flexion/extension in correctly identifying symptom status were 77% and 92%, and 27% and 90% respectively. The high specificity values indicate that there is relatively little error in identifying non-painful subjects when AROMs are not painful.

Recently, Placzek *et al.* [81] reported significantly lower values for cervical extension in chronic headache sufferers compared with controls. This implicates increased shortness of the anterior cervical musculature as part of the postural adaptation associated with chronic headache. Stolk-Hornsveld *et al.* [92] reported significant reductions in all cervical ranges of motion with the exception of forward flexion in CH subjects versus those with other types of headaches. This corroborates the validity of 'reduced ranges of neck motion' as a criterion of CH diagnosis.

On the other hand, Persson and Carlsson [37] found no differences in cervical ROMs between groups of patients with neck pain with or without headache. However, these subjects may all have had reduced ROMs, thereby leaving little room for differences between the subgroups. Grimmer *et al.* [80] reported reduced extension in frequent versus infrequent female CH subjects; however, this difference was not significant after age adjustment. This is important, as AROMs have been shown to reduce progressively after the third decade of life [93].

Several classic prognosis studies [94–96] have reported that AROMs are reduced in chronic whiplash-injured patients. Osterbauer *et al.* [97] recently reported that 10 WAD (whiplash-associated disorder) cases had a combined AROM of 234°, considerably less than the normal 360°. After 6 weeks of conservative treatment, total AROM increased to 297°. Hagstrom and Carlsson [98] compared 30 WAD cases with 30 normal subjects and found reduced AROM in all ranges.

In a recent study, Vernon [99] objectively measured AROM in a sample of 44 chronic WAD patients (all of whom reported headache symptoms) and found moderately high correlations (p = 0.001–0.0001) between all range of motion scores and the subjects' self-rated disability scores (using the neck disability index (see below)). This is the first demonstration of a link between validly measured aspects of WAD-related impairments with levels of disability suffered by these patients. Interestingly, AROM scores were not correlated with age and duration of complaint, leading to the notion that chronic WAD sufferers reach a stable plateau of self-rated disability and impaired ranges of neck motion. In contrast, Jordan *et al.* [100] compared self-rated disability scores (using the Copenhagen Neck Functional Disability Scale (see below)) with active neck extension and found no significant correlation.

Cervical muscular function

Cervical strength testing has recently been reported for neck pain and headache subjects. Vernon *et al.* [101] reported significantly lower strength values in all cervical ranges among chronic neck pain/whiplash sufferers (almost all of whom also complained of headaches) compared with controls. Most importantly, the ratio of flexion:extension strength was much lower (28% v 69%) in the pain group, implicating the importance of flexor muscle weakness in this condition.

Grimmer *et al.* [80] reported that reduced cervical extensor and flexor strength predicted increasing headache frequency in women, but not men. Placzek *et al.* [81] reported reduced extensor and flexor strength as well as reduced endurance of the anterior cervical musculature in women with chronic headaches compared with controls.

To summarize this section of the chapter, it is hypothesized by many of these authors that the separate factors of chronic pain, postural decompensation, reduced ranges of motion and reduced muscular strength and endurance of the cervical spine as a whole interact together in a self-promoting or vicious cycle of progressive mechanical dysfunction, resulting in greater persistence of neck pain. It is also hypothesized that the focus of these regional dysfunctions is the intersegmental tissues, whose dysfunction we now discuss.

Segmental considerations

Static palpation for tenderness and misalignment

Conventional manual palpation can provide the clinician with information about myofascial and joint dysfunction. Careful manual assessment can identify misalignments between upper cervical segments (particularly the position of the C1 TVPs, the C2 spinous process and the C0–C3 posterior articulations). Tissue texture changes include tightened muscles, rotated spinous process of C2 [33] and the taut, tender bands of trigger points. Tender points can be located by pressure over any of the soft tissues and bony insertion sites. Tenderness on palpation of the tissues of the craniovertebral and paraspinal region is the most commonly reported sign of cervical dysfunction in headache subjects. Virtually every relevant author has reported on the subject, from Lewit [102] who reported on 'pain over the posterior arch of atlas', to Sachse *et al.* [103] who reported similar findings of suboccipital and scapular tenderness, to Graff-Radford *et al.* [14] and Jaeger

Table 7.4 Studies of manual tenderness assessment in neck pain and headaches

Author(s)	Findings	Location
Lebbink *et al.* [134]	Neck muscle soreness and stiffness as well as previous neck injury were more common in 164 headache sufferers than 108 controls.	Neck muscles
Jensen *et al.* [135]	Studied 14 muscle sites bilaterally in normals; used Langemark *et al.*'s method of scoring. Norms reported. Older subjects had lower TTS values while females had higher TTS scores.	Cranial and large neck muscles
Jensen *et al.* [136]	TTS scores in TTH and migraine headache sufferers compared. TTHs had lower overall scores. TTHs with headache that day had higher TTS than matched non-headache group.	Cranial and large neck muscles
Hatch *et al.* [138]	Headache subjects had at least one tender muscle more often than controls; TTS in Headaches greater than controls; EMG findings not correlated with tenderness.	Four cranial muscles Two posterior cervical muscles
Watson and Trott [139]	PTHAs had more tenderness findings than controls, particularly in upper cervical spine.	Neck paraspinal muscles
Mercer *et al.* [140]	Headache subjects had higher values of tenderness than controls.	Neck paraspinal muscles
Levoska *et al.* [141]	Test-retest correlation of manual palpation of scapular muscles was high; inter-rater reliability only fair.	Scapular muscles
Levoska *et al.* [142]	Neck pain sufferers had high number of tender points than controls.	Neck paraspinal muscles
Neck paraspinal muscles	Hubka and Phelan [143] Inter-rater reliability of segmental TTS scores were highly correlated (kappa = 0.68).	Neck paraspinal muscles
Sandmark and Nisell [144]	Cervical tenderness was most sensitive (82%) and specific (79%) for neck pain patient discrimination.	Neck paraspinal muscles
Nilsson (145)	TTS scores in neck pain patients, high inter-rater reliability.	Neck paraspinal muscles
Sandrini *et al.* [157]	Mean TTS scores higher in ETTH and CTTH subjects than controls	Trapezius
Persson and Carlsson [158]	TTS scores higher in CH *v* controls	Suboccipital, neck paraspinal and scapular muscles
Stolk-Hornsveld *et al.* [159]	Segmental tenderness on passive motion at C1–C4 higher in CH *v* other headache types. Good inter-rater reliability	Suboccipital, neck paraspinal and scapular muscles

[58] who reported on the numerous cervical tender points which they proposed served to perpetuate myofascial head pain.

Sjaastad *et al.* [6–8] reported on the high prevalence of tenderness at C2–C3. This finding eventually became a hallmark of 'cervicogenic headache'. Bouquet *et al.* [57] reported on 24 cervicogenic headache sufferers, 21 of whom had an ipsilateral trigger point at C2–3. They also commented on a frequently noted finding of an enlarged spinous process of C2, which they proposed was due to static rotational misalignment at that level. In Jaeger's report on 11 patients with cervicogenic headache, tenderness and misalignment around the transverse process of C1 were the most frequently noted findings.

The findings of more recent reports which have employed the standardized methods of tender point analysis in headache subjects which were described above are listed in Table 7.4.

While procedures for manual palpation permit the location (i.e., the identification) of tender points and, to some degree, an assessment of the severity of tenderness present at that point, they are limited in the degree to which such quantification of severity can be accomplished. To address this deficiency, numerous instruments have been devised which would allow for controlled and measurable force application, thereby permitting discrete quantification of the degree of tenderness. Since the object of greatest concern in myofascial and joint dysfunction is the deeper somatic tissues, devices which permit pressure stimuli 'pressure algometers' have become widely used. Fischer's work, in particular, [40,41] enabled the standardization of this type of investigation. According to his protocol, side-to-side differences of 1 kg/cm^2 or absolute tender point values less than 2.5 kg/cm^2 in the cervical region indicate an active tender point. Table 7.5 lists studies which employed a pressure algometer to assess cranio-cervical tenderness in headache and neck pain subjects.

Motion palpation

One of the components of cervicogenic dysfunction most commonly cited by practitioners of manual therapy is disturbance of motion at individual spinal motion segments. This phenomenon has been variously termed 'subluxation' or 'fixation' (in chiropractic circles), 'joint' or 'somatic dysfunction' (in osteopathic circles) and 'joint blockage' in manual medicine circles. The common feature of these terms is that they refer to *hypomobility* of the joints.

The procedures used to assess hypomobility are variations of manual palpation techniques of either the active, passive or accessory motions of the individual spinal motions. These procedures have been devised and described by many experts in the manual therapy disciplines, from Gillet [104], Liekens [105], Faye [106], Grice [107], and Fligg [108] in chiropractic, to Lewit [109] and Mennell [110] in manual medicine. The generic term for these procedures is 'segmental motion palpation'.

The inter-examiner reliability of these procedures is unclear. Several authors have reported poor findings [111,112], but there are many methodological flaws in these studies, including the use of asymptomatic students as subjects, the use of inexperienced students as examiners and the use of multiple replications of the procedures, such that the minor intervertebral derangements meant to be found were, temporarily, removed. In Watson and Trott's well-conducted study [78], multiple outcomes of segmental dysfunction, including segmental motion palpation, were employed to assess cervical headache subjects. They reported on the reliability of posterior-to-anterior glide palpation in 12 of their subjects examined on two occasions by the same examiner. Their kappa reliability values ranged from 0.67 to 1.00, depending on the segment.

More recently, Strender *et al.* [113] reported poor inter-examiner reliability for segmental motion assessment in 50 subjects, half of whom complained of neck or shoulder pain. On the other hand, Jull *et al.* [114] reported very high rates of agreement between several pairs of examiners in their ability to detect the presence or absence of any 'treatable upper cervical dysfunction'. Agreement levels as to the exact segment of dysfunction were somewhat lower, but still acceptable (70% overall agreement). The C1–2 segment showed the highest frequency of joint dysfunction.

With regard to the validity of the notion of spinal joint hypomobility in cervical headache patients, several studies have used both non-controlled and controlled comparisons. Jull [115–117] compared motion palpation findings in headache and non-headache subject. Hypomobility was found at C0–C1, C1–C2 and C2–C3 in 60%, 40% and 55% of headache subjects and 5%, 12% and 22% of non-headache subjects, respectively. These findings were later confirmed in a study comparing motion palpation findings (with tenderness) compared with anaesthetic blockades to zygapophyseal joints in neck pain and headache subjects [117]. The sensitivity of motion palpation was reported as 100%. Jull

Table 7.5 Studies of pressure algometry in neck pain and headache

Author(s)	Findings	Location
Reeves *et al.* [146]	High correlation coefficients for intra- and inter-examiner reliability. Average value for C0–C1 = 3.0 kg/cm²; for trapezius = 3.5 kg/cm².	Occipital and suboccipital
Jensen *et al.* [135]	Highly consistent values bilaterally and over 3–week interval in normals.	Temporalis muscles
Drummond [147]	High intra-examiner reliability; headache subjects had lower algometer values than normals; no difference between TTH and migraine headache.	Scalp and upper cervical muscles
List *et al.* [148]	High reliabilty coefficients; algometry scores highly correlated with manual palpation findings; TMJ pain subjects had lower values than normals.	Temporalis and suboccipital
Langemark *et al.* [149]	Temporalis algometry negatively correlated with headache intensity and to TTS on manual palpation. High correlation between temporal and occipital sites.	Cranial muscles
Takala [150]	High intra- and inter-rater reliability in normal subjects; women had lower algometry values than men; lower values in subgroup with minor neck pain and headache.	Scapular muscles
Hogeweg *et al.* [151]	Good reliability in normals; cervical points have lower algometry values than lumbar points.	Spinal muscles
Bovim [152]	Lower algometry values in cervicogenic headache group *v* migraine, TTH and controls. CH group had lower values in posterior cranial area and on the affected side.	Cranial and suboccipital muscles
Chung *et al.* [153]	Electronic pressure algometer showed good reliability and test-retest consistency in normals.	TMJ and neck muscles
Jensen *et al.* [154]	Algometry values lower in TTH *v* controls.	Cranial muscles
Kosek *et al.* [155]	Algometry in normals showed good 1-week consistency; lower values in upper part of body.	Whole body
Levoska *et al.* [141,142]	Reliability high in neck pain and normals; pain group had lower values.	Scapular muscles
Mazzotta *et al.* [160]	PPT values signif. lower in ETTH *v* controls.	Temporalis
Sandrini *et al.* [157]	PPT values significantly lower in ETTH and CTTH *v* controls.	Frontalis and trapezius
Stolk-Horsnveld *et al.* [161]	High levels of inter-rater reliability. Sensitivity and specificity for CH *v* controls = 82% and 62%.	Suboccipital and neck parapsinal muscles
Bendtsen *et al.* [156]	Reported on an electronic finger pressure pad for palpating tenderness. High levels of inter-examiner reliability.	Cranial muscles

et al. [114] also reported high levels of agreement between examiners' motion palpation findings which were obtained *without* pain cues from their headache subjects and the subjects' subsequent report of pain during each procedure at each cervical segmental level. In other words, joint dysfunction can be validly determined without the subject providing pain-related feedback. Much greater levels of significant joint dysfunction were found in the upper cervical segments of cervical headache subjects than in controls in this study.

Jensen *et al.*'s treatment study [118] of 19 post-traumatic headache patients reported on the findings of hypomobility before and after treatment with a short course of spinal manipulation. Fourteen of the subjects had at least one level of joint blockage in the upper cervical and upper thoracic region, while four had blockage only in the upper cervical region, for a total of 18/19 with upper cervical hypomobility. The most frequently blocked segment was C1–C2.

In Vernon *et al.*'s study [56], 54% of tension-type headache sufferers had hypomobility at two upper cervical segments while 30% had all three levels affects at least unilaterally. In the group of migraine headache sufferers, these figures were 42% and 42%, respectively. In both groups, a total of 84% had at least two upper cervical segments demonstrating hypomobility.

In Watson and Trott's study [78], far more headache subjects than controls demonstrated painful segmental hypomobility, with the most frequent blockage at C0–C1.

Treleaven *et al.* [79] reported on 12 subjects with post-traumatic headache compared with an age- and sex-matched control group. Joint dysfunction (with tenderness) was rated as mild, moderate or marked. Ten of 12 headache subjects had at least one segment demonstrating marked hypomobility in the upper cervical spine. Much more significant joint dysfunction in the headache group was noted between C0–C3 in the headache group compared with the control group.

Stodolny and Chmielewski [89] reported that all 31 of their 'cervical migraine' cases had significant joint dysfunction at C0–1 on manual palpation. Over 80% of subjects had at least two cervical segments demonstrating joint dysfunction, which is remarkably similar to the findings of Vernon *et al.* [56] in TTH and migraine subjects.

Self-rated questionnaires

The neck disability index

The first instrument designed for assessing self-rated disability due to neck pain, in particular, was the neck disability index (NDI) [119]. Designed as a modification of the Oswestry Low Back Pain Disability Index (OLBPDI) [120], the NDI is a 10-item questionnaire with well-established psychometric properties such as high test-retest reliability, good internal consistency and good sensitivity to change. Hains *et al.* [121] recently established a single factor structure to the index as well as reporting that no response bias could be found among the items.

Riddle and Stratford [122] have recently added to the psychometric profile of the NDI by determining three important values for its use in clinical and research settings. These are: 'variation around a measured value', minimal detectable change (MDC) and minimal clinically important difference (MCID). The former of these values addresses the error margin inherent in any single use of the NDI, typically in a practice setting. This value was found to be 5 NDI points, at a 90% confidence interval. To paraphrase Binkley [123] in her recent review article, 'if the error associated with a 50-point scale (such as the NDI) is 5 points, with a 90% confidence interval, the interpretation of this is that given a score of 20/50, a clinician can be 90% sure that the true score lies between 15 and 25' [123, p. 10].

According to Riddle and Stratford [122], the MDC and the MCID values are both 5 NDI points. This means that the sampling error of the instrument limits the range of minimal detectable change in a patient's status to 5 NDI points. However, as a result of its use in a cohort of neck pain patients, they determined that the minimal clinically important difference is also 5 NDI points. Several studies have reported mean change scores well beyond that level [124,125].

In a recent study, of 44 chronic WAD claimants [99], Vernon reported on additional psychometric features of the NDI. Firstly, this sample's responses were in almost identical rank order as the initial sample [119]. The items 'headache', 'lifting', 'recreation' and 'reading' were still among the five most highly rated items, confirming their importance in chronic WAD. Secondly, NDI scores were not well correlated with age and sex, as in the original work, but in this new sample, duration of complaint was also not well correlated ($r = 0.17$, NS). This was explained as follows, 'whiplash-injured patients who go on to experience chronic difficulties may reach a plateau of pain, impairment and self-rated disability, the complex of which (may remain) approximately static from that time onwards' [99, p. 211].

Thirdly, two subsets of items – namely, 'symptoms' (four items) and 'activities' (six items) were compared with one another, with a moderate, but significant level of correlation ($r = 0.55$, $p = 0.05$). The lack of strong correlation may mean that these two subsets may offer unique information on the WAD-sufferers' perception of the effect of their condition on their activities of daily living (ADLs).

Finally, NDI scores in this sample were correlated with scores on a newer 'generic' instrument for self-rating of disability, the disability rating index [126]. The two questionnaires correlated very well ($r = 0.89$, $p = 0.001$). This finding further confirms the construct validity of the NDI as a measure of physical disability.

The neck pain questionnaire (NPQ)

In 1994, Leak *et al.* [127] reported on their development of the Northwick Park Neck Pain Questionnaire (NPQ). The authors reported that, as with Vernon and Mior [119], they used the Oswestry Low Back Pain Disability Questionnaire (OLBPDQ) as a basis for their instrument. No report of the methodology for adapting the OLBPDQ was given.

The NPQ contains nine items that are scored from 0 to 4 for a total score out of 36. The items consist of the following: pain intensity, sleeping, numbness, duration, carrying, reading/television, work, social life and driving. These items represent a mix of symptoms as well as activities thought to be important to neck pain patients. Of these 'activity items', all but one ('carrying' *v* 'lifting') had already been incorporated in the NDI, published 3 years earlier. Both instruments also retained the 'pain intensity' item of the original OLBPDQ.

Forty-four subjects completed an NPQ at their original consultation while 31 completed a second NPQ 3–5 days later. Thirty-five of these subjects also completed NPQs at 4 and 12 weeks later. No formal treatment was offered in the study, but many subjects did receive some form of treatment.

Short-term repeatability was reported as high, with a Pearson's coefficient of $r = 0.84$ and kappa = 0.62. Inter-item agreements ranged from $\kappa = 0.53$ to 0.76. Internal consistency was not formally tested, but was graphically depicted as adequate.

Initial NPQ scores did not correlate well with age, sex, duration or previous history of neck pain. While NPQ scores did not change significantly over the 3–month study interval, they did correlate well with a separate question rating the subject's perception of improvement. This was cited as an indicator of 'sensitivity to change'. Subsets of subjects who either received physiotherapy or performed home exercises had what was described as 'significant improvement' in their NPQ scores.

Given the similarities between the NDI and the NPQ, this author considers Leak *et al.*'s report to be, essentially, a replication study of the NDI. That the same set of psychometric properties was reported – namely, high levels of test-retest reliability, internal consistency and sensitivity to change, as well as poor correlations with age, sex and duration of complaint is therefore not surprising and confirms the original report [119]. To this author's knowledge, no additional studies on the NPQ have been reported since 1994.

The Copenhagen Neck Functional Disability Scale (CNFDS)

The CNFDS was devised by Jordan *et al.* [128] as an attempt to improve the existing questionnaires (NDI and NPQ) for assessing disability due to neck pain. Jordan *et al.* asserted that, since both previous instruments incorporated some items related to 'symptoms' (pain, numbness and duration in the NPQ; pain, headache and concentration in the NDI), these questionnaires lacked some precision for measuring solely the disability due to neck pain itself. This assertion was based on the theory that pain, disability and impairment are separate but inter-related constructs.

The CNFDS contains 15 items with a three-point scale (yes = 0, occasionally = 1, no = 2) for a maximum of 30 points. Many of the item constructs are similar to those in the NDI (sleep, personal care, lifting, reading, headaches, concentration and recreation), while three additional items focus on psychosocial issues.

Jordan et al. reported very high test-retest reliability ($r = 0.99$), excellent internal consistency (Cronbach's alpha = 0.89) and no significant correlation between initial scores and age or sex. Additionally, initial CNFDS scores were highly correlated with patients' global assessment of their condition ($r = 0.83$) and moderately correlated with doctors' global assessments ($r = 0.56$). Initial scores also correlated highly with a separate 11-point pain ratings for neck and arm pain, which somewhat deflates the authors' original premise of a clinically important distinction between self-ratings of pain and disability.

Finally, the authors reported good sensitivity to change in a larger sample of subjects enrolled in a clinical trial for neck pain [100]. At 6, 24 and 52 weeks of this trial, changes in pain scores correlated with changes in CNFDS scores at $r = 0.49$, 0.48 and 0.54 respectively.

Table 7.6 provides a comparison of the different items in each of these instruments.

The headache disability inventory

This 25-item scale was developed by Jacobsen et al. [129] to assess the impact of recurrent headaches on daily function. The items are organized into two scales: 'emotional' and 'functional'. Good stability of scores has been reported over 1-week and 8-week intervals. Unfortunately, Jacobsen et al. [129] reported very poor sensitivity to change in a sample of treated patients. As well, they reported that change in HDI was not well correlated with change in frequency of headaches. As such, the HDI is likely useful in the initial work-up of a patient in order to assess their self-perception of the daily burden imposed by their headache condition, but it may not be useful in monitoring the clinical outcome of a patient under treatment.

Activities of daily living (ADL)

A series of validated questions to monitor the impact of headaches on activities of daily living has been developed by von Korff et al. [130]. These ADL-related questions employ a relatively long interval of 6-months' time. For clinical usage, the intervals of time might be shortened.

Table 7.6 Item comparison of neck disability scales

Instrument (date of publication) Items	NDI (1991)	NPQ (1994)	CNFDS (1998)
1	pain[2]	pain[2]	sleeping[3]
2	personal care[2]	sleeping[3]	daily activities[1]
3	lifting[2]	numbness[1]	daily activities[3]
4	reading[3]	duration[1]	dressing[2]
5	headache[2]	carrying[1]	washing[2]
6	concentration[2]	reading/TV[3]	at home1
7	work[3]	work[3]	lifting[2]
8	driving[2]	social[2]	reading[3]
9	sleeping[3]	driving[2]	headaches[2]
10	recreation[2]		concentration[2]
11			recreation[2]
12			resting[1]
13			family[1]
14			social[2]
15			'future'[1]

3 = item found in all three instruments; 2 = item found in two instruments; 1 = item found in only one instrument.

- How many days in the past 6 months have you been kept from your usual activities (work, school or housework) because of headaches?
- Using the following 0–10 scale, where 0 = 'no interference' and 10 = 'unable to carry out any activities'
- In the past 6 months, how much have your headaches interfered with your daily activities?
- In the past 6 months, how much have your headaches interfered with your ability to take part in recreational, social or family activities?

- In the past 6 months, how much have your headaches interfered with your ability to work (including housework)?

Holroyd *et al.* [131] have recently reported that these questions loaded most highly on a separate factor labelled 'headache disability' in the responses of their headache sample. Scores from the 'disability' scale were not highly correlated with 'pain intensity scores', indicating that self-rated disability is a separate construct in the experience of headache sufferers and should be assessed separately by clinicians and researchers.

ID# _____   Week # _____

Diary for 2000 ____ ____   to 2000 ____ ____   **HEADACHE STUDY**
          mm   dd   mm   dd

Check all that apply	Mon	Tue	Wed	Thu	Fri	Sat	Sun
Did you have a headache today?							
How bad was your headache? 0 = no pain, 10 = worst pain	0 1 2 3 4 5 6 7 8 9 10	0 1 2 3 4 5 6 7 8 9 10	0 1 2 3 4 5 6 7 8 9 10	0 1 2 3 4 5 6 7 8 9 10	0 1 2 3 4 5 6 7 8 9 10	0 1 2 3 4 5 6 7 8 9 10	0 1 2 3 4 5 6 7 8 9 10
The headache was on one side.							
The headache was on both sides.							
Did your headache affect your work or daily activities?							
Did you take any medication for your headache today?							
If so, how many pills did you take?							

Figure 7.1 *Example of a headache diary*

The dizziness handicap inventory (DHI)

This instrument was developed in 1990 [132] as a 25-item scale to assess the impact of dizziness and vestibular problems on daily life. The DHI is composed of three subscales: functional, emotional and physical. The original paper reported good test-retest reliability and internal consistency. DHI scores were found to correlate well with increasing frequency of dizziness episodes and with scores from balance tests [132].

HEADACHE MONITORING

The headache diary

The primary instrument for monitoring headache activity is the headache diary. Numerous versions of such diaries exist, depending on the particular interest of the research involved [133]. For typical clinical use, the once-daily diary-recording format is optimal. An example of such a diary is shown in Figure 7.1. This type of diary permits calculations of the following parameters: frequency of headache days per week/month; headache severity for any particular day or averaged over any interval; peak headache severity per any interval (i.e., worst headache in a month); medication usage. Some diaries record the duration of headaches, but, often, the use of analgesic medications will shorten the duration, thereby providing false impressions of the true duration of ongoing headaches.

For clinical purposes, it is often sufficient to monitor the frequency and average severity of headaches. The desirable outcome of clinical management would be a reduction in both of these parameters. This is typically the kind of outcome that has been reported in clinical trials of prophylactic treatments for TTH or CH.

REFERENCES

1. Silberstein SD. Tension-type headaches. *Headache* 1994;**34**:s2–7.
2. Leonardi M, Nusicoo M, Nappi G. Headache as a major public health problem: current status. *Cephalalgia* 1998;**18**:66–69.
3. Waters WE. The Pontypridd headache survey. *Headache* 1974;**14**:81–90.
4. Diamond S, Baltes BJ. Management of headache by the family physician. *Am Fam Phys* 1972;**5**:68–76.
5. Ad Hoc Committe on Classification of Headache. Classification of Headache. *Arch Neurol* 1962:613–6.
6. International Headache Society. Classification and Diagnostic Criteria for Headache Disorders, Cranial Neuralgias and Facial Pain. *Cephalalgia* 1988;Suppl.7.
7. Pryse-Phillips W, Findlay H, Tugwell P, Edmeads J, *et al*. A Canadian population survey on the clincal, epidemiologic and societal impact of migraine and tension-type headache. *Can J Neurol Sci* 1992;**19**:333–339.
8. Schwartz BS, Stewart F, Simon D, Lipton RB. Epidemiology of tension-type headache. *JAMA* 1998;**279**:381–383.
9. Ramussen BK. Epidemiology of headache. *Cephalalgia* 1995;**15**:45–68.
10. Gobel H, Peterson-Braun M, Soyka D. The epidemiology of headache in Germany: a nationwide survey of a representative sample on the basis of the headache classification of the international headache society. *Cephalagia* 1994;**14**:97–106.
11. Honskaalo M-L, Kaprio J, Keikkila K, Sillanpaa M, *et al*. A population-based survey of headache and migraine in 22,809 adults. *Headache* 1993;**33**:403–412.
12. Edmeads J, Findlay H, Tugwell P, Pryse-Phillips W, *et al*. Impact of migraine and tension-type headache on life-style, consulting behaviour, and medication use: a Canadian population survey. *Can J Neurol Sci* 1993;**20**:131–137.
13. Wober-Bingol C, Wober C, Karwautz A, Schnider P, *et al*. Tension-type headache in different age groups at two headache centers. *Pain* 1996;**67**:53–58.
14. Graff-Radford SB, Reeves JL, Jaeger B. Management of chronic head and neck pain: effectiveness of altering factors perpetuating myofascial pain. *Headache* 1987;**27**:186–190.
15. Waalen DP, White TP, Waalen JK. Demographic and clinical characteristics of chiropractic patients:a five year study of patients treated at the Canadian Memorial Chiropractic College. *J Can Chiro Assoc* 1994;**38**:75–82.
16. Kelner M, Wellman B. Who seeks alternative health care? A profile of the users of five modes of treatment. *J Alt Comp Med* 1997;**3**:127–140.
17. Hurwitz EL, Coulter ID, Adams AH, Genovese BJ, *et al*. Use of chiropractic services from 1985 through 1991 in the United States and Canada. *Am J Public Health* 1998;**88**:771–776.

18. Vernon HT. Spinal manipulation and headaches of cervical origin. *J Manip Physiol Therap* 1989;**12**:455–468.

19. Vernon HT. Spinal manipulation and headaches of cervical origin: a review of literature and presentation of cases. *J Man Med* 1991;**6**:73–79.

20. Vernon HT. Spinal manipulation and headaches: an update. *Top Clin Chiro* 1995;**2**:34–46.

21. Vernon HT. The effectiveness of chiropractic manipulation in the treatment of headache: an exploration in the literature. *J Manip Physiol Therap* 1995;**18**:611–619.

22. Vernon HT. Cervicogenic headache. In *Foundations of Chiropractic: Subluxation* (ed. M. Gatterman), St Louis: Mosby, pp. 306–318, 1988.

23. Sjaastad O, Saunte C, Hovdahl H, Breivek H, *et al*. Cervicogenic headache: an hypothesis. *Cephalalgia* 1983;**3**:249–256.

24. Sjaastad O, Fredrickson TA, Stolt-Neilsen A. Cervicogenic headache, C2 rhizopathy and occipital neuralgia: a connection. *Cephalalgia* 1986;**6**:189–195.

25. Fredrickson TA, Hovdahl H, Sjaastad O. Cervicogenic headache: clinical manifestations. *Cephalalgia* 1987;**7**:147–160.

26. Pollmann W, Keidel M, Pfaffenrath V. Headache and the cervical spine: a critical review. *Cephalalgia* 1997;**17**:801–816.

27. Vincent M, Luna RA. Cervicogenic headache: Josey's cases revisited. *Arq Neuropsiquiatr* 1997;**55**:841–848.

28. Bartschi-Rochaix W. *Migraine cervicale: das encephale syndrom nach halswirbeltrauma.* Bern: Huber, 1949.

29. Hunter CR, Mayfield FH. The role of the upper cervical roots in the production of pain in the head. *Am J Surg* 1949;**48**:743–751.

30. Campbell AMG, Hoyd IK. Atypical facial pain. *Lancet* 1954;**ii**:1034–1038.

31. Pfaffenrath V, Dandekar R, Mayer E, Hermann G, *et al*. Cervicogenic headache: results of computer-based measurements of cervical spine mobility in fifteen patients. *Cephalalgia* 1990;**10**:295–303.

32. Leone M, D'Amico D, Moschiano F, Farinotti M, *et al*. Possible identification of cervicogenic headache among patients with migraine: an analysis of 374 headaches. *Headache* 1995;**35**:461–464.

33. Bogduk N, Marsland A. On the concept of third occipital headache. *J Neurol Neurosurg Psychiatr* 1986;**49**:775–780.

34. Bogduk N. Cervical causes of headache and dizziness. In *Modern Manual Therapy of the Vertebral Column* (ed. GP Grieve), Edinburgh: Churchill Livingstone, pp. 289–302, 1986.

35. Lord SM, Barnsley L, Wallis BJ, Bogduk N. Third occipital nerve headache: a prevalence study. *J Neurol Neurosurg Psychiatr* 1994;**57**:1187–1190.

36. International Association for the Study of Pain (IASP). Cervicogenic Headache. In *Classification of chronic pain. Descriptions of chronic pain syndromes and definitions of pain terms* (eds. H Merskey, N Bogduk), 2nd edn. Seattle, WA: IASP Press, pp. 94–95, 1994.

37. Persson LCG, Carlsson JY. Headache in patients with neck-shoulder-arm pain of cervical radicular origin. *Headache* 1999;**39**:218–224.

38. Sjaastad O, Fredriksen TA, Pfaffenrath V. Cervicogenic headache: diagnostic criteria. *Headache* 1990;**30**:725–726.

39. Leone M, Domenico D, Grazzi L, Attanasio A, *et al*. Cervicogenic headache: a critical review of the current diagnostic criteria. *Pain* 1998;**78**:1–5.

40. Pfaffenrath V, Kaube H. Diagnostics of cervicogenic headache. *Funct Neurol* 1990;**5**:159–164.

41. Nilsson N. The prevalence of cervicogenic headache in a random sample of 20–59 year olds. *Spine* 1995;**20**:1884–1888.

42. Edmeads J. Headaches and head pains associates with diseases of the cervical spine. *Med Clin North Amer* 1978;**62**:533–41.

43. Vernon HT. Vertebrogenic headache. In *Upper Cervical Syndrome: Chiropractic Diagnosis and Management* (ed. HT Vernon), Baltimore: Williams and Wilkins, 1988.

44. Kapandji IA. *The Physiology of the Joints: The Trunk and Vertebral Column.* Edinburgh: Churchill Livingstone, 1974.

45. Bogduk N, Corrigan B, Kelly P, Schneider G, *et al*. Cervical headache. *Med J Aust* 1985; **143**:202–207.

46. Gobel S. An EM analysis of the transsynaptic effects of peripheral nerve injury subsequent to tooth pulp extirpations on neurons in laminae I and II of the medullary dorsal horn. *J Neurosci* 1984;**4**:2281–2290.

47. Kerr FW. Structural relation of the trigeminal spinal tract to upper cervical roots and the solitary nucleus in the cat. *Exp Neurol* 1961;**4**:134–148.

48. Travell JG, Simons DG. *Myofascial Pain and Dysfunction. The Trigger Point Manual.* Baltimore: Williams and Wilkins; 1983;

49. Dreyfuss P, Michaelsen M, Fletcher D. Atlanto-occipital and lateral atlanto-axial joint pain patterns. *Spine* 1994;**19**:1125–1131.

50. Feinstein B, Langton J, Jameson R, Schiller I. Experiments on pain referred from deep somatic tissues. *J Bone Joint Surg* 1954;**36A**:981–987.

51. Bogduk N, Marsland A. The cervical zygapophysial joints as a source of neck pain. *Spine* 1988;**13**:610–617.

52. Dwyer A, April C, Bogduk N. Cervical zygapophyseal joint pain patterns I: a study in normal volunteers. *Spine* 1990;**15**:453–457.

53. Aprill C, Dwyer A, Bogduk N. Cervical zygapophyseal joint pain patterns II: a clinical evaluation. *Spine* 1990;**15**:458–461.

54. Barnsley L, Lord S, Wallis BJ, Bogduk N. The prevalence of chronic cervical joint pain after whiplash. *Spine* 1995;**20**:20–26.

55. Lord SM, Barnsley L, Bogduk N. The utility of comparative local anaesthetic blocks vs placebo-controlled blocks for the diagnosis of cervical zygapophysial joint pain. *Clin J Pain* 1995;**11**:208–213.

56. Vernon HT, Steiman I, Hagino C. Cervicogenic dysfunction in muscle contraction and migraine headache:a descriptive study. *J Manip Physiol Ther* 1992;**15**:418–429.

57. Bouquet J, Boismaire F, Payenville G, Leclerc D, *et al*. Lateralization of headache: possible role of an upper cervical trigger point. *Cephalalgia* 1989;**9**:15–24.

58. Jaeger B. Cervicogenic headache: a relationship to cervical spine dysfunction and myofascial trigger points. *Cephalalgia* 1987;(Suppl 7):398–399.

59. Langemark M, Jensen K, Jensen TS, Olesen J. Pressure pain thresholds and thermal nociceptive thresholds in chronic tension-type headache. *Pain* 1989;**38**:203–210.

60. Bovim G. Cervicogenic headache, migraine and tension-type headache:pressure-pain threshold measurements. *Pain* 1992;**51**:169–173.

61. Bendtsen L, Jensen R, Jensen NK, Olesen J. Pressure-controlled palpation: a new technique which increases the reliability of manual palpation. *Cephalalgia* 1995;**15**:205–210.

62. McCarthy DJ, Gatter RA, Phelps P. Dolorimeter for quantification of articular tenderness. *Arthritis Rheum* 1964;**8**:551–559.

63. Merskey H, Spear FG. Reliability of pressure algometry. *Br J Soc Clin Psychol* 1964; **3**:130–136.

63. Fischer AA. Pressure threshold measurement for diagnosis of myofascial pain and evaluation of treatment *results*. *Clin J Pain* 1987; **2**:207–214.

65. Fischer AA, Chang CH. Temperature and pressure thresholds over trigger points. *Thermology* 1986;**1**:212–215.

66. Reeves JL, Jaeger B, Graff-Radford SB. Reliability of pressure algometer as a measure of myofascial trigger point sensitivity. *Pain* 1986;**24**:313–321.

67. Jensen K, Anderson HO, Olesen J, Lindblom U. Pressure pain threshold in human temporal region: evaluation of a new pressure algometer. *Pain* 1986;**24**:322–3.

68. Kosek E, Ekholm J, Nordemar R. A comparison of pressure pain thresholds in different tissues and body regions. *Scand J Rehab Med* 1993;**25**:117–124.

69. Wallace HL, Jahner S, Buckle K, Desai N. The relationship of changes in cervical curvature to visual analogue scale, Neck Disability Index scores and pressure algometry in patients with neck pain. *J Chiro Res Clin Invest* 1994; **9**:19–23.

70. Vernon HT, Aker PD, Burns S, Viljakaanen S, *et al*. Pressure pain threshold evaluation of the effect of spinal manipulation in the treatment of chronic neck pain. *J Manip Physiol Ther* 1990;**13**:13–16.

71. Bogduk N. The clinical anatomy of the cervical dorsal rami. *Spine* 1982;**13**:26–29.

72. Terrett A. Neck-tongue syndrome and spinal manipulative therapy. In *Upper Cervical Syndrome: Chiropractic Diagnosis and Treatment* (ed. HT Vernon), Baltimore: Williams and Wilkins, 1988.

73. Hack GD, Koritzer RT. Anatomic relation between the rectus capitus posticus minor muscle and the dura mater. *Spine* 1995;**20**:2484–2486.

74. Elvidge AR, Choh-Luh L. Central protrusion of cervical intervertebral disc involving the descending trigeminal tract. *Arch Neurol Psychiatr* 1950;**63**:455–466.

75. Sessle BJ, Hu JW, Yu X. Brainstem mechanisms of referred pain and hyperalgesia in the orofacial and temperomandibular region. In *New Trends in Referred Pain and Hyperalgesia* (eds. L Vecchiet, D Albe-Fessard, U Lindblom, MA Giamberardino), Amsterdam: Elsevier, 1993.

76. Awalt P, Lavin NL, McKeough M. Radiographic measurements of intervertebral foramina of cervical vertebra in forward and normal head posture. *J Cranio Practice* 1989;**7**:275–285.

77. Darnell MW. A proposed chronology of events for forward head posture. *J Cranio Practice* 1983;**1**:50–54.

78. Watson DH, Trott PH. Cervical headache: an investigation of natural head posture and upper cervical flexor muscle performance. *Cephalalgia* 1993;**13**:272–282.

79. Treleaven J, Jull G, Atkinson L. Cervical musculoskeletal dysfunction in post-concussional headache. *Cephalalgia* 1994;**14**:273–279.

80. Grimmer K, Blizzard L, Dwyer T. Frequency of headaches associated with the cervical spine and relationships with anthropometric, muscle performance and recreational factors. *Arch Phys Med Rehab* 1999;**80**:512–521.

81. Placzek JD, Pagett BT, Roubal PJ, Jones BA, *et al*. The influence of the cervical spine on chronic headache in women: a pilot study. *J Man Manip Therap* 1999;**7**:33–39.

82. Nagasawa A, Sakakibara T, Takahashi A. Roentgenographic findings of cervical spine in tension-type headache. *Headache* 1993;**33**:90–95.

83. Zachman Z, Traina A, Keating JC, Bolles ST, *et al*. Inter-examiner reliability and concurrent validity of two instruments for the measurement of cervical ranges of motion. *J Manip Physiol Therap* 1989;**12**:205–210.

84. Cassidy JD, Lopes AA, Yong-Hing K. The immediate effect of manipulation versus mobilization on pain and range of motion in the cervical spine: a randomized controlled trial. *J Manip Physiol Therap* 1992;**15**:570–575.

85. Tucci SM, Hicks JE, Gross EG, Campbell W, *et al*. Cervical motion assessment: a new,simple and accurate method. *Arch Phys Med Rehab* 1986;**67**:225–230.

86. Rheault W, Albright B, Byers C, Franta M, *et al*. Intertester reliability of the cervical range of motion device. *J Ortho Sports Therap* 1992;**15**:147–150.

87. Capuano-Pucci D, Rheault D, Aukai J, Bracke M, *et al*. Intratester and intertester reliability of the cervical range of motion device. *Arch Phys Med Rehab* 1991;**72**:338–340.

88. Youdas JW, Carey JR, Garrett TR. Reliability of measurements of cervical range of motion: comparison of three methods. *Phys Ther* 1991;**71**:98–106.

89. Stodolny J, Chmielewski H. Manual therapy in the treatment of patients with cervical migraine. *J Man Med* 1989;**4**:49–51.

90. Kidd RF, Nelson R. Musculoskeletal dysfunction of the neck in migraine and tension headache. *Headache* 1993;**33**:566–569.

91. Sandmark H, Nisell R. Validity of five common manual neck pain provoking tests. *Scan J Rehab Med* 1995;**27**:131–136.

92. Stolk-Hornsveld F, Gijsbert TJ, Duquet W, Stoekart R, *et al*. Impaired mobility of cervical spine as a tool in the diagnosis of cervicogenic headache (abstr). *Cephalalgia* 1999;**19**:436.

93. Dvorak J, Antinnes JA, Panjabi M, Loustalot D, *et al*. Age and gender related normal motion of the cervical spine. *Spine* 1992;**17**:S393–S398.

94. Hildingsson C, Toolanen G. Outcome after soft-tissue injury of the cervical spine: a prospective study of 93 car accident victims. *Acta Orthop Scand* 1990;**61**:356–359.

95. Hohl M. soft tissue injuries of the neck in automobile accidents: factors influencing prognosis. *J Bone Joint Surg* 1974;**56A**:1675–1682.

96. Gargan MF, Bannister GC. The rate of recovery following whiplash injury. *Eur Spine J* 1994;**3**:162–164.

97. Osterbauer PJ, Derickson KL, Peles JD, DeBoer KF, *et al*. Three dimensional head kinematics and clinical outcome of patients with neck injury treated with spinal manipulative therapy: a pilot study. *J Manip Physiol Therap* 1992;**15**:501–511.

98. Hagstrom Y, Carlsson J. Prolonged functional impairments after whiplash injury. *Scand J Rehab Med* 1996;**28**:139–146.

99. Vernon HT. Correlations among ratings of pain, disability and impairment in chronic whiplash-associated disorder. *Pain Res Manag* 1997;**2**:207–213.

100. Jordan A, Bendix T, Nielsen H, Hansen FR, *et al*. Intensive training, physiotherapy or manipulation for patients with chronic neck pain: a prospective, single-blind, randomized clinical trial. *Spine* 1998;**23**:311–319.

101. Vernon HT, Aker P, Aramenko M, Battershill D, *et al*. Evaluation of neck muscle strength with a modified sphygmomanometer dynamometer: reliability and validity. *J Manip Physiol Therap* 1992;**15**:343–349.

102. Lewit K. Ligament pain and anteflexion headache. *Eur Neurol* 1971;**5**:365–378.

103. Sachse J, Erhardt E. Phenomenological investigation in migraine patients. *Man Med* 1982;**20**:59–64.

104. Gillet H. *Belgian Chiropractic Research Notes*. 10th edn. Huntington Beach, CA: Motion Palpation Institute, 1970.

105. Gillet H, Liekens M. A further study of spinal fixations. *Ann Swiss Chiro Assoc* 1969;**4**:41–46.

106. Faye LJ. *Spine II. Motion Palpation and Clinical Considerations of the Cervical and Thoracic Spine*. Huntington Beach, CA: Motion Palpation Institute, 1986.

107. Grice AS. A biomechanical approach to cervical and dorsal adjusting In *Modern Developments in the Principles and Practice of Chiropractic*, (ed. S Haldeman), New York: Appleton-Century-Crofts, pp. 331–358, 1980.

108. Fligg B. Motion palpation of the upper cervical spine. In *The Upper Cervical Syndrome: Chiropractic Diagnosis and Treatment*, (ed. H Vernon), Baltimore, MD: Williams and Wilkins; pp. 113–123, 1988.

109. Lewit K. *Manipulative Therapy in the Rehabilitation of the Locomotor System*. Oxford: Butterworths, 1991.

110. Mennel JM. *Joint Pain*. Boston: Little, Brown, 1964.

111. DeBoer KF, Harmon R, Tuttle CD, Wallace H. Reliability study of the detection of somatic dysfunctions in the cervical spine. *J Manip Physiol Therap* 1985;**8**:9–16.

112. Mior SA, King RS, McGregor M, Bernard M. Intra- and inter-examiner reliability of motion palpation in the cervical spine. *J Can Chiro Assoc* 1985;**29**:195–199.

113. Strender L-E, Lundin M, Neil K. Interexaminer reliability in physical examination of the neck. *J Manip Physiol Ther* 1997;**20**:516–520.

114. Jull G, Zito G, Trott P, Potter H, *et al*. Interexaminer reliability to detect painful upper cervical joint dysfunction. *Aust J Physiol* 1997;**43**:125–129.

115. Jull GA. Clinical observations of upper cervical mobility. In *Modern Manual Therapy of the Vertebral Column* (ed. GP Grieve), Edinburgh: Churchill-Livingstone; pp. 312–315, 1986.

116. Jull GA. Manual diagnosis of C2–C3 headache. *Cephalalgia* 1985;**5**(Suppl 5):308–309.

117. Jull GA, Bogduk N, Marsland A. The accuracy of manual diagnosis of cervical zygapophysial joint pain syndrome. *Med J Aust* 1988;**148**:233–236.

118. Jensen OK, Nielsen FF, Vosmar L. An open study comparing manual therapy with the use of cold packs in the treatment of post-traumatic headache. *Cephalalgia* 1990; **10**:241–250.

119. Vernon H, Mior S. The Neck Disability Index: a study of reliability and validity. *J Manip Physiol Ther* 1991;**14**:409–415.

120. Fairbank JCT, Couper J, Davies JB, O'Brien JP. The Oswestry Low Back Pain Index. *Physiotherapy* 1980;**66**:271–273.

121. Hains F, Waalen J, Mior S. Psychometric properties of the Neck Disability Index. *J Manip Physiol Ther* 1998;**21**:75–80.

122. Riddle DL, Stratford PW. Use of generic versus region-specific status measures on patients with cervical spine disorders: a comparison study. *Phys Ther* 1998;**78**:951–963.

123. Binkley J. Measurement of functional status, progress and outcome in orthopedic clinical practice. *Orthop Div Res* 1998;**1**:7–17.

124. Vernon HT, Piccininni J, Kopansky-Giles D, Hagino C, *et al*. Chiropractic rehabilitation of spinal pain: principles, practice and outcomes data. *J Can Chirop Assoc* 1995;**39**:147–153.

125. Giles LGF, Muller R. Chronic spinal pain syndromes: a clinical pilot trial complaring acupuncture, a non-steroidal anti-inflammatory drug and spinal manipulation. *J Manip Physiol Ther* 1999;**22**:376–381.

126. Salen BA, Spangfort EV, Nygren AL, Nordemar P. The Disability Rating Index: an instrument for the assessment of disability in clinical settings. *J Clin Epidemiol* 1994;**47**:1423–1434.

127. Leak AM, Cooper J, Dyer S, Williams KA, *et al*. The Northwick Park Neck Pain Questionnaire: devised to measure neck pain and disability. *J Rheumatol* 1994;**33**:469–474.

128. Jordan A, Manniche C, Mosdal C, Hindsberger C. The Copenhagen Neck Functional Disability Index: a study of reliability and validity. *J Manip Physiol Ther* 1998;**21**:520–527.

129. Jacobson GP, Ramadan NM, Aggarwal SK, Newman CW. The Henry Ford Hospital headache Disability Inventory (HDI). *Neurology* 1994;**44**:837–842.

130. Von Korff M, Stewart WF, Lipton RB. Assessing headache severity. *Neurology* 1994; **44**:S40–S46.

131. Holroyd KA, Malinoski P, Davis MK, Lipchik GL. The three dimensions of headache impact: pain, disability and affective distress. *Pain* 1999;**83**:571–578.

132. Jacobson GP, Newman CW. The development of the Dizziness Handicap Inventory. *Arch Otolaryngol Head Neck Surg* 1990;**116**:424–427.

133. Blanchard EB, Andrassik F. *Management of Chronic Headaches: A Psychological Approach*. New York: Pergammon Press, pp. 44–53, 1985.

134. Lebbink J, Spierings EL, Messinger HB. A questionnaire survey of muscular symptoms in chronic headache: and age and sex-controlled study. *Clin J Pain* 1991;**7**:95–101.

135. Jensen R, Rasmussen BK, Pedersen B, Lous I, *et al*. Cephalic muscle tenderness and pressure pain threshold in a general population. *Pain* 1992;**48**:197–203.

136. Jensen R, Rasmussen BK, Pedersen B, Olesen J. Muscle tenderness and pressure pain threshold in headache: a population study. *Pain* 1993;**52**:193–199.

137. Jensen OK, Nielsen FF, Vosmar L. An open study comparing manual therapy with the use of cold packs in the treatment of post-traumatic headache. *Cephalalgia* 1990;**10**:241–250.

138. Hatch JP, Moore PJ, Cyr-Provost M, Boutness N, *et al*. The use of electromyography and muscle palpation in the diagnosis of tension-type headache with and without pericranial muscle involvement. *Pain* 1992;**49**:175–178.

139. Watson DH, Trott PH. Cervical headache: an investigation of natural head posture and upper cervical flexor muscle performance. *Cephalalgia* 1993;**13**:272–282.

140. Mercer S, Marcus D, Nash J. Cervical musculoskeletal disorders in migraine and tension-type headache. *Phys Ther* 1993;**73**:105 (abstr)

141. Levoska S, Keinanen-Kiukaanniemi S, Bloigu R. Repeatability of measurement of tenderness in the neck-shoulder region by dolorimeter and manual palpation. *Clin J Pain* 1993;**9**:229–235.

142. Levoska S. Manual palpation and pain threshold in female office employees with and without neck-shoulder symptoms. *Clin J Pain* 1993;**9**:236–241.

143. Hubka MJ, Phelan SP. Interexaminer reliability of palpation for cervical spine tenderness. *J Manip Physiol Ther* 1994;**17**:591–595.

144. Sandmark H, Nisell R. Validity of five common manual neck pain provoking tests. *Scan J Rehab Med* 1995;**27**:131–136.

145. Nilsson N. Measuring cervical muscle tenderness: a study of reliability. *J Manip Physiol Therap* 1995;**18**:88–90.

146. Reeves JL, Jaeger B, Graff-Radford SB. Reliability of pressure algometer as a measure of myofascial trigger point sensitivity. *Pain* 1986;**24**:313–321.

147. Drummond P. Scalp tenderness and sensitivity to pain in migraine and tension headache. *Headache* 1987;**27**:45–50.

148. List T, Helkimo M, Falk G. Reliability and validity of a pressure threshold meter in recording tenderness in the masseter muscle and the anterior temporalis muscle. *J Cranio Pract* 1989;**7**:223–229.

149. Langemark M, Jensen K, Jensen TS, Olesen J. Pressure pain thresholds and thermal nociceptive thresholds in chronic tension-type headache. *Pain* 1989;**38**:203–210.

150. Takala E. Pressure pain threshold on upper trapezius and levator scapulae muscles: repeatability and relation to subjective symptoms in a working population. *Scand J Rehab Med* 1990;**22**:62–68.

151. Hogeweg JA, Langereis MJ, Bernards ATM, Faber JAJ, *et al*. Algometry: measuring pain threshold, method and characteristics in healthy subjects. *Scand J Rehab Med* 1992;**24**:99–103.

152. Bovim G. Cervicogenic headache,migraine and *tension*-type headache:pressure-pain threshold measurements. *Pain* 1992;**51**:169–173.

153. Chung S, Un B, Kim H. Evaluation of pressure pain threshold in head and neck muscles by electronic algometer: intrarater and interrater reliability. *J Cranio Pract* 1998;**10**:28–34.

154. Jensen K, Anderson HO, Olesen J, Lindblom U. Pressure pain threshold in human temporal region: evaluation of a new pressure algometer. *Pain* 1986;**24**:322–323.

155. Kosek E, Ekholm J, Nordemar R. A comparison of pressure pain thresholds in different tissues and body regions. *Scand J Rehab Med* 1993;**25**:117–124.

156. Bendtsen L, Jensen R, Jensen NK, Olesen J. Pressure-controlled palpation: a new technique which increases the reliability of manual palpation. *Cephalalgia* 1995;**15**:205–210.

157. Sandrini G, Antonaci F, Pucci E, Bono G, *et al*. Comparative study with EMG, pressure algometry and manual palpation in tension-type headache and migraine. *Cephalalgia* 1994;**14**:451–457.

158. Persson LCG, Carlsson JY. Headache in patients with neck-shoulder-arm pain of cervical radicular origin. *Headache* 1999;**39**:218–224.

159. Stolk-Hornsveld F, Gijsberts TJ, Duquet W, Stoeckart R, *et al*. Pain provocation tests for C0–C4 in the diagnosis of cervicogenic headache (abstr.) *Cephalalgia* 1999;**19**:436.

160. Mazzotta G, Sarchielli P, Gaggioli A, Gallai V. Study of pressure pain and cellular concentration of neurotransmitters related to nociception in episodic tension-type headache patients. *Headache* 1997;**37**:565–571.

161. Gijsbert TJ, Stolk-Hornsveld F, Duquet W, Stoeckart R, *et al*. Reliability and validity of pressure algometry as a tool in the diagnosis of cervicogenic headache. *Cephalalgia* 1999;**19**:435–436.

Chapter 8

Tension-type and cervicogenic headaches: Part 2 A systematic review of complementary/ alternative therapies*

Howard T. Vernon, Cameron McDermaid, Carol Hagino

INTRODUCTION

Tension-type headache (TTH) is the most prevalent form of adult benign headache. Recent population-based studies have estimated its prevalence as 35–40% of the adult population in Western societies [1–3]. TTH contributes to a large burden of disability, resulting in lost workdays, diminished quality of life, and considerable healthcare costs to both governments and institutional payers [3,4]. Individual sufferers share in these costs, because the predominant approach to treatment of TTH is the use of over-the-counter analgesic medications [4] for symptomatic relief. Table 8.1 displays the criteria for the diagnosis of TTH from the International Headache Society classification and Diagnostic Criteria for Headache Disorders, Cranial Neuralgias and Facial Pain [5].

Cervicogenic headache (CH) is a recently validated type of headache [5–7], although its existence has been proposed by investigators in the manual medicine field for many decades [8,9]. Nilsson's study [10], using the criteria established by the International Headache Society (IHS) [5] reported the prevalence of cervicogenic headache in a Scandinavian population to be approximately 16%. There is still some confusion in the clinical profiles of TTH and CH. The IHS-based definition of CH is given in Table 8.1.

Reprinted from: *Comp Ther Med* 1999;**7**:142–155 with permission.

A number of systematic reviews and meta-analyses have been reported on treatments for headache [11–17]. The interventions studied in these reviews have been confined to pharmacological therapies and cognitive/behavioural therapies. The majority of these reviews have been for treatments of migraine-type headache. Bogaards and ter Kuile's recent meta-analytic review of treatments for 'recurrent tension headache' [13] confined itself to the following categories of intervention: pharmacological, cognitive therapy, relaxation therapy, EMG biofeedback therapy and combinations, although some complementary/alternative therapies (CATs) such as acupuncture and physiotherapy were regarded as control or 'pseudo-placebo' treatments. No primary complementary/alternative therapies were included. This chapter presents a systematic review of all randomized clinical trials of CATs for tension-type and cervicogenic headaches.

Since the publication of Eisenberg's important article describing the usage of CAT by Americans [18], interest in the topic within orthodox medical circles has grown and the use of these therapies in society has increased considerably. Utilization rates by sufferers of TTH of CAM (complementary/alternative medicine) therapies are poorly understood. Several studies cite the proportion of patients seeking chiropractic care for headache to be approximately 3–10% of patients in practice [19,20].

Table 8.1 Criteria for tension-type headache and cervicogenic headache from the IHS classification [7]

(1) Tension-type headache:
A. At least 10 previous headache episodes fulfilling criteria B-D.
B. Headache lasting from 30 minutes to 7 days.
C. At least two of the following criteria:
   1. Pressing/tightening (non-pulsatile) quality
   2. Mild or moderate intensity (may inhibit, but does not prohibit activity)
   3. Bilateral location
   4. No aggravation by walking, stairs or similar routine physical activity.
D. Both of the following:
   1. No nausea or vomiting (anorexia may occur)
   2. One of photo- or phonophobia may be present, but not both.

(2) Cervicogenic headache:
A. Pain localized to the neck and occipital region. May project to forehead, orbital region, temples, vertex or ears.
B. Pain is precipitated or aggravated by special neck movements or sustained postures.
C. At least one of the following:
   1. Resistance to or limitation of passive neck movements.
   2. Changes in neck muscle contour, texture, tone or response to active and passive stretching and contraction.
   3. Abnormal tenderness of neck muscles.
D. Radiological examination reveals at least one of the following:
   1. Movement abnormalities in flexion/extension.
   2. Abnormal posture.
   3. Fractures, congenital abnormalities, bone tumours, rheumatoid arthritis or other distinct pathology (not spondylosis or osteochondrosis).

LITERATURE SEARCH

A literature search was conducted of Medline (English-language, 1966 to mid-1998), Psych-Info and CINHAL databases. The Medline search strategy is given in Table 8.2. Once these searches were obtained, supplementary

Table 8.2 Medline search strategy

1. randomized controlled trial.pt.
2. controlled clinical trial.pt.
3. randomized controlled trials.sh.
4. random allocation.sh.
5. double blind method.sh.
6. single blind method.sh.
7. 1 or 2 or 3 or 4 or 5 or 6
8. (animal not human).sh.
9. 7 not 8
10. clinical trial.pt.
11. exp clinical trials/
12. (clin$ adj25 trial$).ti,ab.
13. 13 ((singl$ or doubl$ or trebl$ or tripl$) adj25 (blind$ or mask$)).ti,ab.
14. placebos.sh.
15. placebo$.ti,ab.
16. random$.ti,ab.
17. research design.sh.
18. of/10–17
19. 18 not 8
20. 19 not 9
21. comparative study.sh.
22. 22 exp evaluation studies/
23. follow up studies.sh.
24. prospective studies.sh.
25. (control$ or prospective$ or volunteer$).ti,ab.
26. or/21–25
27. 26 not 8
28. 26 not (9 or 20)
29. 29 9 or 20 or 28
30. exp headache/
31. headache.ti,ab.
32. headache/ci
33. 30 or 31
34. 33 not 32
35. exp alternative medicine/
36. exp plants, medicinal/
37. exp plant oils/
38. exp plant extracts/
39. exp formularies, homeopathic/
40. ((complementary or unconventional or folk or alternative) adj25 (med$ or ther$ or treat$ or care)).ti,ab.
41. exp holistic health/
42. exp physical therapy/
43. (physical ther$ or physiother$).ti,ab.
44. exp osteopathy/ or exp osteopathic medicine/
45. (chiropract$ or naturopath$ or osteopath$ or homeopath$ or acupunct$).ti,ab.
46. or/35–45
47. 29 and 34 and 46
48. limit 47 to english language
49. 47 not 48

searches of citation and reference lists in other systematic literature reviews, as well as author queries were done.

Inclusion criteria

From the total initial citation lists, a screening process was undertaken by the senior author to identify the study design as one of the following: clinical trial, case series, case report or letter to the editor. Only randomized controlled trials (RCTs) were retained for analysis in this report. Relevant RCTs were defined as prospective studies with a sample of adult headache sufferers in which at least two groups were randomly allocated to receive one or more interventions. Studies involving exclusively migraine, cluster or organic types of headache were excluded. A small number of studies included both tension (-type) and migraine groups and were included in the review. In some reports, older terminology such as 'muscle contraction' or 'tension' headache was used, and this was accepted for our review.

Studies included in the review involved those reporting typical clinical outcomes related to headache activity (i.e., Headache index, severity, frequency and medication usage). Studies which employed only physiological outcomes (EMG measurements only, blood chemistry and eye function), without clinical measures were not included in this review. As noted above, any studies which employed non-CAM therapies were not reviewed.

Quality scoring

Data abstraction and quality reviews were independently conducted by two reviewers (CM and CH), using a standardized abstraction form and a quality review protocol modified from van Tulder *et al.* [21]. (Operational definitions for the quality review are available from the authors on request.) This quality review protocol was deemed most appropriate for our purposes as it was devised for reviewing clinical trials of non-medical treatments for spinal pain. As such, items pertaining to medications (dosages, side effects, monitoring via blood samples, etc.), which would be relevant to drug trials and which appear in other quality review schemes

[12,22], were excluded to prevent quality decrements from unfairly being applied to the CAT studies.

The reviewers were not blinded to the source of the citations. While there is evidence that a difference may exist between blinded and unblinded reviews, the differences demonstrate little consistency in direction of bias or its magnitude [23].

The reviewers included one clinician as well as a non-clinician methodologist. The reviewers' scores were assessed for consistency with the intraclass correlation coefficient. The standard error of the mean of the difference scores was calculated to determine the absolute level of difference between the reviewers' scores.

Evidence tables were constructed to include author(s), year of publication, study duration, sample size, headache type (as well as use of IHS classification) and a review of the outcome of the trial, specifically whether a positive or negative result was obtained when comparing the experimental to the comparative or control treatment(s). No statistical pooling was attempted.

The quality review protocol contains 18 items answered by *yes/no/don't know* scores. The latter two response categories were collapsed, making the scoring dichotomous. No weighting factor was used. Scores therefore range from 0–18, and were converted to percentages for ease of interpretation and reporting. A rating of 0–40% was deemed to indicate 'poor' quality; ratings of 40–60% were deemed 'moderately high' and ratings above 60% were deemed to indicate 'high' quality.

RESULTS

The Medline search resulted in 444 citations; 349 of these were excluded immediately because they were irrelevant to our study; they involved migraine headaches; or they involved studies of behavioural or cognitive-type treatments of any type of headache. This left 95 citations related to CAM treatments, 73 of which were non-RCT reports (case series, case reports, reviews, letters and abstracts); therefore, 22 RCTs were identified in this search. The PsychInfo and CINHAL searches revealed no additional RCTs. Citation searches revealed one additional RCT [24].

One RCT [25] was identified in the recent literature. Five additional reports did not deal directly with clinical outcomes but were investigations of physiological effects [26–29] or, in one case, did not involve symptomatic subjects [30]. They were excluded from the review.

The 24 studies included in this review were organized into groups according to the primary modality of treatment. This was straightforward for studies involving acupuncture, spinal manipulation and homeopathy. The category of 'physiotherapy' was less straightforward. Studies investigating electrical therapies alone and as the primary modality were placed in the 'electrotherapy' category. Studies included in the 'physiotherapy' category involved multiple modalities, including electrotherapy in some. Table 8.3 gives the breakdown of number of RCTs by treatment category. The largest group involves studies of acupuncture, with no other group having more than five distinct trials. In the manipulation group, one of the trials was reported twice, with different sample sizes. We conducted quality reviews on each of these reports separately.

Twenty-two of the trials involved tension headache subjects. Only two reports (one trial) [31,32] involved CH. Only one study involved post-traumatic headache (PTTH) subjects [33]. Subjects in these three trials received spinal manipulation as compared to soft tissue therapy (for the CH trials) or ice therapy (in the PTTH trial).

The quality raters' scores achieved a reliability coefficient of 0.72 (p = 0.0015). Scores were not statistically significantly different from one another (t = -1.5, p = 0.14) and the 95% CI of the mean difference between scores was 1.9–0.3. Given this level of consistency, we averaged the two raters' scores for a final trial quality score.

Table 8.3 RCTs by type of treatment

Treatment	No of studies
Acupuncture	8
Manipulation	6
Electrotherapy	4
Physiotherapy	3
Massage	1
Homeopathy	1
Other	1
Total:	24

Results of the quality reviews

Acupuncture trials

The quality scores for the eight acupuncture trials ranged from 44 to 69, with an average score of 58 and a median score of 61. The quality scores for the four high quality trials ranged from 61–69%. These trials were published within the years 1979 to 1996. The total number of subjects reported in these trials is 99, with an average of about 25 subjects per trial. Three of these trials [24,34,35] were sham-controlled, with an average treatment duration of 52.5 days. The other trial [36] compared acupuncture with physiotherapy. Tavola *et al.* [35] reported a 'negative' outcome, in that the acupuncture treatment was no better than the placebo, while Ahonen *et al.* [36] reported significant improvement in the acupuncture and physiotherapy groups, with no difference between the two groups. Two trials [24,34] reported a significant difference favouring acupuncture over sham placebo with regard to the frequency of headaches, but these two trials have a combined total of 39 subjects, thus precluding any definitive conclusions.

The quality scores for the other four trials ranged from 44 to 50 (moderately high quality) [37–40]. They were published from 1984 to 1991. The total number of subjects in these reports was 173, with an average of 43 per trial. Only one of these studies was sham controlled [39], while one used a no-treatment control [40]. The average duration of treatment was 99 days. Three of these studies reported a positive benefit in that acupuncture was shown to be better than sham-control for frequency [39], better than no-treatment control [40] and better than medication [38]. On the other hand, Johansson *et al.* [40] did not demonstrate differences between acupuncture and an occlusal splint for TMJ-related tension headache and Carlsson *et al.* [37] reported that subjects receiving physiotherapy obtained greater benefit than acupuncture.

In summary (see Tables 8.4 and 8.5), the total number of TTH subjects reported in the literature receiving acupuncture is 264. The treatment durations of these studies range from 6 to 12 weeks. Five (63%) of these studies were controlled (4/5 employed sham

Table 8.4 Evidence table for high quality acupuncture studies

Authors	Headache type	Sample size	Study duration	Treatment groups (n)	Results	Side-effects	Quality scores
Tavola *et al.*, 1992 [40]	Tension-type headache (IHS)	30	60 days	(1) Acup = 15 (2) Sham = 15	Pre – Post Tx reduction F (1) 44.3 % (2) 21.4% NS Pre – Post Tx reduction S (1) 58.3% (2) 27.8% NS	Not mentioned	69
White *et al.*, 1996 [29]	Episodic tension-type headache (IHS)	10 (Pilot study)	45 days	(1) Acup = 4 (2) Sham = 5	Post – Tx F (1) 9/28 wks HA-free (2) 3/36 wks HA-free	None	69
Borglum-Jensen *et al.*, 1979 [39]	Not specified (non-migraine)	29	60 days	(1) Acup = 19 (2) Sham = 10	Pre – Tx F: (1) 34.6 (17) /60 days (2) 26.9 (16) Post – Tx F: (1) 25.7(17) (2) 23 (15) $p<0.05$	None	64
Ahonen *et al.*, 1984 [41]	'Myogenic headache'	22	30 days	(1) Acup = 12 (2) Sham = 10	Pre – TX F: (1) (2) daily 6 5 >1/wk 0 1 1/wk 0 1 <3/mo 0 0 Post – Tx F: (1) (2) daily 5 3 >1/wk 2 5 1/wk 3 1 <3/mo 2 1 NS	Not mentioned	61
Totals or average		91	48 days				66

(n) = sample size in each treatment group; (IHS) = inclusion based on criteria of the International Headache Society Classification [9];
Treatment types: ACUP = acupuncture, SHAM = sham placebo treatment, SPLINT = occlusal splint, CONTR = no-treatment control, P/T = physical therapy or physiotherapy, MEDS = medication, MANIP = chiropractic spinal manipulation, STT = soft tissue therapy, AMIT = amitriptyline, RELAX = relaxation therapy, TENS = transcutaneous electrical nerve stimulation, ELEC. STIM. = electrical stimulation, LO- = low level, BIOF = biofeedback, ATTEN. = attention control.
Outcomes: Tx = treatment; HA = headache; S = severity; F = frequency; mm = millimetres on a visual analogue scale; /wk = per week; wk = week(s); mo = month; (1), (2)... = treatment group; for 'severity': mod. = moderate; sev = severe; v. sev. = very severe
for 'frequency': sev = several; for 'global relief': hi= high, mod = moderate, min= minimal; improv. = improvement; ≥ = statistically significantly better than; = means: not statistically significantly better than.
Statistical significance: NS = not significant, * = 0.05, ** = 0.01, *** = 0.001

controls). Two of four higher quality studies reported negative results, although, with the small sample sizes in all of these trials, the likelihood of a type II error is quite high. Acupuncture has been shown in at least one study (low quality) to be more beneficial than medication over a 3–month period, and equivalent to an occlusal splint in the treatment of TMJ-related tension-type headache. Acupuncture does not appear to be more effective than a course of physiotherapy.

Spinal manipulation trials

Three RCTs of spinal manipulation for TTH [25,41,42], two for cervicogenic headache

Table 8.5 Evidence table for lower quality acupuncture studies

Authors	Headache type	Sample size	Study duration	Treatment groups (n)	Results	Side-effects	Quality scores
Hansen and Hansen, 1985 [44]	Chronic tension headaches	18	105 days (crossover)	(1) Acup = 9 (2) Sham = 9	Pre – Tx F[1]: (1) = 42.2 (2) = 40.7 Post – Tx F: (6 weeks) (1) = 26.4* (2) = 35.2 Post -Tx F: (12 weeks[2]) (1) = 30.1 (2) = 30.9* 1 = primary measure is 'Period Index' 2 = groups crossed-over	1 subject had aggravation of pain from needling	50
Johansson *et al.*, 1991 [45]	Muscle tension headache	45	120 days	(1) Acup = 15 (2) Splint = 15 (3) Contr	Pre – Tx S: (1) 52 mm (2) 55 mm (3) 50 mm Post – Tx S: (1) 27 mm* (2) 29 mm* (3) 56 mm NS between (1) and (2)	Not mentioned	50
Carlsson *et al.*, 1990 [42]	Chronic tension-type HA (IHS)	62	60–90 days	(1) Acup = 23 (2) P/T = 29	Pre – Tx S: (%) (1) (2) none 3 0 mild 3 3 mod. 17 29 sev. 59 58 v. sev.17 10 Post –Tx S: (%) (1) (2) none 9 7 mild 9 38 mod. 39 41 sev. 35 14 v. sev. 9 0 * *** Pre – Tx F: (%) (1) (2) none 0 0 1–2/mo 7 0 1/wk 7 7 sev/wk 31 36 daily 55 58 Post – Tx F: (%) (1) (2) none 0 0 1–2/mo22 17 1/wk 26 38 sev/wk 13 14 daily 39 31 ** ***	None	50

Table 8.5 Continued

Authors	Headache type	Sample size	Study duration	Treatment groups (n)	Results	Side-effects	Quality scores
Loh *et al.*, 1984 [43]	'Muscle tension' = 7 migraine = 31 mixed = 10	48	120 days	(1) Acup = 41 (2) Meds = 36	(1) improv. level great = 9/41 mod slight = 8/41 none = 14/41 (2) improv. level great = 3/36 mod = 1/36 slight = 5/36 none =27/36 (Subjects may have received both Txs in series)	Not mentioned 7/41	44
Total or average		173	105 days				48

(n) = sample size in each treatment group; (IHS) = inclusion based on criteria of the International Headache Society Classification [9];
Treatment types: ACUP = acupuncture, SHAM = sham placebo treatment, SPLINT = occlusal splint, CONTR = no-treatment control, P/T = physical therapy or physiotherapy, MEDS = medication, MANIP = chiropractic spinal manipulation, STT = soft tissue therapy, AMIT = amitriptyline, RELAX = relaxation therapy, TENS = transcutaneous electrical nerve stimulation, ELEC. STIM. = electrical stimulation, LO- = low level, BIOF = biofeedback, ATTEN. = attention control.
Outcomes: Tx = treatment; HA = headache; S = severity; F = frequency; mm = millimetres on a visual analogue scale; /wk = per week; wk = week(s); mo = month; (1), (2)... = treatment group; for 'severity': mod. = moderate; sev = severe; v. sev. = very severe
for 'frequency': sev = several; for 'global relief': hi= high, mod = moderate, min= minimal; improv. = improvement; ≥ = statistically significantly better than; = means: not statistically significantly better than.
Statistical significance: NS = not significant, * = 0.05, ** = 0.01, *** = 0.001

[31,32] and one for 'post-traumatic headache' [33] were identified. The quality scores ranged from 56–80%, with a mean score of 67.5%.

Table 8.6 reviews these trials. No trial included an exclusively sham or placebo-type control group, so that the 'efficacy' of spinal manipulation treatment cannot yet be determined. With respect to determining the effectiveness of spinal manipulation, comparative treatments include soft tissue mobilization [41], resting briefly [41], ice pack [33], amitriptyline [42] and soft tissue therapy [25,31,32]. A total of 286 subjects were included in these reports.

There is some inconsistency with regard to the diagnostic classifications used in these studies. The report by Hoyt *et al.* [41] involved a single manipulative session provided to nine subjects with a concurrent 'muscle contraction' headache (versus 13 other control subjects).

Jensen *et al.*'s [33] study was conducted on a small group of subjects with 'post-traumatic headache'. Boline *et al.*'s [42] and Bove and Nilsson's [25] studies were the only ones to explicitly include 'tension-type headache' according to the IHS criteria [5]. The former study included a 6-week intervention phase and a 4-week follow-up, while the latter study involved 4 weeks of treatments with no follow-up phase. Nilsson's study [31,32] was the only one conducted on subjects with cervicogenic headache.

As no high quality studies exist which employed an exclusive placebo or sham-control group, the efficacy of SMT for TTH-like or cervicogenic headache cannot be determined. Four high quality studies do exist which compare SMT to other forms of therapy, although two of them have relatively small sample sizes. Three of these studies

Table 8.6 Evidence table for spinal manipulation studies

Authors	Headache type	Sample size	Study duration	Treatment groups (n)	Results	Side-effects	Quality scores
Hoyt *et al.*, 1979 [46]	'Muscle contraction'	22	1 =10	(1) Manip (2) Mob = 6 (3) Rest = 6	Post – Tx S: (1) –48% *** (2) 0 (3) 0	Not mentioned	56
Jensen *et al.*, 1981 [38]	Post-traumatic	19	2	(1) Manip = 10 (2) Ice = 9	Post – Tx S: (1) –30.7/100 ** (2) +6.7/100	Not mentioned	60
Nilsson, 1995 [36]	Cervicogenic	39	6	(1) Manip = 20 (2) STT = 19	Post – Tx F: (1) –3.4 (–59%) (2) –2.1 (–45%) Post – Tx S: (1) –15 (–45%) (2) –10 (–24%)	Not mentioned	64
Nilsson, 1997 [37]	Cervicogenic	53	6	(1) Manip = 28 (2) STT = 25	Post – Tx F: (1) –3.2 * (–69%) (2) –1.6 (–37%) Post – Tx S: (1) –17* (–36%) (2) –4.2 (–17%)	Not mentioned	72
Boline *et al.*, 1995 [42]	Tension-type headache (IHS)	126	12	(1) Manip = 70 (2) Amit = 56	Post – Tx F: (1) –3.8/28 (2) –4.0/28 Follow-up F: (1) –1.0** (2) +5.0 Post – Tx S: (1) –1.3/20 (2) –1.8/20** Follow-up S: (1) –.5 ** (2) +2.0	(1) 4.3% neck stiffness (2) 82.1% dry mouth, drowsy, or weight gain	75
Bove and Nilsson, 1998 [30]	Tension-type headache (IHS)	75	8	(1) Manip +STT = 38 (2) Sham + STT = 37	Post – Tx F: (1) –1.5 hr (2) –1.9 hr Post – Tx S: (1) No change (2) No change	Not mentioned	80
Total or average		286	6				68

(n) = sample size in each treatment group; (IHS) = inclusion based on criteria of the International Headache Society Classification [9];
Treatment types: ACUP = acupuncture, SHAM = sham placebo treatment, SPLINT = occlusal splint, CONTR = no-treatment control, P/T = physical therapy or physiotherapy, MEDS = medication, MANIP = chiropractic spinal manipulation, STT = soft tissue therapy, AMIT = amitriptyline, RELAX = relaxation therapy, TENS = transcutaneous electrical nerve stimulation, ELEC. STIM. = electrical stimulation, LO- = low level, BIOF = biofeedback, ATTEN. = attention control.
Outcomes: Tx = treatment; HA = headache; S = severity; F = frequency; mm = millimetres on a visual analogue scale; /wk = per week; wk = week(s); mo = month; (1), (2)... = treatment group; for 'severity': mod. = moderate; sev = severe; v. sev. = very severe
for 'frequency': sev = several; for 'global relief': hi= high, mod = moderate, min= minimal; improv. = improvement; ≥ = statistically significantly better than; = means: not statistically significantly better than.
Statistical significance: NS = not significant, * = 0.05, ** = 0.01, *** = 0.001

report a benefit of SMT. In these studies SMT is more effective than ice pack applications and soft tissue therapy in post-traumatic and cervicogenic headache. SMT appears to be as effective as amitriptyline in producing short-term benefit for TTH; however, there may be a longer-term benefit with SMT once the treatments are withdrawn. In one study, the addition of SMT to a group already receiving therapeutic levels of deep massage did not improve outcomes in TTH sufferers beyond the level obtained by a group receiving the massage and a placebo treatment. This study is the only one to report no additional benefit from SMT.

Electrotherapy studies

Four RCTs were obtained which investigated electrotherapy as the sole modality. Three studied transcutaneous electrical nerve stimulation (TENS) and one used a form of 'cranial electrotherapy'. The latter study and two of the TENS studies [43–45] were placebo-controlled, while the other study [46] compared TENS to relaxation therapy, biofeedback and a combination of all three treatments. The quality scores for these studies ranged from 39–61%, with an average score of 50%. Only one study achieved a rating that would qualify it as of 'high' quality [43]. The studies by Reich [46] and Solomon *et al.* [45] included both tension-type and migraine sufferers, while the studies by Airaksinen and Pontinen [44] and Solomon and Guglielmo [45] involved only tension-type headache. Airaksinen and Pontinen [44] investigated the short-term changes in pressure pain threshold at 'trigger points' in TTH sufferers (presumably as a measure of pain relief for concurrent headache), while the other three studies investigated the prophylactic benefit of a series or programme of treatments. A total of 507 tension headache subjects were included in these four studies (see Table 8.7).

At least one high quality RCT and two others of moderately high quality demonstrate that electrotherapy is more efficacious than placebo in the treatment of TTH. One moderately high quality study demonstrated that TENS is at least as effective as other cognitive/behavioural therapies in reducing headache activity, although patient variables

such as the duration of headache complaint and the number of treatments rendered have an impact on individual patient response.

Physiotherapy trials

Three RCTs were identified involving multi-modality physiotherapy treatment programmes. The quality scores for these trials ranged from 33–58% (low-to-moderately high quality). The study with the highest rating (Carlsson *et al.* [47]) compared physiotherapy treatment with acupuncture. In this trial, 'physiotherapy' consisted of a variety of patient-initiated modalities, including relaxation techniques, stretching, TENS and ice therapy, as well as education regarding muscle tension and how to control it 'autogenically'. Both treatments produced positive benefit in mood state and overall health function as well as in the intensity and frequency of headaches. Physiotherapy produced greater gains in mood state and in headache intensity.

In both other studies [48,49], the physiotherapy modalities employed included TENS, heat, massage and ultrasound therapy to the painful areas, trigger-point therapy, exercise therapies, biofeedback and education. In Jay *et al.*'s study [48] all subjects received amitriptyline medication. They reported that subjects receiving the additional physiotherapy treatments fared better than those receiving only the medication. Only the study by Marcus *et al.* [49] employed a control procedure consisting of education and 'skin-cooling' biofeedback. They reported that the combined physiotherapy group 'was more likely to experience significant headache relief' than the attention control group (72.7% *v* 28.6%, p<0.03).

In all three studies (see Table 8.8) various combinations of these 'physiotherapeutic' and 'cognitive/behavioural' therapies (as well as medications, in one study) were employed, making the determination of the effect of each of these components impossible. A total of 147 subjects were included in these three studies (two additional reports by Carlsson *et al.* [28,29] were on the same group of subjects and were excluded from this review).

The evidence from the three studies on TENS adds to the evidence of the studies reviewed above under 'electrotherapy'. There are no high quality studies to support the

Table 8.7 Evidence table for electrotherapy studies

Authors	Headache type	Sample size	Study duration	Treatment groups (n)	Results	Side-effects	Quality scores
Reich, 1989 [51]	Muscle contraction headache (Migraine also incl. but not analysed here)	331	at least 15 weeks Tx 36 months follow-up	(1) Relax (2) Tens (3) Biof (4) Comb	Post – Tx S: (At discharge) (1) –1.5/5 (2) –2.1/5 (3) –2.4/5*** (4) –2.1/5 Post – Tx F: (At discharge) (1) –20 hr (2) –22 hr (3) –30 hr*** (4) –22 hr	Not mentioned	44
Solomon et al., 1989 [48]	Tension headache	100	6–10 weeks	(1) Cranial Elec. stim = 50 (2) Sham = 50	Post – Tx S: (1) –2.1 (35%)* (2) –1.2 (18%) Global relief: (%) (1) (2) hi 12 4 mod 24 12 min 26 20 none 38 63 **	(1) 10.5% (2) 12.7% most frequent = irritation at electrode site	61
Airaksinen and Pontinen, 1992 [49]	Chronic tension headache	14 (self control)	1 week, 2 sessions	(1) Elec. Stim. = 14 (2) Sham = 14	Pre – post Pressure thresholds: (kgs) (1) pre = 2.83 (.16) post = 3.46 (.21)* (2) pre = 3.34 (.2) post = 3.48 (2.1)	Not mentioned	39
Solomon and Guglielmo, 1985 [50]	Migraine = 21 muscle contraction = 33 combined = 8	62	one treatment	(1) Active TENS = 18 (2) Lo-TENS = 18 (3) Sham = 22	Percent showing clinically significant improvement (Muscle contraction headache) (1) = 55% (2) and (3) = 10%	Not mentioned	56
Total or average		507					50

(n) = sample size in each treatment group; (IHS) = inclusion based on criteria of the International Headache Society Classification [9];

Treatment types: ACUP = acupuncture, SHAM = sham placebo treatment, SPLINT = occlusal splint, CONTR = no-treatment control, P/T = physical therapy or physiotherapy, MEDS = medication, MANIP = chiropractic spinal manipulation, STT = soft tissue therapy, AMIT = amitriptyline, RELAX = relaxation therapy, TENS = transcutaneous electrical nerve stimulation, ELEC. STIM. = electrical stimulation, LO- = low level, BIOF = biofeedback, ATTEN. = attention control.

Outcomes: Tx = treatment; HA = headache; S = severity; F = frequency; mm = millimetres on a visual analogue scale; /wk = per week; wk = week(s); mo = month; (1), (2)... = treatment group; for 'severity': mod. = moderate; sev = severe; v. sev. = very severe

for 'frequency': sev = several; for 'global relief': hi= high, mod = moderate, min= minimal; improv. = improvement; ≥ = statistically significantly better than; = means: not statistically significantly better than.

Statistical significance: NS = not significant, * = 0.05, ** = 0.01, *** = 0.001

Table 8.8 Evidence table for physiotherapy studies

Authors	Headache type	Sample size	Study duration	Treatment groups (n)	Results	Side-effects	Quality scores
Carlsson et al., 1990 [33]	Chronic tension headache	62	60–90 days	(1) P/T = 29 (2) Acup = 23	Post – Tx F: (1) reduced, P<0.001 (2) reduced, P<0.01 Post – Tx S: (1) –25 mm @ 4–9 weeks +1 mm @7–12 months *** (2) –1 mm @ 4–9 weeks +12 mm @ 7–12 months	Not mentioned	58
Marcus et al., 1995 [54]	Migraine = 36% tension = 28% combined 36% (IHS)	25	60 days	(1) P/T +Biof = 11 (2) Atten control = 14	Post – TX F: (1) –8.3 days (2) –2.7 days (sig. ?) Post – Tx S: (1) –88.2% (2) –32.7% Subjects with significant change: (1) 73%* (2) 27%	Not mentioned	55
Jay et al., 1988 [53]	Chronic muscle contraction headache	60	90 days Tx 90 days follow-up	(1) Meds+ Biof (2) +P/T +tens (3) +P/T only	Post – Tx S: WK (1)(2)(3) 1 26 33 24 5 14 1.74 74.3 8 3 1 1.9 24 4 1 61.3 (2) and (3) > (1) (2) = (3)	Not mentioned	33
Total or average		147	80 days				47

(n) = sample size in each treatment group; (IHS) = inclusion based on criteria of the International Headache Society Classification [9];
Treatment types: ACUP = acupuncture, SHAM = sham placebo treatment, SPLINT = occlusal splint, CONTR = no-treatment control, P/T = physical therapy or physiotherapy, MEDS = medication, MANIP = chiropractic spinal manipulation, STT = soft tissue therapy, AMIT = amitriptyline, RELAX = relaxation therapy, TENS = transcutaneous electrical nerve stimulation, ELEC. STIM. = electrical stimulation, LO- = low level, BIOF = biofeedback, ATTEN. = attention control.
Outcomes: Tx = treatment; HA = headache; S = severity; F = frequency; mm = millimetres on a visual analogue scale; /wk = per week; wk = week(s); mo = month; (1), (2)... = treatment group; for 'severity': mod. = moderate; sev = severe; v. sev. = very severe
for 'frequency': sev = several; for 'global relief': hi= high, mod = moderate, min= minimal; improv. = improvement; ≥ = statistically significantly better than; = means: not statistically significantly better than.
Statistical significance: NS = not significant, * = 0.05, ** = 0.01, *** = 0.001.

efficacy of any other form of 'physiotherapy' in the treatment of TTH. There is some lower quality evidence supporting the effectiveness of combined physiotherapy regimens in treating TTH.

Massage trials

No RCT was found on the effects of manual massage as the primary therapy for non-migrainous headache. The study by Bove and

Nilsson [25] employed deep muscular massage to the trapezius and suboccipital region as a control treatment. Subjects in both groups received this therapy, while they were randomly allocated to *additionally* receive spinal manipulation or sham treatment. As such, before 1998, no randomized comparison of massage alone versus another treatment has been reported.

Since the completion of our systematic review, a new RCT of a type of massage for TTH was published. Hanten *et al.* [50] randomly divided 60 TTH sufferers into three equal groups: active craniosacral massage (whose putative purpose is to mobilize the temporo-parietal sutures), resting cervical stretch and resting control. The treatments were applied for 10 minutes during a subject's headache. Pain intensity and affect scores were significantly reduced in the active massage group compared with the two other groups. Unfortunately, in this design, both the treaters and the subjects were not blinded as to the nature of the therapy; therefore, a significant placebo effect of the treatment cannot be ruled out.

Homeopathy trials

Only one RCT was identified for homeopathic treatments of TTH. Walach *et al.* [51] reported on 98 subjects, about half of whom had chronic tension-type headaches and who were randomly allocated to receive either an individualized homeopathic remedy or an inert, indistinguishable placebo for 12 weeks. This trial achieved a quality score of 86%, which was the highest in our series, chiefly as a result of the high methodological rigour that included an appropriate sample size and double-blinded, placebo controls. This trial reported no difference between the two groups on any important clinical variables related to headache activity.

Other remedies

One clinical trial was retrieved which investigated the use of an analgesic/counter-irritant ointment ('Tiger Balm') in the treatment of tension headache [52]. This study achieved a high quality rating of 72%. Fifty-seven tension headache subjects were randomly allocated to receive Tiger Balm, topical placebo or parac-etamol (1000-mg dose) as a treatment for a concurrent headache. Both Tiger Balm and paracetamol produced greater pain relief than placebo in a single headache episode (p <0.05) for up to 3 hours, with no difference between these two.

One study was found on the effects of 'therapeutic touch' on TTH [53]; it achieved a quality score of 47%. The therapeutic benefit is purported to derive from the 'therapeutic intent' of the therapist. No manual contact is applied in this therapy. This trial involved the application of either true or 'placebo' therapeutic touch to 60 randomly allocated tension headache subjects who were experiencing a headache concurrently. Subjects in the 'experimental group' obtained twice as much pain relief as those in the control group immediately and 4 hours after the 5-minute intervention.

Methodological deficiencies

Table 8.9 presents the results of the quality ratings per item of the rating checklist, based upon agreement between raters for *no* or *don't know*. Those items scoring higher than 30% represent critical deficiencies in this body of studies, most of which relate to internal validity.

DISCUSSION

CAM therapies for tension-type and cervicogenic headache appear to operate within several intersecting theoretical models. The more general of these involves the amelioration of pain states by activation of putative endogenous anti-nociceptive processes [54–56]. The mechanism by which these therapies may work could be described as 'systemic', and could include acupuncture and homeopathy, as well as some of the relaxation techniques employed within 'physiotherapy'. These latter therapies are consistent with cognitive and behavioural therapies that have demonstrated effectiveness [14,16,17,57].

A second mechanism appears to involve treatments targeted to the cervical spine or cranial muscles as putative sources of headache pain. The notion that headache pain may arise from the cervical spine is generally

Table 8.9 Percentage of trials with deficiencies (based on reviewer agreement) (modified from van Tulder *et al.* [26])

Item	Percentage of trials
Eligibility criteria specified	0
Random allocation	4
Groups similar at baseline	25
Interventions explicitly described	4
Provider blinded	50
Co-interventions described and limited	29
Compliance monitored	25
Patient blinded	24
Assessor blinded	8
Outcome measures relevant	4
Adverse effects monitored	33
Drop-out rate described and acceptable	25
Short-term follow-up	0
Long-term follow-up	42
Timing of outcome assessments	4
Sample size described	4
Intention-to-treat	58
Point estimates and variability	8

well accepted today, based upon the work of Kerr [58], Sjaastad and colleagues [6,7] and Bogduk and colleagues [59–63]. This work has contributed to acceptance of a category of headache known as 'cervicogenic' [5)] The degree to which problems in the cervical spine may contribute to tension-type headache is still unresolved, from both theoretical and nosological perspectives. Cervical musculo-ligamentous dysfunction has been demonstrated in tension-type headache sufferers [63]. Despite the controversy, spinal manipulation, mobilization, massage, electrotherapy and other 'physiotherapeutic' procedures such as exercise and postural education appear to target the soft tissues of the cervical spine and the cranio-cervical junction which may be producing referred head pain.

The other regional mechanism involves therapies directed to the cranial area, including electrotherapy to cranial skin and muscles as well as topical creams applied to the cranial skin whose purpose is to reduce local pain and muscle spasm. Another putative mechanism involves mobilization of the cranial bones as in craniosacral therapy.

Of these latter mechanisms, the first two may be described as 'local' and appear to involve either the amelioration of possible referred cranial pain from cervical sources or the reduction of local cranial pain by counterirritation. As well, these therapies might theoretically exert a relaxant effect on local musculature. Craniosacral therapy is controversial in that its exact mechanism is uncertain. Despite the professed intention of 'mobilizing cranial bones', this therapy may exert a relaxant effect on cranial muscles.

These mechanisms are described for the sake of providing a theoretical basis for CATs. The reader is referred to primary sources for more complete descriptions of the proposed theoretical mechanisms, and any corroborating evidence, underlying these therapies.

The findings of our review demonstrate that randomized clinical trials of CAM therapies for non-migrainous headache do exist, and that some of them have been conducted and reported at a sufficiently high level of quality. There are some who claim that it is not possible to investigate the benefit of CAM therapies with RCTs, in that, in requiring an appropriate level of standardization and methodological rigour, compromises to the treatment context which may invalidate the results obtained are created [15]. While this may be true to some extent, it would appear that this is not an absolute circumstance. In fact, several of the trials have successfully incorporated sham/placebo treatments in order to investigate the efficacy of the primary treatment.

It has also been shown that investigators in these areas can develop well-designed, high-quality studies and recruit appropriately large samples of subjects interested in participating. As this development evolves, the database of outcomes for at least some of these treatment approaches should become large enough to conduct meta-analyses so that more robust evidence-based decisions can be made by practitioners.

It is noteworthy that one therapy, electrotherapy to cranial muscles, would appear to have sufficient strength of evidence to support its use in treating TTH. Additionally, for another therapy, homeopathy, there is at least one high quality trial whose results might recommend against its use in TTH on the basis that is was found to be no better than placebo. For the other therapeutic modalities, the evidence base either contains too few trials or contains trials resulting in contradictory findings that preclude any definitive summary.

The methodological deficiencies cited in Table 8.9 indicate the areas where future clinical trials should be improved. Careful selection of headache subjects according to explicit inclusion and exclusion criteria following the IHS classification guidelines [5] should be employed. Provider and subject blinding may be difficult to achieve in studies of CAM treatments, but every effort should be made to blind the treatment allocation from all parties not directly involved in the treatment, particularly the assessors. The issue of long-term follow-up must be dealt with in future trials in order to establish the true value of these treatments to society at large and their impact on the healthcare system.

CONCLUSION

Twenty-five published randomized controlled trials of acupuncture, spinal manipulative therapy, electrotherapy, physiotherapy, massage, homeopathy and 'other therapies' for TTH and CH have been reviewed in this chapter.

Interpretation of the evidence reviewed here should be done with caution since it is based solely on the RCT literature. Evidence ratings that utilized more levels of evidence may have yielded different results, but we were interested in determining evidence ratings based on the 'gold standard' of the randomized controlled trial. Pooling of trial data would be the most desirable representation of the evidence; however, the small number of trials in each category, as well as the variability in outcome measures in the trials precluded this type of analysis at present.

Quality issues that require attention in further trials include: similar groups at baseline, description of co-interventions, compliance monitoring, subject blinding (where possible), monitoring of adverse effects, describing dropouts, collecting long-term follow-up, and using intention-to-treat analysis.

REFERENCES

1. Schwartz BS, Stewart WF, Simon D, Lipton RB. Epidemiology of tension-type headache. *JAMA* 1998;**279**:381–383.
2. Rasmussen BK. Epidemiology of headache. *Cephalalgia* 1995;**15**:45–68.
3. Pryse-Phillips W, Findlay H, Tugwell P, Edmeads J, *et al*. A Canadian population survey on the clinical, epidemiologic and societal impact of migraine and tension-type headache. *Can J Neurol Sci* 1992;**19**:333–339.
4. Edmeads J, Findlay H, Tugwell P, Pryse-Phillips W, *et al*. Impact of migraine and tension-type headache on life-style, consulting behaviour, and medication use: a Canadian population survey. *Can J Neurol Sci* 1193;**20**131–137.
5. Classification and Diagnostic Criteria for Headache Disorders, Cranial Neuralgias and Facial Pain. 1st edn. International Headache Society. *Cephalalgia* 1988;**8**(Suppl. 7).
6. Sjaastad O, Fredrickson TA, Stolt-Neilsen A. Cervicogenic headache, C2 rhizopathy and occipital neuralgia: a connection. *Cephalalgia* 1986;**6**:189–195.
7. Sjaastad O, Saunte C, Hovdahl H, Breivek H, *et al*. Cervicogenic headache: an hypothesis. *Cephalalgia* 1983;**3**:249–256.
8. Vernon HT. Spinal manipulation and headaches: an update. *Top Clin Chiro* 1995;**2**:34–46.
9. Vernon HT. Spinal manipulation and headaches of cervical origin: a review of literature and presentation of cases. *J Man Med* 1991;**6**:73–79.
10. Nilsson N. The prevalence of cervicogenic headache in a random population sample of 20–59 year olds. *Spine* 1995;**20**:1884–1888.
11. Pryse-Phillips WEM, Dodick DW, Edmeads JG, Gawel MJ, *et al*. Guidelines for the nonpharmacologic management of migraine in clinical practice. *Can Med Assoc J* 1998;**159**:47–54.
12. Jadad AR, McQuay HJ. Meta-analyses to evaluate analgesic interventions: a systematic qualitative review of their methodology. *J Clin Epidemiol* 1996;**49**:235–243.
13. Bogaards MC, ter Kuile MM. Treatment of recurrent tension headache: a meta-analytic review. *Clin J Pain* 1994;**10**:174–190.
14. Haddock CK, Rowan AB, Andrasik F, Wilson PG, *et al*. Home-based behavioral treatments for chronic benign headache: a meta-analysis of controlled trials. *Cephalalgia* 1997;**17**:113–118.
15. Whitmarsh T. Evidence in complementary and alternative therapies: lessons form clinical trials of homeopathy in heachache. *J Alt Comp Med* 1997;**3**:307–310.
16. Penzien DB, Rains JC, Holroyd KA. A review of alternative behavioral treatments for headache. *Mississippi Psychol* 1992;**17**:8–9.

17. Penzien DB, Holroyd KA. The behavioral treatment of migraine: a meta-analytic review of the literature. *Diss Abs Int* 1987;**47**(DA8629941)
18. Eisenberg DM, Kessler RC, Foster C, Norlock FE, *et al.* Unconventional medicine in the United States. *N Engl J Med* 1993;**328**:246–282.
19. Waalen DP, White TP, Waalen JK. Demographic and clinical characteristics of chiropractic patients: a five year study of patients treated at the Canadian Memorial Chiropractic College. *J Can Chiro Assoc* 1994;**38**:75–82.
20. Coulter ID, Hurwitz EL, Adams AH, *et al. The Appropriateness of Manipulation and Mobilization of the Cervical Spine*, Santa Monica, CA: RAND, 1996.
21. van Tulder MW, Koes BW, Bouter LM. Conservative treatment of acute and chronic non-specific low back pain. *Spine* 1997;**22**:2128–2156.
22. Chalmers TC, Smith H, Blackburn B, Silverman B, *et al.* A method of assessing the quality of a randomized control trial. *Contr Clin Trials* 1981;**2**:31–49.
23. Moher D, Pham B, Jones A, Cook D, *et al.* Does quality of reports of randomised trials affect estimates of intervention efficacy reported in meta-analyses? *Lancet* 1998;**352**:609–613.
24. White AR, Eddleston C, Hardie R, Resch KL, *et al.* A pilot study of acupuncture for tension headache, using a novel placebo. *Acup Med* 1996;**14**:11–15.
25. Bove G, Nilsson N. Spinal manipulation in the treatment of episodic tension-type headache: a randomized controlled trial. *JAMA* 1998;**280**:1576–1579.
26. Nappi G, Facchinetti F, Bono G, Micieli G, *et al.* Plasma opioid levels in post-traumatic chronic headache and trigeminal neuralgia: maintained response to acupuncture. *Headache* 1982;**276**:279
27. Facchinetti F, Nappi G, Savoldi F, Genazzani AR. Primary headaches: reduced circulating beta-lipotropin and beta-endorphin levels and impaired reactivity to acupuncture. *Cephalalgia* 1999;**1**:195–201.
28. Carlsson J, Fahlcrantz A, Augustinsson L. Muscle tenderness in tension headache treated with acupuncture or physiotherapy. *Cephalalgia* 1990;**10**:131–141.
29. Carlsson J, Rosenhall U. Oculomotor disturbances in patients with tension headache treated with acupuncture or physiotherapy. *Cephalalgia* 1990;**10**:123–129.
30. Gobel H, Schmidt G, Soyka D. Effect of peppermint and eucalyptus oil preparations on neurophysiological and experimental algesimetric headache parameters. *Cephalalgia* 1994;**14**:228–234.
31. Nilsson N. A randomized controlled trial of the effect of spinal manipulation in the treatment of cervicogenic headache. *J Manip Physiol Ther* 1995;**18**:435–440.
32. Nilsson N, Christensen HW, Hartvigsen J. The effect of spinal manipulation in the treatment of cervicogenic headache. *J Manip Physiol Ther* 1997;**20**:326–330.
33. Jensen OK, Nielsen FF, Vosmar L. An open study comparing manual therapy with the use of cold packs in the treatment of post-traumatic headache. *Cephalalgia* 1990;**10**:241–250.
34. Borglum-Jensen L, Melsen B, Borglum-Jensen S. Effect of acupuncture on headache measured by reduction in number of attacks and use of drugs. *Scand J Dent Res* 1979;**87**:373–380.
35. Tavola T, Gala C, Conte G, Invernizzi G. Traditional Chinese acupuncture in tension-type headache: a controlled study. *Pain* 1992;**48**:325–329.
36. Ahonen E, Mahlmaki S, Partenen J, Riekkenen P, *et al.* Effectiveness of acupuncture and physiotherapy on myogenic headache: a comparative study. *Acup Electro-Ther* 1984;**9**:141–150.
37. Carlsson J, Wedel A, Carlsson GE, Blomstrand C. Tension headache and signs and symptoms of craniomandibular disorders treated with acupuncture or physiotherapy. *Pain Clin* 1990;**3**:229–238.
38. Loh L, Nathan PW, Scott GD, Zilkha KJ. Acupuncture versus medical treatment for migraine and muscle tension headaches. *J Neurol Neurosurg Psychiatry* 1984;**47**:333–337.
39. Hansen PE, Hansen JH. Acupuncture treatment of chronic tension headache – a controlled cross-over trial. *Cephalalgia* 1985;**5**:137–142.
40. Johansson A, Wenneberg B, Wagerten C, Haraldson T. Acupuncture in treatment of facial muscular pain. *Acta Odontol Scand* 1991;**49**:153–158.
41. Hoyt WH, Shaffer F, Bard DA, Benesler JS, *et al.* Osteopathic manipulation in the treatment of muscle contraction headache. *J Am Osteop Assoc* 1979;**78**:322–325.
42. Boline PD, Kassak K, Bronfort G, Nelson C, *et al.* Spinal manipulation vs amitriptyline for the treatment of chronic tension-type headache: a randomized clinical trial. *J Manip Physiol Therap* 1995;**18**:148–154.
43. Solomon S, Elkind A, Freitag F, Gallagher RM, *et al.* Safety and effectiveness of cranial electrotherapy in the treatment of tension headache. *Headache* 1989;**29**:445–540.
44. Airaksinen O, Pontinen PJ. Effects of electrical stimulation of myofascial trigger points with tension headache. *Acup Electro-Ther* 1992;**17**:285–290.

45. Solomon S, Guglielmo KM. Treatment of headache by transcutaneous electrical stimulation. *Headache* 1999;**25**:12–15.
46. Reich BA. Non-invasive treatment of vascular and muscle contraction headache: a comparative longitudinal clinical study. *Headache* 1989;**29**:34–41.
47. Carlsson J, Augustinsson L, Blomstrand C, Sullivan M. Health status in patients with tension headache treated with acupuncture or physiotherapy. *Headache* 1990;**30**:593–599.
48. Jay GW, Brunson J, Branson SJ. The effectiveness of physical therapy in the treatment of chronic daily headaches. *Headache* 1989;**29**:156–162.
49. Marcus DA, Scharff L, Turk DC. Nonparmacological management of headaches during pregnancy. *Psyshosom Med* 1995;**57**:527–535.
50. Hanten WP, Olson SL, Hodson JL, Imler VL, *et al.* The effectiveness of CV-4 and resting position techniques on subjects with tension-type headaches. *J Man Manip Ther* 1999;**7**:64–70.
51. Walach H, Haeusler W, Lowes T, Mussbach D, *et al.* Classical homeopathic treatment of chronic headaches. *Cephalalgia* 1997;**17**:119–126.
52. Schattner P, Randerson D. Tiger Balm as a treatment of tension headache: a clinical trial in general practice. *Aust Fam Phys* 1996;**25**:216–222.
53. Keller E, Bzdek VM. Effects of therapeutic touch on tension headache pain. *Nurs Res* 1986;**35**:101–106.
54. Gillette RG. Gatterman MI (eds.). *Foundations of Chiropractic: Subluxation. Spinal cord mechanisms of referred pain and neuroplasticity*, St Louis: Mosby Yearbook, 1995.
55. Sandoz R. The physical mechanisms and effect of spinal adjustments. *Ann Swiss Chiro Assoc* 1976;**6**:91–141.
56. Vernon HT, Dhami MSI, Howley TP, Annett R. Spinal manipulation and beta-endorphin: a study of the effect of a spinal manipulation on plasma beta-endorphin levels in normal males. *J Manip Physiol Ther* 1986;**9**:115–123.
57. Blanchard EB, Andrassik F, Ahles TA, Teders ST, *et al.* Migraine and tension headache: a meta-analytic review. *Behav Ther* 1980; **11**:613–631.
57. Kerr FW. Structural relation of the trigeminal spinal tract to upper cervical roots and the solitary nucleus in the cat. *Exp Neurol* 1961;**4**:134–148.
58. Bogduk N, Marsland A. On the concept of third occipital headache. *J Neurol Neurosurg Psychiatryy* 1986;**49**:775–780.
59. Bogduk N. Cervical causes of headache and dizziness. In *Modern Manual Therapy of the Vertebral Column* (ed. GP Grieve), Edinburgh: Churchill Livingstone, pp. 289–302, 1986.
60. Bogduk N, Marsland A. The cervical zygapophysial joints as a source of neck pain. *Spine* 1988;**13**:610–617.
61. Barnsley L, Lord S, Wallis BJ, Bogduk N. The prevalence of chronic cervical joint pain after whiplash. *Spine* 1995;**20**:20–26.
62. Lord SM, Barnsley L, Wallis BJ, Bogduk N. Third occipital nerve headache: a prevalence study. *J Neurol Neurosurg Psychiatryy* 1994;**57**:1187–1190.
63. Vernon HT, Steiman I, Hagino C. Cervicogenic dysfunction in muscle contraction and migraine headache: a descriptive study. *J Manip Physiol Ther* 1992;**15**:418–429.

Chapter 9

Cranio-cervical pain: Medical management

P. J. Rothbart and G. D. Gale

INCIDENCE OF CHRONIC HEADACHE

Chronic headache is defined as a headache occurring more than 15 days a month for 6 months. It occurs in about 5% of the population.

DEFINITION OF CERVICOGENIC HEADACHE

This is a particular kind of headache which was first described as cervicogenic [1] and this clinical description was used in the classification of chronic pain of the International Association for the Study of Pain (IASP) [2]. This described a clinical syndrome of moderate or moderately severe unilateral headache, which does not change sides, involving the whole hemicranium, usually starting in the neck or occipital region and eventually involving the forehead and temple areas, where the maximal pain is frequently located. It often begins intermittently and then becomes continuous. The pain may involve the infraorbital area and may be bilateral. It is commoner in women and often follows neck trauma. Cervicogenic headache may be precipitated by neck movements or by pressure on the occipital nerve.

A problem with this clinical definition was that the features of cervicogenic headache were very variable so that the North American Cervicogenic Headache Society proposed in

September 1995 [3] that it should be defined as referred pain perceived in any region of the head caused by a primary nociceptive source on the musculoskeletal tissues innervated by cervical nerves. Since 1983 many papers have investigated the relationship between neck injury and cervicogenic headache; the authors include Bogduk, Sjaastad, Blume, Gawel and Rothbart.

INCIDENCE OF CERVICOGENIC HEADACHE

This has been difficult to determine because of inconsistencies of the application of diagnostic criteria so that it may be misdiagnosed as tension-type headache or migraine. However, in our clinic we see about 600 new chronic headache patients a year and an estimated 80% of these are diagnosed as having cervicogenic headache clinically, many of whom go on to have it confirmed with diagnostic nerve blocks.

PHYSIOLOGY OF CERVICOGENIC HEADACHE

The muscles supporting the cervical vertebrae and attaching to the base of the skull, ligaments (including anterior and posterolongitudinal and alar ligaments) zygapophyseal joints and annulus fibrosis of the intervertebral discs are all well supplied with sensory cervical nerves the pathways of which have been described by Bogduk [4–7].

In the upper neck these nerves travel via the C1 to C4 nerves to the dorsal horn at the appropriate level. Nerve impulses are then transmitted to the ipsilateral and contralateral spinal thalamic tracts. The impulse is then passed through the thalamus to the cortex and this is the usual model of how nociceptive pain is perceived.

HOW NECK PAIN IS PERCEIVED AS HEADACHE

The trigeminal or fifth cranial nerve is responsible for sensory innervation of the face and the head, excluding the occipital area. Its sensory afferent neurones enter the brainstem to terminate by synapsing in the trigeminal nucleus which is also known as the trigeminocervical ganglion which extends caudally through the brainstem and becomes contiguous with the dorsal columns down to about the C3 level.

The three upper cervical nerves enter the dorsal columns and synapse in the trigeminocervical ganglion. From these, secondary neurons carry the impulses centrally to the thalamus and cortex but the brain is unable to differentiate the impulses arising in the cervical region from those arising in the head and face region, so cervical pain is felt as a referred pain in the head and face. It appears that the brain has a preference for interpreting pain as arising in the head and face rather than the neck where the impulses are actually generated.

CLINICAL PRESENTATION OF CERVICOGENIC HEADACHE

Symptomatology may be very varied in cervicogenic headache but frequent features are as quoted above for its clinical definition. Common features are that it becomes severe and continuous, always worse on the same side of the head, but may be on both sides and is related to neck movements. Increased headache on flexion suggests a pain generator in the discs and on extension in the zygapophyseal joints (as they are pressed together) or by compression by lateral flexion to the affected side. Bogduk has shown that a common cause of cervicogenic headache is zygapophyseal joint injury [6].

However, the clinical diagnosis of cervicogenic headache can present problems because its symptomatology may resemble that of migraine, tension-type headache or even cluster headache which upsets the classification of these conditions according to the International Headache Society's (IHS) classification of these conditions [8].

Although migraine is now considered to arise from brain activity which then stimulates intracranial structures such as meninges innervated by the trigeminal nerve, it may also arise in a post-traumatic form from injured cervical structures. In these cases treatment of the neck injury may ease the migraine by reducing its severity below the threshold for pain.

REGARDING NECK INJURY

With the advent of the motor age, the velocity of collisions has increased and the structure of the human cervical spine predisposes it to injury when excessive acceleration/deceleration forces are applied to the head. This contrasts with the case of the howler monkey of South America who has evolved a very strong cervical spine where animals have been seen to sustain an 80-foot fall and then get up and walk away, apparently uninjured.

Should X-rays of the neck be performed, it is recommended that to obtain maximal information erect lateral, oblique and flexion and extension views should be obtained. Neck injuries not severe enough to cause fractures often cause or exacerbate biomechanical disorder of the spine so that the gravitational line and the flexion and extension of individual joints should be noted. The gravitational line runs vertically through the odontoid and lies over the body of the seventh cervical vertebra normally. When the neck is injured, anterior carriage of the head often results, so that this can be measured by the horizontal distance between the gravitational line and the anterior superior part of the body of the seventh cervical vertebra in the erect lateral X-ray view. Other features of injury often are loss of the normal cervical lordosis resulting in alordosis or even kyphosis and absent flexion or extension of joints from the occiput to C7 should be noted.

Table 9.1 Symptoms often seen in the post-traumatic syndrome

Headaches
Tiredness
Light-headedness
Difficulty with concentration
Dizziness
Memory difficulties
Trouble expressing thoughts
Blurring of vision
Double vision
Bothered by bright lights
Ringing in the ears
Hearing loss
Balance difficulties
Staggering
Change in handwriting
Dropping things
Lack of ambition
Loss of interest in sex
Depression
Clumsiness
Irritability
Fear or anxiety associated with the accident such as driving a car
Fear of leaving the house
Other unusual fears
Sleep disturbance
    Trouble falling asleep
    Trouble staying asleep
    Early rising in the morning
    Need for too much sleep
Bad dreams, usually about accidents of life-threatening experiences
Appetite change
Craving for junk food
Weight change
    Loss
Seizures

Score: Total positive responses related out of 28

REGARDING DIAGNOSIS OF CERVICOGENIC HEADACHE, NECK AND ASSOCIATED INJURIES

This involves history, examination and investigations. The time of onset of the headache and its characteristics should be noted and the relationship with neck trauma. In 'whiplash' cases there may be injuries to structures attached but not fixed to the cranium.

REGARDING TMJ INJURY AND POST-TRAUMATIC SYNDROME

These are the jaw and the brain. Enquiry should therefore be made about potential TMJ problems regarding TMJ pain, clicking, locking and mouth opening. The identification of minor brain injury after whiplash has been a controversial area because of the lack of 'objective' evidence, but its presence as identified by a constellation of symptomatology has become increasingly recognized as post-traumatic syndrome in recent years [9,10]. The constellation of symptoms suggesting post-traumatic syndrome are shown in Table 9.1 [11].

REGARDING HEADACHE

Headache characteristics may help to differentiate between different aetiologies. A headache that is worse on neck movements or occipital pressure suggests cervicogenic origin. The effect of posture on headache may be important. If it is worse on lying down, this suggests intracranial aetiology such as meningitis in the acute headache. If it is worse on standing up, this may suggest low CSF pressure headache. Some cervicogenic headaches become worse on lying down and this is probably due to stressing of neck mechanics; it often results in patients waking in pain at night or in the early morning. For similar biomechanical reasons, chiropractic adjustments may make cervicogenic headache better or sometimes worse.

PHYSICAL EXAMINATION OF THE PATIENT WITH CERVICOGENIC HEADACHE AND SPINAL PAIN

This should be comprehensive at the first visit.

Musculoskeletal system

Gait and posture should be observed. Patients with musculoskeletal pain often change position frequently; this is known as antalgic behaviour. In examining standing posture, the observer should stand behind the patient and look for anterior carriage of the head, prominence of the T1–T2 spines, symmetry of the shoulders and hips and the characteristics of the thoracic kyphosis and the lumbar lordosis. Palpation should be used to determine tenderness and muscle spasm in the back. Tenderness should be looked for in the sacroiliac joints and the joints of the shoulder girdle.

With the patient sitting, the neck should be examined, noting anterior carriage of the head and shoulder asymmetry. Neck range of movements should be examined. Decreased flexion suggests disc problems and decreased extension or neck pain on extension suggests zygapophyseal joint injury or arthritis.

Neck palpation may detect early muscle spasm or later wasting either of which may occur after neck injuries. Paracervical and scalene muscles are often swollen and tender in cervicogenic headache cases. The greater and lesser occipital nerves should be palpated and this may stimulate headache going through to the eye, forehead and temple in some cases of cervicogenic headache. Palpation should then be applied over the zygapophyseal joints which are usually accessible at C2–7 bilaterally and their degree of tenderness assessed. A good correlation between cervical tenderness and positive diagnostic blocks has been noted but this observation has only been properly documented in one paper [12].

A full neurological examination should be performed. Should signs of impairment be found it may suggest intracranial pathology. A whiplash patient seen recently had unilateral diminished hearing and on computed tomography (CT) of the brain, was found to have a large acoustic neuroma. Cardiovascular, respiratory and gastrointestinal examination should also be performed and unexpected findings sometimes occur, notably of the blood pressure and the liver.

OTHER INVESTIGATIONS

In the brain

The CT or magnetic resonance imaging (MRI) or X-rays of the skull should be ordered if intracranial pathology is suspected.

In the neck

X-rays are useful to show disorder of biomechanics, principally anterior carriage of the head, alordosis and aberrant kinematics as described earlier. Apart from this, X-rays, CT, MRI and myelograms have limited value because they only show the shape of structures but do not relate pain to pathology. These tests may show degenerative disc disease but since this is often present in a symptomatic individual, it may not be the cause of cervicogenic headache. So pathology may be present but not the cause of the pain.

Tests are therefore required to relate pain to pathology. These are:

1. Diagnostic facet blocks at the zygapophyseal joints of the neck require the use of the X-ray imaging:

   This test makes use of the fact that the nerve supply of the zygapophyseal joints is highly localized. The cervical 2/3 joint is entirely supplied by a branch of the third cervical (occipital) nerve. The 3/4 cervical joint is supplied by a medial branch of the posterior primary ramus of the C3 nerve and a branch from the C4 nerve. Similarly the lower cervical joints are supplied by branches from the cervical nerves above and below the joints.

   Local anaesthetic is used to block these nerves in such a small volume (0.5 ml) that it remains in the location of the nerves. If this results in abolition of the neck pain or headache for 1 hour or more, then it is inferred that the pain generator was in the joint or joints that were blocked. To exclude false positives, the blocks are performed twice, using lignocaine and bupivacaine and are only accepted as positive if the pain relief is longer with bupivacaine. Barnsley found in whiplash victims using this double-blind differential local anaesthetic block a 54% prevalence of symptomatic joints. This is therefore the commonest source of neck and head pain in whiplash patients.

2. The C2 nerve diagnostic block.

   Under X-ray control with the patient prone, a long needle is placed using a posterior approach close to the atlanto-occipital joint, which is in close proximity to the C2 nerve and 0.5 ml of local anaesthetic is injected there. If this relieves pain, it is inferred that the pain generator is in the cervical two-nerve distribution [13].

3. Occipital nerve blocks.

   The occipital nerve is the main sensory part of the C2 nerve and supplies the back of the head. Its entry at the dorsal horn of the spinal cord is an important relay area for pain impulses. If occipital nerve blocks relieve the patient's headache, it is suggestive of cervicogenic headache.

4. Provocative and relieving discograms:

   As discussed above, X-rays, CTs and MRIs are not helpful in determining if disc injury is the cause of cervicogenic headache. Schellhas has shown that provocative discograms were a better prediction of discogenic pain than the MRI [14].

   The provocative discogram involves injecting contrast medium into the suspected disc and a positive result is indicated by the stimulation of pain concordant in location with the patient's original pain. The pain is then relieved by injecting a small amount of local anaesthetic if the relieving test is positive.

TREATMENT OF CERVICOGENIC HEADACHE AND NECK PAIN

Since about 90% of whiplash patients recover in the first year, it may not matter greatly what treatment they receive because they are destined to recover anyway. However, they usually receive 'rehabilitation' with stretching and exercise.

It is for the other 10% of patients with persistent pain that therapy should be given. Among the possible options are:

1. If cervical diagnostic blocks are positive, then surgical facet intervention or neurotomy may be performed. The results are quoted as being 60–80% successful. The pain sometimes returns in 9 months if the nerves regenerate but the procedure may then be repeated.

2. If the C2 nerve diagnostic block is positive, there are two options:
   i. C2 nerve ganglionectomy which is more successful when the headache is a post-traumatic occipital lancinating type of pain [15].
   ii. Occipital denaturation, which is an operation to burn small nerves in the occipital region with about 50 radiofrequency lesions on the affected side but does not destroy the greater occipital nerve because this causes a wide area of numbness but may still be painful. Occipital denaturation was developed by Dr Horst Blume who has reported a good success rate with it [16,17].

3. If provocative discograms are positive this indicates discogenic pain. In the past, discotomy and fusion have been performed for this, but results have often proved unsatisfactory, particularly when more than one disc is involved because the headache may not be relieved or returns shortly thereafter. Moreover, the surgery is traumatic and not without risk.

So a new procedure has been developed. Unfortunately, this can only be used for thermocoagulation of the nucleus polposus of lumbar discs. This is because the cervical disc has a different anatomy from the lumbar disc and does not appear to have a nucleus polposus. Some physicians, however, have thermocoagulated the small fibres on the outside of the posterior aspect of the disc near the nerve root. However, this is still experimental [18].

When surgery is not an option, pain palliation should be considered.

1. *Medication.* Drugs include antidepressants, non-steroidal anti-inflammatory drugs, aspirin derivatives, antiepileptic drugs and opioids.

   Among antidepressant drugs the older drugs such as amitriptyline are more effective and can be started at a dose of 10 mg at night and then increased as tolerated if necessary up to 100 or 150 mg. It often reduces pain and may also reduce depression.

   Opioids are now widely used and the slow release preparations are preferred such as MS Contin because they are less likely to lead to addictive behaviour. The prescribing physician has to carefully monitor the drug use to minimize the potential for abuse or diversion of these drugs.

2. The use of *palliative nerve blocks* has been shown to improve the quality of life and the activities of daily living and reduce depression in patients with severe cervicogenic headache even though the pain relief may only be obtained for 1–3 days. When

blocks are performed the beneficial effects on the patient's life last much longer than the actual period of pain relief [19–22].

3. *Cognitive therapy* has a place in the management of cervicogenic headaches and neck pain. This helps the patient to manage his pain because not all pain can be relieved. Methods include cognitive therapy pain management, meditation, hypnosis and biofeedback.

4. *Physical therapy* should be used in conjunction with the other methods of pain control. Chiropractic manipulation has been found to be very helpful in some patients but can cause increased pain in others. Heat, cold and massage are very safe and often helpful, but cervical traction has had variable results and has sometimes increased neck pain.

REFERENCES

1. Sjaastad O, Saunte C. Unilaterality of headache. Hauge's studies revisited. *Cephalalgia* 1983; **3**:201–205.
2. Merskey H, Bogduk N (eds.). *Classification of Pain: Descriptions of Chronic Pain Syndromes and Definitions of Pain Terms*, 2nd edn, Seattle: International Association for the Study of Pain, p. 64, 1994.
3. Personal communication with Bogduk N.
4. Bogduk N. The clinical anatomy of the cervical dorsal rami. *Spine* 1982;**7**:319–330.
5. Bogduk N. Headache and the cervical spine. An editorial. *Cephalalgia* 1984;**4**:7–8.
6. Bogduk N, Marsland A. The cervical zygapophyseal joints as a source of neck pain. *Spine* 1988;**13**:610–617.
7. Bogduk N. Windsor M, Inglis A. The innervation of the cervical intervertebral discs. *Spine* 1988;**13**:2–8.
8. Headache Classification Committee of the International Headache Society. Classification and Diagnostic Criteria for Headache Disorders, Cranial Neuralgias and Facial Pain, *Cephalalgia, An International Journal of Headache*, 1988;**8**(Suppl):7.
9. Sadwin A. Rothrock, Mandel S. Sadwin D. In: *O'Leary L. Post-Traumatic Syndrome in Minor Head Trauma* (eds. S Mandel, RT Sataloff, SR Shapiro), Berlin: Springer Verlag, pp. 142–158, 1993.
10. Young WB, Packard RC. Post-traumatic headache and post-traumatic syndrome. In *Headache* (eds. PJ Goadsby, SD Silberstein), Boston: Butterworth-Heinemann, Vol 15: 253–277, 1997.
11. Saper JR. *Post-Traumatic Headaches and Syndrome*. 1999 Syllabi on CT-ROM. American Academy of Neurology, 1999.
12. Jull G, Bogduk N, Marsland A. The accuracy of manual diagnosis for cervical zygapophyseal joint pain syndromes. *Med J Aust* 1988; **148**:233.
13. Bogduk N. Local anesthetic blocks of the second cervical ganglion: a technique with application to occipital headache. *Cephalalgia* 1981;**1**:41–50.
14. Schellhas KP, Smith MD, Cooper R, *et al.* Cervical discogenic pain, prospective correlation of magnetic resonance imaging and discography in asymptomatic subjects and pain sufferers and pain sufferers. *Spine* 1996;**21**(3).
15. Lozano AM, Vanderlinden G, Bachoo, R Rothbart. P Microsurgical C2 Ganglionectomy for chronic intractable occipital pain. *J Neurosurg* 1998;**89**:359–65.
16. Blume HG: Radiofrequency denaturation in occipital pain;results in 450 cases. *Appl Neurophysiol* 1982;**45**:543–548.
17. Blume HG, Atac M, Golnick J. Neurosurgical treatment of persistent occipital myalgia-neuralgia syndrome. In *Updating in Headache* (eds. V Pfaffenrath, PO Lundberg, O Sjaastad), Berlin, Heidelberg, New York: Springer, pp:24–52, 1985.
18. Personal communication with Blume HG.
19. Groenbaek E. Cervical anterolateral microsurgery for headache. In *Updating in Headache Headache* (eds. V Pfaffenrath, PO Lundberg ,O Sjaastad), Berlin Heidelberg New York: Springer, pp.17–23, 1985.
20. Caputi CA, Firetto V. Therapeutic blockade of greater occipital and supraorbital nerves in migraine patients. *Headache* 1997;**37**:174–179.
21. Bartschi-Rochaix W. Headaches of cervical origin. In *Handbook of Clinical Neurology* (eds. PJ Vinden, GW Bruyn), Vol 5, Chap 17. Amsterdam: North Holland Publishing, pp. 192–20, 1968.
22. Pilot study submitted for publication.

Chapter 10

Psychological aspects of head and neck pain

Jaan Reitav and Gregory Hamovitch

INTRODUCTION

This chapter will provide readers with an overview of developments in psychological approaches to head and neck pain. We will also introduce readers to a range of questionnaires that have been developed specifically for assessing the pain experiences of patients, and for evaluating the impact of pain treatments from the patient's perspective. Wherever we have found them, we include tests designed specifically for patients with head and neck pain, or which have norms for this group.

Pain is an area with a rich variety of questionnaires that can help in answering important clinical questions, and which are not restricted in this way. The authors will introduce the most useful of them and direct readers to where they can get more information should they want to acquire the tests, to use them in their practice settings, and to further develop their clinical understanding of these sometimes difficult patients.

This chapter is organized to review three different themes. Firstly, we review how psychological factors entered the mainstream of clinical management of pain patients, and then describe for other members of the multidisciplinary health team the general perspective that a broad biopsychosocial model provides to understanding these patients. Secondly, we review the contribution of psychological factors to the understanding of headache and whiplash injury. Much of the understanding of psychological factors in whiplash injury comes from research conducted by physicians and has been published in journals outside the psychological literature. For psychologists we bring together a diverse body of information on whiplash injury from the medical literature. Finally, we will review the most useful clinical psychometric tools for working with these patients to provide an understanding of when to use them, and of their main strengths and weaknesses. This should be of interest to all who work with patients with head and neck pain. For the purposes of this review, we will focus primarily on two types of head and neck pain: persistent benign headaches and whiplash-associated pain symptoms.

Nevertheless, it is instructive to consider that conditions like cancer are recognized to involve pain in almost half of patients early in the disease, and as many as three-quarters of patients by the latter stages [1]. There are guidelines for assessment and treatment for these patients, yet there continue to be barriers for effective management of these patients. Barriers to effective treatment include misconceptions about pain among both health professionals and patients, failure of physicians to employ standardized assessment techniques like formal assessment measures and, even, lack of knowledge among family members. Indeed, there is evidence that treating physicians routinely underestimate the amount of pain experienced by these patients, as well as having difficulty identifying quality-of-life issues, and both of these impact on the adequacy of treatment provided [1].

When dealing with clinical conditions that have little or no laboratory test results confirming their presence (like benign headache and whiplash injury), and with no standard guidelines for care, the tendency to overlook or minimize the pain symptoms is likely to be greater. Although no empirical study of these issues exists for patients with headache and whiplash injury, it is likely that it would advocate for better education, more formalized assessment procedures, and treatment that addresses the individual needs of each patient.

BIOPSYCHOSOCIAL MODEL OF PAIN

A number of reviews and articles have advanced the biopsychosocial model as the most appropriate context within which to understand chronic pain phenomena in general [2–4]. According to this model, all pain is a personal experience influenced by a combination of the physical pathology, the person's attention to it and its meaning, all of which are influenced by our previous learning history and by the responses of those around us. The biopsychosocial model views illness as the result of a complex interaction of biological, psychological and social variables. The focus of this broader model is therefore on all three classes of variables, in contrast with the biomedical model's emphasis on disease process (biological variables) alone.

While biomedical factors appear to initiate the report of pain in most cases, it appears that psychosocial and behavioural factors maintain or exacerbate pain levels and influence each individual pain patient's adjustment and disability. As Turk [3] states, 'the experience of pain is a complex amalgam maintained by an interdependent set of biomedical, psychosocial, and behavioural facts, whose relationships are not static but evolve and change over time. The various interacting factors that affect an individual with chronic pain suggest that the phenomenon is quite complex and requires a biopsychosocial perspective' (p. 24).

To illustrate the empirical evidence supporting this perspective, Turk and Okifuji [5] evaluated the contributions of physical, operant, cognitive and affective factors to individual differences in pain behaviours for fibromyalgia patients. Among the tests used were the Center for Epidemiologic Studies Depression Scale and the West Haven-Yale Multidimensional Pain Inventory (see: Instruments). Hierarchical regression analyses revealed that the physical, cognitive and affective factors were all significantly related to observed pain behaviours. Furthermore, this set of factors accounted for 53% of the variance in observed pain behaviour. The authors concluded that pain behaviours should be conceptualized as behavioural manifestation of pain based on a complex interaction of various psychological and physical factors.

As an alternative to the biomedical model, the biopsychosocial model emerged from Melzack and Wall's [6] proposal of a new theory to account for many perplexing clinical findings among pain patients. We will begin with a review of gate control theory, and then return to considering cognitive and social factors in chronic pain, as well as emotional states and the experience of pain. Although we have done this to highlight some key issues it is important to keep in mind that these phenomena occur together and interact with each other, and in that sense cannot be separated from each other. In fact cognitive, emotional, social and biological factors are so intertwined as to make separating them out illogical for understanding a given person's pain experience. Yet it is helpful to understand how each makes a unique contribution to the pain experience. As evident from the sections that follow, quality of life considerations are also intricately interwoven within the biopsychosocial model of pain.

Gate control theory

Pain research and clinical practice changed permanently 35 years ago after the publication of Melzack and Wall's [6] article proposing a 'gate control theory' of pain. This article ended an era of dichotomous thinking, in which physical and physiological events were split off from psychological phenomena. What Melzack and Wall proposed was that an organic process, the relay of pain signals at the dorsal horn, could be influenced by psychological processes. This was not because of psychological wish or conjecture, but because anatomy made it impossible to function otherwise. The theory also provided a testable hypothesis of how pain phenomena worked, and has led to the development of a more multidisciplinary approach to the treatment of pain.

Most important is Melzack and Wall's characterization of pain phenomena as 'a rich variety of experiences and responses' which are constantly evolving on the basis of physiological and psychological processes. As they put it, the pain experience represents the end product of 'an abstraction of information that is sequentially re-examined over long periods of time by the entire somesthetic system.' They took pain from the mechanistic world of exact and neurally fixed underlying connections and reflex arcs into the era of probabilistic modelling and of Heisenberg's principle, wherein conscious examination of a pain phenomenon is not possible without changing the underlying phenomenon itself.

Melzack and Wall postulated that function follows form, or that the pain experience is decided by converging influences: the intensity of the pain signal from the periphery and the descending signals, usually inhibiting, from the central cortex. What they found to be true in the dorsal horn is that incoming pain signals are routinely modified by signals coming from the cortex, including the conscious brain. This process of central modulation of physical signals has generated a great deal of research and has been updated and elaborated, but not refuted [7].

The dorsal horn was the first anatomical gate at which signals of emotion and thought, both of which are changing and 'non-physical', could be seen to have an impact on the visceral experience of pain. Over 30 years of research have not discredited their hypothesis; in fact we can now see the same potential for modulation built into the nociceptive system at many levels and with many different mechanisms of action [8]. It is also important to understand that this involvement of central neural processing can either increase or decrease the original pain signal from the periphery.

However, the fact that a gate exists for psychological signals to moderate the experience of pain is not proof that it is used, under what circumstances it is used, and whether it amplifies or inhibits the pain signal. What

Melzack and Wall outlined were new, and clinically relevant, possibilities but ones that would have to be demonstrated as relevant for a given pain patient. Since Melzack and Wall's work, it is difficult to argue that psychological processes can't influence pain experience. Establishing that they do influence the experience of a particular patient, or of a whole class of patients such as those with head and neck pain, must be established through empirical investigation.

Cognitive and social factors in chronic pain

Much of the psychological literature highlights the role of assessing and treating cognitive-behavioural phenomena. The behavioural approach emphasizes the need to study behaviour empirically and focuses not on abstract mental constructs, but on concrete behaviours and the stimuli in the environment surrounding these behaviours. Behavioural learning theorists argue that all learning is the result of connections between stimuli and responses. Cognitive-behavioural theorists acknowledge the role of behavioural factors as well, but emphasize the internal cognitive processes in learning and recognize the importance of internal events, such as thoughts and emotions, in the development and maintenance of pain and pain-related conditions.

The cognitive-behavioural approach is most commonly used by psychologists in understanding and working with pain patients, and includes considerations such as the individual's perception of control of pain, self-efficacy, catastrophizing coping skills and even optimism. Turk [9] concluded his review of the role of psychological factors in chronic pain with the following: 'In summary, patients come to treatment with diverse sets of attitudes, beliefs, expectancies, and coping resources, including social supports that will influence all aspects of their current circumstances, adaptations, and response to treatment. It would seem prudent to (a) attempt to identify pain patients' idiosyncratic beliefs, (b) address those beliefs that are inaccurate and potentially maladaptive, and (c) to match treatments to patients' biomedical and psychosocial differences (p.888).'

A more recent review of the low back pain literature [10] continues to remind us that the conceptualization of pain and its progression into chronic disability has evolved from unidimensional models to more integrative, biopsychosocial models that take into account the biological, psychosocial, social and economic factors that can contribute to the low back pain experience. These themes will be revisited in our discussion of whiplash injury.

Social factors that impact on a person's pain experience are also diverse [3]. They can include cultural and ethnic factors involved in how we are taught to communicate the experience of pain to others. They also include the fact that how other people respond to us while we are in pain can itself perpetuate our pain communications, or attenuate them. This can happen because those with whom we interact around these experiences can reinforce or punish our pain behaviour. They can therefore play an important part in helping the pain patient rehabilitate towards higher functioning, or to dissuade them from making every effort to increase their functionality.

Emotional states and the experience of pain

Emotional factors are involved in pain perception almost by definition. When the International Association for the Study of Pain (IASP) developed its taxonomy of pain, it endorsed a distinction be made between perception and sensation in pain evaluation [11]. They suggested that the term 'pain' be reserved for the perception of pain, and the term 'nociception' be used for describing the sensory stimuli capable of being perceived as pain.

Nevertheless, the roles of important affective determinants of pain, like frustration, anger and depression, are relatively underrepresented in the psychological literature on chronic pain. A refreshing contribution is the recent review of the affective dimensions of the pain experience by Price [12]. Price makes the cogent point that one cannot have a theory of the affective components of pain without first having an adequate model of affects generally. He goes on to review the recent theoretical developments in this area, and proposes that the affective responses of the pain patient can be characterized as occurring on two levels.

The first stage involves the spontaneous affective experiences of the individual. This comprises the moment-to-moment unpleasantness of pain, as well as other emotional feelings that pertain to the present or short-term future. Aside from the sensory input, psychological and physiological signals (such as general arousal, autonomic responses and focus of attention) will influence the pain's unpleasantness. Price proposed that the emotional state that accompanies the immediate unpleasantness of pain represents a synthesis of internal physiological activation, in relation to meanings of the pain and to the context of the pain.

Even the most immediate affective response can be 'powerfully and selectively modulated by... contextual factors such as the degree of threat present', and 'the perception of threat, either to one's body or consciousness or both, is common to all instances of pain-related affect.' In this context, he points out that the intensity of immediate pain unpleasantness *could* be modulated by cognitive factors, such as expectation. It is the particular mixture of desires associated with coping, and expectations related to these desires, that partly co-determine the magnitude and quality of immediate pain unpleasantness. In this context the person's sense of self-efficacy will predict their pain tolerance, but have no effect on their pain perception.

Price goes on to define a second stage of pain affect. This second stage of pain related affect is based on 'more elaborate reflection and relates to memories and imagination about the implications of having pain, such as the way pain may interfere with different aspects of one's life, the difficulty of enduring pain over time, and concern for the long term consequences.' This stage of pain is equated with the trait part of the state-trait continuum. As this component relates to how the pain affects one's long-term future, and time is required for the development of more complex meanings and future implications, this aspect of pain affect is not expected to be seen in the immediate period after injury. Price goes on to define three key components of this longer-term affective response. The first is the increasing realization that pain will continue to interrupt one's ability to function. The second is that pain is now a constant burden, and one that will have to be endured for a long time. The third is that the persistent pain means that something permanently harmful has happened, or could happen.

Price suggests that personality traits as well as effects of age and cultural factors can be understood in the context of the second stage of pain affect. In this regard, the prominent negative effects of many chronic pain patients reflect their selective focusing on negative outcomes, feeling very uncertain about influencing their circumstances, and feeling trapped by pain for an interminable time. Although every chronic pain patient can feel frustration, anxiety, depression and anger, the longer-term prevalent feelings experienced by a particular patient will depend on their particular way of understanding themselves, their pain and their future.

PSYCHOLOGICAL FACTORS AND HEADACHE

The relevance of psychological factors in headache

Numerous reviews of clinical management across the past decade have emphasized that psychological factors often have a significant role in the genesis and maintenance of headache problems [13,14]. For a range of headache conditions, clinical management requires recognition of psychological factors, being able to screen for them, and assessing their impact on treatment progress. Packard [15] instructed that psychological factors need to be considered after head trauma or persistent post-traumatic headache, and the same comment has been made in assessing migraine [16], and tension-type headaches [17].

Samuels [18] conducted a review of headache syndromes and their treatment. He concluded that headache is the second most common reason people go to their family doctor, and the primary reason for consulting a neurologist, because they fear that they may have a brain tumour. In discussing treatment issues, this neurologist emphasized that a doctor must be able to tell the patient that he or she 'does not have a brain tumour.' He

added that if the doctor is not able to tell the patient exactly that, then '*it is unlikely that they will be able to help anyone with headache.*' In other words, if the physician is not mindful of the person's anxiety about their symptom, medical treatment alone will not be effective. The doctor must consider the psychological aspect of that person's headache in everyday practice.

Passchier *et al.* [19] investigated the health-related quality of life (HRQL) of headache patients who were consulting their general practitioner. The patient cohort consisted of 147 adults aged 20–50, with migraine, tension headache, or both. They related HRQL to the perceptual and emotional components of headaches. HRQL was measured by the Nottingham Health Profile (NHP). The perceptual components included intensity, frequency, and duration of the pain, and were measured with a headache diary. The emotional components were measured with five visual analogue scales for tension, depression, frustration, anger and fear. While there were no differences in HRQL between the headache groups, each headache patient group had a lower HRQL than the healthy reference group on the NHP dimensions of pain, sleep, energy and social isolation. Not surprisingly, the greater the patient's emotional pain, the more problems he or she had with physical mobility and social isolation. Neither the type of headache nor the headache index was related to the HRQL of the patient. Therefore, emotional components can be considered key factors in the day-to-day work with patients suffering from headache.

Multidisciplinary health teams should become more sensitized to looking out for the factors involved in management of these patients. Whenever emotional factors are thought to influence pain behaviour, some testing to establish which factors are prominent should be routine. For example, if patients display a high level of distress, or if they are focused on getting medications, self-medicating, or searching for healthcare services, further investigation should be explicitly considered. In some patients a high level of distress can be discerned from dramatizations of pain behaviours or of failures to respond to treatments provided. In all these instances, further testing with the tools described later would be indicated.

Psychiatric co-morbidity with headache

There is a difference between altered psychological and emotional processes and actual psychiatric disorders. Often the difference is only a matter of degree. For example, everybody will feel down or depressed from time to time. In most cases, these moods do not constitute a psychiatric condition. However, there is a continuum of possibilities here, with actual psychiatric disorder being at the far end of the continuum. Bearing this in mind, an important clinical question has been whether the emotional turmoil that almost all persistent pain sufferers will feel periodically constitutes an actual psychiatric disorder.

Penzien *et al.* [20] reviewed the literature on psychiatric morbidity and headache, and concluded that about seven out of 10 chronic headache patients show clear evidence of maladaptive behaviour patterns, even psychopathology. The authors note that these headache patients do not necessarily manifest a level of psychopathology that would be clinically diagnosed as a disorder according to DSM-IV criteria [21]; just that the integrity of their functioning is compromised by the existence of the recurrent headaches. Such patterns will impact on their quality of life (discussed below). Previous studies by Kindler *et al.* [22,23] found that 35 out of a series of 177 females with chronic headache complaints (1 in 5), and 18 of 51 males (1 in 3), had significant elevations on MMPI profiles. In other words, 23% of the group showed patterns of responses typical of psychopathology, which is about equal to the 24% prevalence rate for psychiatric conditions in a multinational study of the population of patients attending general practitioners' offices [24].

Wade *et al.* [25] investigated the contribution of more stable personality traits, and therefore presumably pre-existing psychological traits, on the overall MMPI profiles obtained for 59 chronic pain patients (not headache). They found that only the most severely distressed profiles were associated with their measures of stable personality attributes (e.g., neuroticism and extraversion). These authors concluded that for most patients, elevations found on measures of psychological distress reflect more the individual's endorsement of somatic items associated with their underlying pain condition. For a minority of more distressed patients, elevations can reflect broader emotional and behavioural tendencies which predate the chronic pain. This finding highlights the importance of using tools that have been standardized on a chronic pain population, and even more preferably, patients within homogeneous groups of headache conditions.

Penzien *et al.* also cautioned that many headache sufferers may score higher on scales of depression, such as the Beck Depression Inventory, as their *physical* headache symptoms lead to endorsing some depression items positively. This raises the important point that, for many of these patients, there are multiple coexisting symptoms, some physical and some psychological, and the clinical conclusions one arrives at usually require a level of sophistication in assessing both domains. The multidisciplinary health-team member is urged to communicate with others and develop this expertise by routinely using certain tests to understand the norms of pain-patient responses on these tests.

Although headache patients generally cannot be said to be at risk for developing psychiatric symptoms, Williams *et al.* [26] reported that there were different rates of psychopathology among different subgroups of headache patients. They found that the highest elevations were for patients with post-traumatic and conversion headaches, slight elevations for tension-type and combined headaches, with migraine and cluster-headache patients having the least distressed profiles. Robinson *et al.* [27] also found no general relationships between five different diagnostic categories of headache patient and the MMPI profiles for a series of 485 headache sufferers, a finding again corroborated by Kurlman *et al.* [28].

Penzien *et al.* [20] concluded that for evaluation of recurrent headache sufferers it is useful to employ some screening tools for psychopathology, to evaluate a range of psychosocial factors and attend to drug use and other behavioural factors. Suggestions for specific tools in these areas are elaborated later.

Quality of life

After years of being the poor cousin, the role of supportive care in working with pain patients is increasingly recognized as important. Included in this recognition has been the need to make explicit the long-held understanding in health care that the most important goal is optimal patient functioning and wellbeing. This effort to make more explicit the timeless value of medical care has evolved over the past 25 years and has come to be labelled 'quality of life' research [29]. Quality of life is understood to be subjective as well as multidimensional. Its subjectivity is such that it is best measured from the patient's perspective. Its multidimensionality is such that the measurement of quality of life requires the investigator to inquire about a range of areas of the patient's life, including physical wellbeing, functional ability, emotional wellbeing, social wellbeing and spiritual wellbeing. In relation to the goals of this chapter we will review the recent quality-of-life literature as it applies to pain patients in general as well as patients suffering from a range of headache conditions.

Pain and quality of life

Skevington [30] examined the impact of pain on quality of life (QOL) in 320 healthy adult subjects and patients who had been selected from all major categories of illness. A new, multidimensional, multilingual generic profile designed for cross-cultural use in health care (the WHOQUOL) was used to assess quality of life (QOL). Results indicated that pain and discomfort have a significant impact on perceptions of general QOL related to health. Furthermore, the presence of pain affected perceptions of five of the six domains of QOL. Spirituality, religion and personal beliefs were the exception. When assessing QOL, negative feelings were most closely associated with reports of pain and discomfort than any other facet of quality of life.

Henriksson [31] used a semistructured interview format to assess quality of life of 40 Swedish and American white women (aged 16–57 years) diagnosed with fibromyalgia. Results of this study indicated that the contradiction between the patient's perception of illness and the lack of objective findings was stressful. The women in this study reported feeling rejected, misunderstood and disbelieved. Their daily routines were disrupted, conflicts between life roles led to additional stress and the women experienced a loss of ability to perform valued activities. As clinicians we have to take from this that patients need early and adequate information and that consequences of our patients' condition must be acknowledged and taken into consideration in order to minimize secondary economic and psychosocial consequences.

In the same way in which Becker *et al.* [32] found that 58% of the patients were found to have a depressive or anxiety disorder, the authors also examined the pain epidemiology and health-related quality of life (HRQL). The subjects in this study were 150 chronic non-malignant pain patients (aged 23–89 years) who had been referred to a multidisciplinary pain centre. HRQL was evaluated with a medical outcome measure, a hospital anxiety and depression scale, and a psychological general wellbeing scale. The results of this study indicated that physical, psychological and social wellbeing were severely reduced among this group of patients. Statistically significant but modest correlations were found between pain severity and HRQL. Psychological and social wellbeing was closely correlated. Compared with the normal population, the chronic pain patients had used the health-care system five times more often in the years before referral. This study, like many others, confirms the multidimensional impact of chronic pain and demonstrates that HRQL of chronic non-malignant pain patients is among the lowest observed for any medical condition.

Solomon [33] summarized the impact migraine has on the life of the migraine sufferer. He distinguished between a general health-related quality of life questionnaire, and one that is specific to the disease being studied. Measures of general quality of life, like the SF-36, have shown significant limitations in all eight domains of wellbeing and functioning measured by this instrument. Indeed, chronic headaches were found to cause significantly more impairment of function than diabetes, hypertension, osteoarthritis and low back pain. In addition, results suggested that each of the common headache disorders (migraine, tension-type, cluster) had its own unique pattern of disruption. Solomon concluded that future studies should employ headache-specific QOL questionnaires. More recently, a newer breed of QOL instruments have been developed which assess limitation in physical, social, psychological and behavioural domains, and link these restrictions with the importance of the individual classes of activities. This results in a more meaningful understanding of what areas are limited and how important they are for the individual, and therefore what areas to focus treatment efforts on.

In an earlier study Solomon *et al.* [34] investigated whether QOL differs among headache diagnoses. Two hundred and eight consecutive headache patients (aged 17–80 years) within a multispecialty-group headache clinic, were studied in an interview survey using the Medical Outcomes Study Short Form Health Survey. The study included all six health components of the SF-20. 'Patients with cluster headache had a significantly higher (worse) pain score and higher percentage of patients with poor health due to pain than patients with migraine headache. There were fewer cluster patients with poor health associated with physical functioning than tension-type or mixed headache patients. Poor health associated with social functioning was greater for cluster and tension-type headache than for migraine. There was a significantly higher percentage of tension-type headache patients with poor health associated with mental health than patients with migraine.'

Osterhaus *et al.* [35] compared the health-related QOL of adult patients suffering from migraines with adults in the general population reporting no chronic conditions and with patients suffering from osteoarthritis, hypertension, diabetes and clinical depression. Two to 6 months after taking part in a clinical trial 546 subjects (90% female) completed the SF-36 Health Survey, a migraine severity measurement scale, and demographic information. After adjusting for co-morbid conditions, survey scores were significantly lower in migraine sufferers relative to age and sex-adjusted norms for subjects with no chronic conditions. Some health dimensions were more affected by migraine than other chronic conditions, while others were less affected. Measures of bodily pain, role disability due to

physical health and social functioning discriminated best between the three groups. Consistent with a number of the articles reviewed here, the subjects who reported moderate to very severe migraines scored significantly lower on five of the SF-36 scales than did the subjects with no chronic conditions.

All the studies above confirm the significantly negative impact that pain has on the QOL of the patients we all see in practice. They also suggest that failing to take account of psychosocial factors may both retard and limit the rehabilitation of these patients. The studies reviewed suggest that this is particularly true for patients with headache type pain. In short, chronic pain patients in general report significantly poorer QOL than non-chronic pain populations. Within the chronic pain population headache sufferers report significantly greater limitations in all eight domains of wellbeing and functioning than other chronic patients. Each of the headache subtypes (tension, migraine and cluster) have different patterns suggesting that treatment results would probably be optimized by implementing very individualized and specialized treatment plans.

Effects of coping

The way a given patient deals with a persistent pain problem is very instructive in understanding the maintenance of the pain condition and in individualizing the treatment programme. Passive coping patterns tend to be maladaptive and ineffective. A passive pattern of coping is often associated with poor self confidence and could be the result of a number of different factors, such as poor advice, poorly designed treatment programme, personality structure or social reinforcement for the passive behaviour. An adaptive approach to the same persistent pain could include active strategies for influencing pain intensity, or at least distracting one's attention from it. These patients tend to feel more self confident and are usually willing to try new approaches to further manage their pain and improve their quality of life. Understanding coping patterns is very helpful in clinical treatment, and has generated considerable research.

Burckhardt *et al.* [36] studied the pain-coping strategies of 71 female patients with fibromyalgia compared with other patients. In particular they investigated whether pain-coping strategies are predictive of pain, fatigue, poor sleep and QOL. These patients were tested before and after 6 months of treatment. Results showed that they used a multiplicity of pain-coping strategies. Increased use of any positive strategy is associated with better functioning and fewer symptoms. On the other hand, catastrophizing, depression and lack of perceived ability to control and decrease pain predicted increased pain, fatigue, and poor sleep, and, as we would expect, a resulting negative impact on QOL. This results of both this and the Skevington study support the value of psychological interventions with these patients. By increasing effective pain-coping strategies and perceived control and decreasing negative thinking, catastrophizing and depression, psychological interventions should have a positive impact on QOL and patients' overall sense of wellbeing.

Ward *et al.* [37] tested a stress-coping model of relationships between patients' beliefs about pain, coping (analgesic use), pain severity, analgesic side-effects, and three QOL outcomes. One hundred and eighty-two men and women (aged 31–84 years) with cancer completed valid and reliable self-report measures of relevant variables. The authors found that beliefs were significantly related to analgesic use. Analgesic use was inversely related to pain severity, but was not related to side-effect severity. Analgesic use was inversely related to impairments in QOL before controlling for pain and side-effect severity, but not after these two variables were controlled. Both analgesic side-effects and pain severity were related to impaired QOL outcomes which included difficulty performing life activities, depressed mood and poor perceived health status.

Myers *et al.* [38] investigated appraisal and coping strategies of tension-type headache sufferers and headache-free controls. The results of their studies suggest that individuals with tension-type headache report higher levels of subjective stress than headache-free controls when they make baseline ratings of stress, and that this elevation cannot be attributed to the anticipation of a future stressful event.

There is very little research that appears to answer the cart and horse question. That is, do patients with premorbidly low QOL experience chronic pain in a less adaptive way, or does the pain condition itself result in low QOL scores? Penzien [20] concluded that there are no specific personality traits that characterize headache sufferers or that predispose certain individuals to develop a headache syndrome and experience poorer quality of life. We think it safe to say that, in most cases, the pain condition is the horse and the reduced QOL is the cart. This being said, we believe it also safe to assume that the two are very synergistic and that, once the patient experiences chronic pain, QOL issues need to be addressed as a component of treatment.

Referral decisions

Penzien [20] highlighted warning signs that should lead to involving a psychologist in treatment. These include the development of psychiatric symptoms, memory problems, exaggerated pain behaviours, high stress, poor coping abilities, family dysfunction and decline in psychosocial functioning. Most of these warning signs are psychological and relate to poor initial coping skills, problematic pre-existing personality features or the development of psychopathological symptoms under the impact of chronic headaches. Other factors relate to complicating environmental and social features, and require the contribution of a psychologist as part of the treatment plan.

PSYCHOLOGICAL FACTORS AND WHIPLASH-ASSOCIATED DISORDERS

Recent reviews have emphasized a variety of psychological factors being important to managing whiplash injury [39,40]. Probably the most complete review of the syndrome, its assessment, management and outcome is the monograph *Cervical Flexion-Extension/Whiplash* by Teasell and Shapiro [41], supplemented by an important recent update by Mayou and Radanov [42] entitled *Whiplash Neck Injury*. The monograph by Teasell and Shapiro is especially useful as it embodies a multidisciplinary approach to clinical whiplash injury: there is a systematic discussion of the clinical features of the condition [43], a detailed discussion of headache [44], as well as the common psychological consequences of whiplash [45] and the importance of addressing both physical and psychological factors in treatment [46]. Also, the monograph provides a complete discussion of the question of how litigation complicates the clinical picture [47] and the related question of prognosis [48].

While the monograph was published before the Quebec Task Force into Whiplash Disorders [49], Mayou and Radanov's [42] review begins with the authors making the point that whiplash is the description of a process of injury, not a diagnosis. The clinical manifestations of whiplash are whiplash-associated disorders (WAD) which have been defined by the Quebec Task Force Review (1995) as occurring in four grades. The authors make the additional point that clinically, 'whiplash' (Grades I and II) should be clearly separated from conditions in which there is head injury that has caused alterations in consciousness (Grades III and IV). Although the conclusions proposed by the Quebec Task Force are debated [50], it is the best diagnostic nosology currently in use for assessing these patients.

Mayou and Radanov discuss epidemiology, aetiology, and clinical features and natural history, and draw conclusions about clinical management and assessment. They take the view that a comprehensive and multidisciplinary perspective is required for clinical management of the condition, emphasizing that, as in so many other physical conditions like low back pain and concussion, 'the interaction of physical, psychological, and social variables determines ways in which physical symptoms are perceived, and [the] effects on behaviour and quality of everyday activities' (p. 462). In this context they note the particular lack of attention given to the need for standardized psychological and QOL assessment with these patients.

Both reviews also consider treatment suggestions for whiplash patients. They conclude that appropriate treatment includes a consistent approach combining information, active rehabilitation exercises, acknowledgement of the unpleasantness of the acute symptoms and acceptance of gradually increased movement and everyday activity. The monograph by Teasell and Shapiro specifically addresses the importance of coordinated treatment of the psychological issues [46],

while Mayou and Radanov note that psychological treatments have been advocated, but not widely used. Mayou and Radanov conclude that 'A relatively poor outcome is substantially predicted by a wide range of psychological and social variables. . . [that] need assessment and may benefit from intervention' (p. 472).

Despite this consensus in the most complete recent reviews, there have been some recent articles which question the involvement of psychological factors in WAD. This next section reviews the research evidence establishing psychological factors in WAD with prospective study of large clinical cohorts in more detail, and then addresses the specific doubts that have been raised by some authors.

Prospective studies of psychological factors in whiplash

The past 5 years have seen the publication of a series of prospective studies of WAD patients in England and Switzerland, each of which has followed the evolution of the symptom picture among these patients, and considered what factors account for the different rates of recovery among patients, and which predicted poor outcome 1, 2 and 5 years later.

Mayou and Bryant [39] reported a prospective study interviewing consecutive whiplash patients, all of whom had presented to the emergency department of the hospital after road-traffic accidents. The authors measured reports of neck problems, depression, anxiety, personality factors, post-traumatic symptoms, travel anxiety, disability and use of medical services immediately after the accident, 3 months later and 12 months later. At the 1-year mark follow-up data were available for 57 adult men and women, aged 18–70. Overall, improvement was greatest in the first 3 months. However, a full 40% had continuing neck pain symptoms at one year, with a similar percentage reporting significant psychological symptoms, chiefly anxiety about travel and post-traumatic symptomatology. Almost one in four (21%) had a diagnosable psychiatric condition, although this is almost exactly the proportion that would be found among all patients presenting at medical offices [24].

Mayou and Bryant [39] also looked at the QOL of the subjects. Half the patients continued to describe moderate or severe consequences in at least one of three (work, leisure, family and social relationships) domains at one year. All who had been working before the accident had returned to work. Nevertheless, patients reported limitations in physically active leisure activities, due to pain restriction, and avoidance of social and other leisure activities, as a result of travel anxiety. Both were reported relatively commonly (one in four patients). Moreover, very few of those reporting moderate or greater difficulties at 3 months reported any substantial improvement at one year! Significant correlations were also found between social impairment at a year and the presence of psychiatric symptoms. Finally, the authors noted that in comparison with a parallel group of multiple-injury patients, all hospitalized due to more extensive physical injuries, the whiplash group (neck injury only) showed a tendency towards more anxiety disorders, while the hospitalized group showed more depressive disorders.

Gargan *et al.* [40] studied both physical and psychological factors among 50 consecutive whiplash patients also coming to a district hospital after motor-vehicle accidents in England. The authors found that both the range of neck movement and psychological response (as measured by the General Health Questionnaire – GHQ28) were equally predictive of long term (2-year) outcome, suggesting that a significant component in chronic disability after whiplash injury is psychological. Furthermore, the authors noted that psychological scores immediately after the accident (1 week later) *did not* discriminate between groups. However, by 3 months, results on the psychological tests *did* predict ultimate disability, suggesting that psychological disorders: (1) developed between 1 week and 3 months; (2) were correlated with corresponding physical factors (neck immobility) and therefore not 'purely psychological'; (3) were best characterized as secondary to the pain condition; and (4) were unrelated to litigation status or outcome. The authors suggested that the greatest potential for influencing the natural history of this syndrome is within the first 3-month period.

Radanov's Swiss research group [51,52] reported a prospective study, also at the 2-year post-accident mark, with 117 adult motor-vehicle-accident (MVA) patients. This is a much larger sample size than either of the English studies reviewed above. However, subjects were not consecutive patients arriving at a given hospital. Subjects were recruited as referrals from local general practitioners who saw any patient with a WAD. All of these patients were assessed for whiplash immediately post-MVA. They noted that theirs was a very homogeneous sample, in that all were from the same context – namely, the Swiss countrywide insurance scheme, which the authors stated makes compensation-seeking behaviour improbable. All patients were seen within 2 weeks of their MVA. The whiplash patients were also homogeneous in that the authors excluded patients with fractures, dislocations of the spine or those with head injury or loss of consciousness. They did a comprehensive physical evaluation at the onset of the whiplash injury, and followed the cohort for 2 years. Patients who had not improved by the 2-year point were placed in the dysfunctional group, and were considered to have had a poor outcome, the so-called 'late whiplash syndrome.'

The authors concluded that whiplash is a benign condition with a fairly high recovery-rate. Only 18% of patients exhibited chronic symptomatic presentation at the 2-year mark, and only 4% had not returned to work (elsewhere estimated at 8% [48]). What the authors wanted to know was why did one in five patients not get better? All had access to the same medical services, lived in the same country and dealt with the same insurance system. How could it be that such a large group failed to improve?

Among factors from the *initial* evaluation that proved to be highly related to poor outcome, 2 years later, were a mixture of both physical and psychological factors. Physical factors included whether the head had been inclined or rotated at impact, whether there were immediate symptoms of radicular deficit or of brainstem disturbance, or of X-ray signs of degeneration or osteoarthritis. Psychological factors included worry about illness and disability, presence of anxiety when being in the car, and a variety of non-specific factors including forgetfulness, blurred vision and increased fatigue.

For the patients who did develop late whiplash syndrome, the authors proposed a model that highlighted the involvement of multiple physical factors, with radicular irritation, degenerative changes and pre-existing headache problems being primary predisposing factors. In the first phase of rehabilitation (up to 6 months) sleep disturbances and 'adjustment problems', which might involve psychological difficulties, were highlighted. These authors suggested that it was only 3–6 months *after* the MVA that psychological factors became primary considerations for outcome. These factors included relationship problems, frustrations about unsuccessful treatment and problems with the insurance company.

Most interesting was the fact that the greatest difference between the two groups was observed on the immediate onset of sleep disturbances. The majority (73%) of dysfunctional patients had such problems within 2 weeks of injury, while only a third (31%) of the recovered patients had such a report at initial evaluation. Even more interesting is the fact that this finding was not discussed explicitly by the authors, despite the fact that it was the *single largest difference* between groups.

Also missing from the reports is a regression analysis, to determine whether any of the factors actually predicted outcome in the dysfunctional group at 2 years' time. The absence of such an analysis makes it difficult to evaluate which factors are associated with chronic dysfunction, and which ones are causal. A good example of this is in interpreting the significance of disturbed sleep of most of the poor-outcome group. As disturbed sleep is itself a common final pathway for both psychological and physical dysfunction, it is not clear how to understand and interpret the sleep problems of these patients.

Reitav *et al.* [53] have shown that the purely psychological factor of 3 weeks of examination stress, for students writing their final examinations, was associated with both disrupted sleep for these normal young adults, as well as significantly and substantially decreased musculoskeletal pain thresholds. The authors concluded that anxiety had an important mediating role in both the sleep problems and the reduced thresholds for musculoskeletal pain. Further study examining sleep disruption among WAD patients, investigating both psychological and physical status variables, would be helpful. Of particular note is the

prevalence of anxiety and post-traumatic stress conditions among these patients [39]. Given the potentially powerful mediating role of anxiety in the perception of pain, even among normal subjects, further study of these mediating factors is warranted.

In summary, there has been no prospective study of WAD patients that did not show a significant role for psychological factors. Although studies differ in what measures of specific psychological constructs are employed, all have found the measures they do take to be related to clinical progress and outcome – that is, in all who have to recover from a WAD, psychological factors play a part in how long it takes to recover. On the other hand, it is also clear that psychological factors rarely operate without underlying physical pathology. More recently, Radanov *et al.* [54] have posed a more interesting question: is it possible to isolate psychological factors that represent the entire group who did not improve, in contrast with matched controls who had recovered?

Contrasting improved and not improved patients

Radanov *et al* [54] compared their unselected population of 21 patients who remained symptomatic at the 2-year mark, with an age-, sex- and education-matched group of 21 subjects from the same study *who had improved*. Methodologically, this represents the best prospective study of psychological factors involved in whiplash conducted to date. They measured the overall wellbeing of the patients with a wellbeing scale, as well as a number of personality factors with the Freiburg Personality Inventory. Although neither of these tools is routinely used in North American research, the constructs are familiar. The basic research question is simple: are there any psychological variables which emerge from a contrast of these two groups, that help us to understand how those who improve are different from those who do not?

The wellbeing scale they used would appear to be a self-reported global measure of wellbeing, independent of any specific symptom presentation. Scores above 17 correspond to *t*-scores above 56, and are considered a reflection of impaired wellbeing. Radanov *et al.* reported a main effect caused by group and time, with no interactions qualifying either main effect. For the asymptomatic group who recovered within 6 months of injury *t*-scores began just above the statistical mean (50) at 53.17, were below 50 by 3 months, and remained normal. What is most interesting for this group is that the standard deviation of the group consistently shrank from 11.11 at 3 months, to 8.96 at 6 months, to 6.97 at 2 years. This means that as time passed, all members of the group increasingly converged on this group's lower *t*-score of 44.81.

In contrast, the symptomatic group started well above others and well into the pathological zone, at *t* = 59.5, and even at the 2-year mark had only improved to *t* = 55.4, still averaging very near the cut-off for pathological scores (*t* = 56). Regardless of how or why the measure was constructed, it would seem that this wellbeing measure could be an excellent global early predictor of poor treatment response. High scorers should be considered for psychological evaluation early in the rehabilitation process. An English language version of this scale would help foster further research into this important area.

The scales of the Freiburg Personality Inventory did not show anywhere near as clear a picture, yet are interesting as well. The authors reported that scores above 6 are elevated, or pathological, on this scale. In reviewing all the group means there are only three scales that show that any of the research groups are above the cut-off, and all three are for the symptomatic group. Mean scores in the asymptomatic group never exceeded the cut-off on any scale of the personality test at any of the time periods. This again would suggest that readings above 6 are good measures of pathological results, requiring further study, and could be considered an early warning sign of possible poor prognosis.

Overall, the highest elevations found on any scale were for the closed-mindedness scale which began at 6.43 decreased to below 6 at 6 months, then increased again, to end up at 6.19. However, controls were also high on this scale (starting at 5.81 and remaining just under 6 across all time periods), and standard deviations were higher than on any of the other scales, so there were no significant group differences with a small sample.

The other two variables that showed a pathological score were in the symptomatic group for 'nervousness' and 'passivity' scales. On 'nervousness' the symptomatic group began at 5.38 and increased across time, to reach an average of 6.19 at the 2-year mark. In contrast, the asymptomatic controls began at 4.05 and decreased within the first 3 months, to remain at an even lower 3.33 at 2 years. For this factor, there was a significant group-by-time interaction effect, with the major variability being accounted for by the changes within the first 3 months. In other words, those who recovered showed a diminishing of overall nervousness very quickly, while those who did not recover showed higher levels of nervousness across time, with a pathological level reached only gradually some time after the 6-month mark.

The authors described the nervousness scale as identifying 'subjects prone to develop psychosomatic conditions (elevated scores on this scale, however, may also be observed during the course of a serious somatic illness).' From this description it would appear that nervousness refers to a preoccupation with somatic concerns, rather than physiological anxiety phenomena per se. Further examination of this scale and its relationship to somatization, hypochondriasis and physiological anxiety would be helpful in future studies.

Elevated scores were also found for the symptomatic group, on the 'passivity' scale. Ratings for the symptomatic group started at 5.05 and increased to 6.24 by 2 years, and for the asymptomatic group started slightly lower, at 4.8 and decreased to 3.86 by the 2-year mark. Although these would seem to be reasonably consistent, and diverging, trends, the statistical analysis did not reach significance. This might be because only some of the asymptomatic patients showed the pattern of increasing elevations, while others did not (there was increasing variability within the group across time). Although it did not reach significance, the higher passivity of this group, coupled with the increased nervousness and somatic preoccupation of the group suggests the primary features of the pattern seen in kinesiophobic patients, and should be explored further.

Among the remaining scales of the Freiburg Inventory, there were other comparisons which reached statistical significance, but interpreting these is difficult owing to interaction effects and the fact that the group means remained within the range of what was considered normal on this test. Noteworthy among the scales that showed *no difference between groups* were the 'depression' and 'neuroticism' scales. This would suggest that depressive symptoms are not generally seen among WAD patients, even at the 2-year mark, when compared with matched controls. More importantly, while these patients had not recovered, this was clearly for reasons other than depressiveness. This finding supports a similar conclusion reached by Mayou and Bryant, wherein it was only the more seriously injured, hospitalized, group of whiplash patients for whom depression was a concern.

Radanov *et al.* [54] concluded that neuroticism, as well as psychological symptoms, did not appear to be of primary relevance for the course of recovery from the whiplash condition. What remains puzzling is why no regression analysis was conducted. This would be the appropriate test of predictive validity of antecedent variables, whether physical or psychological. Even with the small sample size, variables with strong predictive potential will emerge. In the absence of regression analysis, comparisons between the two clinical groups, alone, cannot be taken as proof one way or another, of what causes the poor outcome in the symptomatic group. We await further reports from this very prolific and rigorous research group.

The prediction of poor outcome

Only two studies have reported regression analyses, one at 1-year after the accident [39], and the other [55] at 5 years after the accident. All of the 57 neck-injury patients in the Mayou and Bryant study cohort had returned to work by 1 year after the accident, so none of these patients could be considered permanently disabled. Nevertheless, about four in 10 of these patients continued to have neck problems, and a similar proportion had psychological symptoms, chiefly social restrictions, post-traumatic stress and travel anxiety. The authors did regression analyses for continuing neck problems, for psychiatric symptoms, and for social outcome. No common factor

emerged from these analyses. Instead, each outcome measure was predicted by a different set of predictors.

Persisting neck problems were best predicted by immediate report of neck symptoms, as well as sex and driver status, with women passengers being more at risk than men, or drivers of either sex. Anxiety and depression at 1 year were predicted by previous psychiatric history, and post-traumatic disorder and travel anxiety were both predicted by the initial report of 'horrific memories' of the accident. Social outcome was predicted by a history of psychological problems from before the accident, and to a much lesser degree emotional distress immediately after the accident.

These results and this study are very instructive. They clarify that there is no single factor, physical or psychological, that answers all questions of relevance to clinical outcome. Persistent problems for this cohort are independent of litigation issues and require a multidimensional approach in assessment. Specifically, they concluded that management of WAD is often haphazard, and more attention to the anxiety symptoms, and the developing social disabilities of these patients, in the period around 3 months after accident would be clinically indicated.

Mayou and his colleagues [55] then pooled the data for neck-injury only with the multiple-injury patients, to conduct a study of prevalence of continued psychological problems at 5 years post-accident. This long-term outcome study was conducted by questionnaire only, and was only able to locate 111 (64%) of the 171 subjects who had been interviewed in the earlier phases of the research. Eleven of these patients reported continuing major physical problems, although these were almost exclusively (eight) among motorbike riders.

Much more prevalent were continuing problems with quality of life as well as anxiety. Most prevalent were reports of deteriorating enjoyment of leisure activities, with about 40% of all subjects reporting such continued difficulties 5 years later. About half as many (22%) reported additional problems with either enjoyment of social life or work dissatisfaction. Problems with family relationships were much less common, but were reported by a small minority (14%) of the cohort. With all four QOL dimensions, motorbike riders endorsed a higher level of problems in all areas. A regression analysis found that poor social outcome (on any of the four dimensions) was predicted only by current (self-reported) physical problems.

The anxiety variables that were tracked were post-traumatic stress disorder (PTSD) and travel anxiety. Of these two, travel anxiety was more pervasive, with 60% of all subjects being 'concerned' about travel, up to 40% reporting 'minor effects' on travelling, 28% with a probable diagnosable phobic anxiety disorder, and 11% reporting major travel phobia. However, travel anxiety was not predicted by any psychological or physical variables other than the presence of immediate emotional distress at the time of the accident. This would suggest that the presence of a strong anxiety reaction at the time of the accident creates the conditions necessary for generalization of anxiety to all elements of driving and travel. However, the fact that immediate emotional distress only accounted for about 3.5% of the variance in the factor, suggests that this was a necessary, but not sufficient factor, as many of these distressed patients were able to overcome this potential effect through their own informal strategies of improvement.

Post-traumatic stress disorder presents an even more interesting pattern of results. Across the follow-up period a full 20% of subjects presented with PTSD at some point. As a proportion of the subject cohort, the percentage experiencing PTSD remained constant at about 10% of the cohort at each three follow-up points. Eleven subjects had acute onset of PTSD within 3 months, of which eight were still symptomatic at 1 year, but only one at 5 years. (This one subject had suffered a severe accident initially, and had also had an accident both before and after the accident bringing him into the study.) Three additional subjects had an onset of PTSD symptoms between 3 and 12 months, with all improved at 5 years. And eight more subjects had a late onset identified at the 5-year follow-up, with no previous occurrence.

Prediction of PTSD also changed across time. At the 1-year point, symptomatology was predicted primarily by the occurrence of initial frightening, distressing, intrusive memories, but not by other psychological, social or physical measures. At 5 years, PTSD symptoms were still predicted by initial intrusive memories, but so were immediate emotional distress, and self-report of continuing medical problems at 5 years. These three factors accounted for 29% of the variance in the PTSD. The authors note that not all variables that could be of importance to understanding the occurrence of PTSD were incorporated into the study design and further study is definitely warranted. Nevertheless, there appear to be two overlapping subgroups of PTSD patients: the early-onset group responding primarily to the distressing, intrusive memories, and a delayed-onset group responding to distress, intrusive memories and constant reminders of dysfunction such as constant pain, and disability in social and leisure activity; the later factor acting to precipitate the PTSD across time.

The important clinical question this raises for the Swiss studies [51,52,54] is whether any of their symptomatic group would have done better with immediate attention to their sleep and/or psychological problems. The authors were silent on this point, except to say that they favoured the usefulness of a comprehensive multidisciplinary initial assessment of whiplash patients, in order to better understand the operation of the psychological factors in the period 6 months after injury. Taken together with Mayou's [55] results, it is clear that we are only beginning to understand that there are important psychological and psychophysiological processes happening here that ought to explored in more detail, whether with tools like the Well-Being Rating scale and the Freiburg nervousness and passivity scales, or some of the measures described later in this chapter.

Even though it may seem self evident that psychological factors are significant in many areas of patient management, if not yet clearly implicated in chronic pain. We will soon see that it is still too tempting to strip away the psychological factors and return to the simpler model of pure physical causation.

Psychological and medical models

So, are psychological factors of importance from the outset of WAD or not? One recent report has raised the significance of this issue once again. Wallis *et al.* [56] reported on a study of 24 whiplash patients who were at least 3 months post MVA, and presumably not much longer than 6–9 months, although no mean times since accident were reported for the group. The authors were particularly interested in understanding what causes the psychological distress that is triggered by the pain and injury of the accident, and hence how it would best be resolved. They proposed that if the psychological distress were secondary to the patient's chronic pain, then relief of the chronic pain should resolve the psychological distress without any need for psychological treatment.

All their subjects were selected on the basis of diagnosis of a painful cervical zygapophysial joint. 'Patients had to obtain complete relief of their neck pain on each occasion that two different local anaesthetics were administered, but no relief when normal saline was used.' The authors did not clarify how many patients were tested to establish the final cohort of 24 patients, but in another publication [57] they report that 60% of a consecutive series of 68 WAD patients 3 months or more after the accident responded to the surgery. The rest did not.

The subjects selected for the study received either an active neurosurgical treatment, or an operative placebo-control equivalent to relieve their pain condition. Before the experimental procedures all subjects completed a VAS pain rating, the McGill Pain Questionnaire [58], and the SCL–90–R [59] rating of psychological symptoms. The authors wrote that: 'the psychological model would maintain that the pain and psychological distress exhibited by patients with chronic neck pain both stem from a primary psychological disorder.'

What is particularly noteworthy is how the authors define the 'psychological' model. Nobody who works in the behavioural medicine [2] area today would ever suggest that *all* pain *and* psychological distress are the result of a primary psychological disorder. Most WAD patients have a physical mechanism of injury which is the cause of their distress, although not always visible on physical tests; Wallis *et al.*'s proposed 'psychological' model is a straw man which proposes that a psychological model would ignore all peripheral signals and define the pain experience

exclusively on what happens centrally. This would only be true of the 'functional pain' hypothesis advanced in psychiatry at the end of the last century. It is not consistent with modern gate control theory, or with empirical results such as those presented in the prospective studies reviewed earlier.

Wallis *et al.* [56] found that the surgery did resolve the psychological distress reported by these patients on the SCL-90-R. They concluded that their result 'calls into question the present nihilism about chronic pain, which proclaims medical therapy alone to be ineffectual, and psychological co-therapy to be imperative. Co-therapy may be useful if medical therapy cannot provide complete relief of pain, but it is redundant if psychological distress disappears when pain is relieved.' This is a very important clinical finding which would suggest that the psychological sequelae of most WAD patients are indeed secondary to pain, and that these sequelae are self-limiting, when the chronic pain signal is removed.

The need for psychological intervention, surgical intervention or any other kind of intervention, should be indicated by positive findings from a careful assessment, not taken as a given for entire groups of patients. Another question raised by these studies is how resilient this reversal of psychological sequelae is. If subjects come for surgery within 3 months the reversal would be swifter as patterns of negative reinforcement, disillusionment, etc. have not set in. But will the same results be obtained for procedures conducted 6, 12 or 18 months post trauma? The prospective studies [40,54,55] would suggest an increasing difficulty with such reversals, but these studies have not yet been done.

The 'theoretical' question which Wallis *et al.* raised – namely, whether a 'psychological' or a 'medical' model best accounts for the pattern of distress reported by these patients, is not a meaningful question. Aside from the fact that their 'psychological model' is actually a very narrowly defined concept from historical psychiatry, the results from recent English and Swiss studies show conclusively that one cannot reduce all symptomatology reported by patients to biomedical factors within the broader cohort of real patients. This dichotomization is regressive, and unlikely to lead to any clearer understanding of the patients involved, or of the real challenges they pose to healthcare management.

We ask every healthcare provider to be sceptical, and to ask the question 'do psychological factors enter into the pain phenomena that I am dealing with in my patient?' This question must be asked anew with each and every patient treated. Evidence suggests that this question becomes increasingly relevant by about 3 months post accident. Clearly, prospective studies with consecutive series of whiplash patients indicate that ignoring psychological factors means having only part of the clinical picture in chronic WAD patients. Sometimes puzzles can be solved with only part of the pieces, but more often they cannot.

Does 'late whiplash' exist?

There is consensus that whiplash-associated symptoms occur within a day or two of the trauma, and for most patients resolve within 6 weeks of the trauma [41]. However, it was generally accepted that up to one in five did not improve, even after 2 years post accident [52]. These are the so called 'late-whiplash' syndrome patients. Very recently, there has been doubt cast on whether such a syndrome actually exists, or whether late, or chronic, whiplash should be considered a 'compensation neurosis' instead [60].

In 1996, a group of Scandinavian researchers [61] published an often cited study on the relationship between whiplash injury and chronic headaches. They recruited 202 Lithuanian middle-aged adults (78% male) from a consecutive (unselected) police registry of almost 240 adults who had been in rear-end motor vehicle accidents an average of 22 months earlier. Most of the MVAs ranged from minor damage (45%), to moderate damage (44%), but 11% of the cars were reported to be wrecked in the accidents.

The accident group was paired with age- and sex-matched controls, who reported not having been in a vehicle accident. The corresponding, and correct, procedure for the clinical group would have been to similarly exclude *any* 'whiplash' subjects who actually never had symptoms of WAD. However, the investigators did not do this; yet, throughout the report,

they describe all the accident subjects as being in 'the whiplash group.' That is, the investigators offered no clinical evidence that any of these people actually experienced the physical symptomatology associated with whiplash at the time of the accidents [62]. The absence of such proof makes generalizations about 'whiplash', to say nothing of 'late whiplash', pure conjecture. It severely limits the generalizability and clinical utility of their headache findings. Other methodological problems include the fact that the study was retrospective, and all information obtained was questionnaire data.

Frequency and type of headache

The investigators were interested in finding the prevalence, chronicity and type of headache after whiplash. The half of the subjects who reported at least some headache were sent questionnaires that permitted the diagnosis of tension-type headache, migraine or cervicogenic headache. Previous research had suggested that headache as a symptom of late whiplash syndrome is found in 9–25% of patients [44]. Evans [63] observed that most headaches following whiplash injury are tension-type headaches, associated with cervical muscle injury, greater occipital neuritis/neuralgia or temporomandibular joint syndrome.

The researchers first looked for differences in the frequency of headaches between groups. They classified headaches into one of four groups: no headaches, one per month, episodic (1–15) and chronic (>15). The authors focused on the presence or absence dimension, reporting that they found that 50% of the whiplash group complained of headaches; but so did 48.5% of the control group. Although this would suggest no relationship between whiplash and headaches, a χ^2 test of headache frequencies among the four classifications of frequency *was significant* ($P<0.02$) [64]. The authors reported the significant χ^2 in the table, but did not discuss its meaning in the text of the article.

It must therefore be noted that there was a statistically significant difference between the accident cohort and the control group: even if there weren't more patients with headaches, the ones with headaches reported increased frequencies, with *two-thirds more* whiplash patients (55) reporting regular/episodic headaches (1–15 days per month) than controls (33). Also, even though the authors maintained that chronic headaches (>15 days per month) were reported no more frequently among the whiplash group (16) than among the controls (12), again the χ^2 result would not support this characterization. If one adds up the increased number of more frequent headaches (in these two cells), one gets 26, or about 13% of the cohort. This is slightly less than the 20–24% incidence of unresolved cases reported 2–4 years after the accident [65] but, given other methodological concerns regarding unknown prevalence of WAD at the outset, these results can not be taken to rule out the presence of some degree of chronic post-traumatic headaches in their population.

In reviewing the types of headaches reported, the authors concluded there was no difference in the incidence of migraine (13 *v* 15), episodic tension-type headaches (45 *v* 50) or chronic tension-type headaches (8 *v* 10). There was a trend in the number of headaches diagnosed as 'possible cervicogenic headaches', with six pure cases in the whiplash group and only one among the 202 controls ($P = 0.13$). What makes generalization from these results tenuous is the high number of headaches (29 whiplash headaches, and 22 among controls) the authors were not able to classify, using their questionnaire methodology.

The 'unclassified' cases represent three times the number of cases documented for both of the chronic tension-type, and cervicogenic headache classes. Therefore, proper classification of these unclassifiable cases could substantially affect the final outcome of the prevalence of these types of headache. Interestingly, the authors noted that they carried out a number of follow-up phone calls, to clear up 'equivocal' questionnaire responses, but apparently making clearer determinations of diagnosis was not possible. In summary, further methodological improvements are necessary before one can confidently say that there was no difference in the frequency of different types of headaches between conditions.

Methodological questions and cross-cultural study

Radanov [66] recently provided a broad-ranging critique of the methodological

problems with the Lithuanian study. These critiques include the fact that the study was retrospective, included only questionnaires, included a disproportionate number of males and drivers. It must also be noted that the study had only a small number (22) of cases with more severe force involved in the accident. The authors did not attempt to classify a large number of 'unclassifiable' headache cases, or consider whether the incidence of cervicogenic headaches in the whiplash group increased as the severity of accident forces increased. In the absence of proof that the 'whiplash group' are clinical WAD patients, such a review would have been helpful.

The small number of severe accidents in the cohort would suggest that it is premature to conclude, on the basis of these results alone, that clinical WAD can not result in either cervicogenic headache or chronic tension-type headaches. The authors conclude that chronic headache complaints after whiplash are more probably attributable to the medico-legal context present in the Western world, than to the actual trauma or injury itself. We can certainly agree that for these accident subjects chronic headache complaints were not related to their injury. But was their injury actually WAD? It would seem that further prospective research would be necessary to begin to support the kind of conclusions proposed. We are hopeful that the planned prospective follow-up study will address methodological issues and shed some light on these important questions.

It must be noted that this study did more to generate discussion about this important topic than anything in the preceding decade. Readers interested in the research questions, and the cultural and medico-legal questions that were raised by this important study are urged to read the original articles in '*The Rheumatologist And Chronic Whiplash Syndrome*' [66,67] and the subsequent printed discussions in the *Journal of Rheumatology* [68–70]. Most interesting is the emergence of suggestive evidence from Greek and German studies that the incidence of post-traumatic headaches is also reduced in these cultures.

The impact of the medico-legal context

Schrader [61,62] and his colleagues concluded that the lower incidence of headaches among the 'whiplash patients' in their study cohort was because of the medico-legal context specifically. However, this conclusion was reached by inference, and methodological concerns (see above) make it hard to be persuaded that the medico-legal context alone can affect presenting clinical symptomatology to such an extent. A recent study by Cassidy *et al.* [71] demonstrates quite clearly that the medico-legal context certainly does influence claimants' reports of continued difficulties. Cassidy and his colleagues conducted their study when a regional government in Canada changed from a medico-legal context that allowed suing the insurance company for pain and suffering (the tort system of compensation), to a no-fault system where all accident victims received necessary treatment and income replacement benefits during rehabilitation, but no right to sue. The study excluded more severe injuries, for example if patients were in hospital longer than 2 days, had more than one accident or who were not injured in a car (motorcyclists, etc.).

It is important to stress that all other variables remained the same during the data collection periods. As many or more accidents were occurring, and the miles driven also increased. The authors report no changes in how lawyers billed during this time. Also, the broader insurance administration framework within which claims were processed was the same, and presumably did not change their way of processing or adjudicating claims. The only significant change between time periods was the medico-legal context, which essentially removed a legal right of suing and replaced it with better treatment and benefits rights.

The primary outcome measure was the duration of time that accident claims remained open. This is the point at which income replacement payments ceased and a final agreement was reached between the insurer and the claimant. The authors also stress that the time to closure is a common proxy for recovery in studies of insurance claims. They add that this point usually coincides with the end of treatment or the attainment of maximal medical improvement, but no evaluation of final clinical status is provided for any of these patients. For example, it could just be that the insurance company has become more generous in offering the claimants more money to close the claim. The fact that no clinical evaluation

is conducted makes the results less useful for those involved in treating these patients.

The change in medico-legal context turned out to have a huge impact on claims experience. First, there was a 28% reduction in the overall number of claims made, mainly as a result of fewer claims opened by young males. The median time to closure under tort was 433 days, and under no-fault was 194 days [71], which represents a 50% decrease in claims duration. Under both systems, having a lawyer involved was a strong predictor of delayed closure, which makes sense because the job of the lawyer is to advise you to keep your options open. But it also illustrates that the tort system effectively creates a different kind of social context around the patient, one which actively influences the patient to behave differently.

The authors noted other clinical findings of importance. Under both systems, the time to closure was longer for older people, women and those with a higher level of education. In addition, a higher initial baseline score for the intensity of pain and a greater percentage of the body in pain (both self-rated) was associated with a longer time to closure; that is, for all whiplash patients, these factors can be considered factors that aggravate clinical improvement. Older people take longer to recover from many physical problems, so this is entirely expected. Women and the better educated may take longer as pre-existing strength and fitness may be lower. Finally, severity of initial trauma (real or perceived) would also be expected to extend rehabilitation.

There were factors which extended recovery under tort but not no-fault, and others that extended recovery under no-fault but not tort. Clearly, these too merit attention, but interpreting their significance is more difficult. It must be said that owing to the size of the study cohort, none of these can be considered chance findings. Under tort, time to closure was extended by anxiety before the collision, having been employed full time, experiencing reduced or painful jaw movement and reporting concentration difficulties. A jaded interpretation would offer that enough full-time employees who might have been unhappy with their work could have seen tort as an opportunity to change careers. The clinical presentation variables that are not confirmed as significant among the no-fault group suggest that these may be symptoms that claimants could become more self-absorbed in, or even be coached to present with.

Most interesting is the fact that there were variables which extended closure under no-fault when compared with tort. These included being married, having pain or numbness in the arm, having broken bones and having memory problems after the collision. How can we understand the fact that while in this condition recovery times are twice as fast as under tort, these variables become factors which extend rehabilitation? Being married could extend closure as the claimant has other responsibilities and involvements at home that could keep them there longer, and being off work would mean being able to take more time to attend to these matters. The clinical presentation factors could become important as the shorter time to rehabilitate now introduces new factors that effectively put a speed limit on recovery. It is unlikely that these were not important in the tort group, just that they were not visible owing to the much longer periods of recovery (on average 200 days longer).

Overall, the results Cassidy *et al.* present support the view that an insurance system which uses continued presence of symptoms to determine financial compensation actually provides barriers to clinical recovery. The adversarial context can promote the persistence of symptoms in the claimant. 'In the course of proving that their pain is real, claimants may encounter conflicting medical opinions, unsuccessful therapies, and legal advice to document their pain and suffering' [71, p. 1185]. There is little doubt that the social factors impinging on these patients do impact their behaviour and level of symptomatology.

However, we can not conclude that all closed cases are asymptomatic either, or that these patients do not continue to have some difficulties with their functioning or with pain. Similar results have been reported for low-back-pain disability and for similar changes in other jurisdictions, so we can consider this to be a reliable finding. All in all the data presented by Cassidy *et al.* confirm that WAD are real clinical disorders: if they were not, recovery time would have collapsed to near zero. However, they do tend to be benign and self-limiting, as suggested by the Quebec Task Force, but can be significant problems for some patients, based on the seriousness of the original injury and the level of strength and fitness of the patient.

Cassidy *et al.* also showed that the presence of certain factors affected recovery speed throughout the entire follow-up period. Self-reports of greater physical activity were associated with increased recovery speed, and reports of depression among patients slowed down their recovery for the tort group. Among the much shorter recovery times of the no-fault group, changes in the improvement of neck pain was associated with increased recovery speed and depressive symptoms slowed down recovery rates. These results show that even though whiplash can be considered a generally benign condition, both physical and psychological factors appreciably influence the rate at which patients will recover from such conditions. We should also note that this work did not conduct an exhaustive study of all possible psychological factors shown by research to relate to improvement. The presence of anxiety is an important example of a factor not assessed in this study. Overall, we can consider this study to add more weight to the argument that physical and psychological factors, in synergistic interaction with each other, are potent variables in influencing rates of recovery from whiplash-associated disorders.

Permanent disability

Although the many prospective studies reviewed all suggest that complete, or permanent, disability from a whiplash injury is very rare, it can happen. Estimates of rates of complete inability to return to work average around 54% [54]. Those who must conduct disability determinations to assess complete inability to return to work are aware that there are few psychometric tools of much value for this purpose. The best orientation to the complex issues involved in disability evaluations is provided in a series of articles in the 1997 (volume 336) volume of the journal *Clinical Orthopaedics and Related Research*. This volume provides a series of editorial comments on the problems of disability assessment in the context of evaluating low-back-pain disability.

No such discussion has been held about conducting such assessments with whiplash injuries, but it is safe to say the issues are the same.

Of particular note is the editorial by Fordyce [72] entitled 'On the nature of illness and disability.' Fordyce fleshes out the dangers of the physician embracing a strict biomedical model that does not consider the psychological and social components in disability determinations. Specifically, he notes that disability programmes are intended to provide opportunities not guarantees. Society and the individual both have primary responsibility in the successful outcome of these programmes. Moreover, participating parties such as the treating physician and the individual's family have important supportive roles, roles similar to a coach urging the player to put forward his, or her, best effort.

A disability evaluator must assess a number of functions in order to make a determination of disability. As Fordyce eloquently puts it, 'disability pertains to performance or behaviour... [and] performance as a criteria of disability status is complicated further by effort related considerations' (p. 48). In other words, every healthcare provider charged with making a determination on disability status cannot make a final decision without explicitly, or implicitly, evaluating the individual's performance; and therefore without making judgement of the individual's effort during that performance.

Another issue should also be raised in this context. Namely, to make the determination that a claimant is, or is not, able to carry out their work activities, also requires that the disability evaluator give serious thought to the psychological demands of the workplace on that claimant's resources. In some cases, chronic pain, tinnitus or other associated symptoms will significantly interfere with the individual's ability to attend, concentrate or problem-solve, thus preventing them from effectively coping with their work. Where such factors are significant, corollary disability evaluations from a clinical psychologist, or a neuropsychologist would be necessary.

The most widely used approach to disability determination is that outlined by the American Medical Association *Guides to the Evaluation of Permanent Impairment* [73]. These guides take the general perspective that disability evaluation is 'assessed by medical means and is a medical issue.' [73, p. 1]. However, at the start of the chapter reviewing the evaluation of chronic pain, the guides elaborate on how a narrow medical perspective is inappropriate to disability evaluation of pain conditions. Three models of pain are discussed, and the disability evaluator is urged to classify the claimant's condition using all three models. Importantly, evaluating psychological factors is central to all three.

However, the guides do not just make a separate case for pain, compared with all other medical conditions that could be disabling. They go on to make a separate case for evaluating headache conditions, compared to other pain conditions. At the outset the guides suggest that the vast majority of primary headache disorders will not have permanent impairments (although whiplash is not discussed, or alluded to). In addition, the intensity-frequency grid proposed as the correct way of determining impairment due to chronic pain is further elaborated for headache patients. For headache, the assessor is also urged to be cognizant of the fact that there can be significant variability in the persistence of the pain problem. That is, some patients may present with a stable clinical picture, as would be the case for general chronic pain patients, but this is not the only possibility. It is also possible that such patients present with a cyclical pattern, with periods of partial or temporary remission, or that they present with widely fluctuating pain intensities. In summary, the guides consider headache pain to be a valid reason for finding permanent impairment, and more latitude is given the evaluator to make this determination, compared to other chronic pain conditions.

In most disability evaluations the 'performance' evaluation usually takes the form of functional testing of strength, persistence and consistency of efforts. But does this adequately consider the social and psychological components involved in the disability assessment [74]? And what of the possibility that a severe WAD patient with disabling headaches of a cyclical pattern comes for a functional evaluation during a period of remission. The clinical challenges of assessing these patients are formidable, and tackling these in a sensitive yet objective manner is very important. Fordyce observed that the effort that an individual expends in their rehabilitation, and at the disability evaluation, is variable and dependent on psychological, social and contextual forces. Its implication is that every disability evaluator of chronic head and neck pain must assess these factors explicitly.

For all who work in the area of rehabilitation from traumatic injury, it has been clear for a long time that patients rehabilitate at different rates, and some fail to respond to treatment. What are the factors that predict poor response? Bannister and Gargan [48] summarized that among factors that do not correlate with prognosis are immediate, acute symptoms, radiological findings, pre-existing psychiatric condition, pre-existing degenerative changes and litigation status. On the other hand, the 'duration and severity of symptoms, age over 50 years, upper limb radiation and thoracic or lumbar back pain are indicators of a poorer prognosis' (p. 567). The guides themselves make a point that the eight characteristic attributes of chronic pain syndrome patients can often be clinically determined as early as 2–4 weeks after onset of the pain condition. Chronic pain syndrome patients do not fall out of the sky at 6 months. Appropriate treatment includes monitoring for poor treatment response early on.

Martelli *et al.* [75] have recently revisited the issue of establishing which factors will predispose the patient to disability. They presented a vulnerability to disability rating scale, for use with patients who are rehabilitating from a traumatic injury. The scale was developed from work with a Grade III WAD patient, and identifies a mixture of physical, social, psychological and treatment variables which are evaluated in a systematic way. For the individual to be considered 'at risk' for becoming disabled, they must show signs of multiple risk factors. Each of the 11 dimensions can be scored as a 0, 1 or 2, yielding a total score out of 22. Scores above 13 warn the doctor of vulnerability to chronic disability.

The variables that are evaluated are not all psychological variables. Two variables relate to medical status: one to premorbid status and another to collateral injury. Some could be considered related to the patient's motivation to improve. For example, previous treatment failure and medication reliance are both highlighted. A fifth variable weights the duration of time since the injury. While the last three might be considered psychological, they are not necessarily so. The remaining six factors are all psychological factors: one is a vague and inconsistent presentation of complaints, and the others are aspects of current psychological functioning. These factors include severity of current psychological stresses, concurrent psychiatric condition, the individual's victimization perception and two social factors – illness reinforcement and social vulnerability. These factors need to be considered explicitly in all WAD patients who have not begun to respond to appropriate treatment. The results from prospective studies reviewed earlier [39,40,51,54] suggest that such an evaluation should be considered within 3 months of the original trauma.

The vulnerability to disability rating scale has not yet been validated beyond the traumatic brain injury (TBI) case that led to the development of the scale itself. It is noteworthy that the factors selected for the VDRS are not the same factors emerging from the Swiss study [54] of long-term follow-up of a homogeneous sample of WAD Grade II patients. Overall, although we may be far from reaching consensus on the specific factors that are most predictive of vulnerability to disability, there is now more accumulating evidence that psychological factors do play an important part in determining the ultimate status of the individual with chronic head or neck pain.

PSYCHOMETRIC TOOLS FOR CLINICAL ASSESSMENT

There are now hundreds of questionnaires, structured interviews or paper and pencil tools available for evaluating any conceivable aspect of the head and neck pain patient's experiences. What we have tried to do is to provide a sketch of what have seemed to us to be the most useful clinical tools in evaluating dimensions of the pain experience as well as other psychological dimensions of relevance to understanding the pain patient better.

In reviewing the assessment tools outlined below the reader must keep in mind that no assessment tool should ever be used in isolation and that self-report measures that do not have built-in reliability and validity scales may provide limited information. We concur with the conclusions of Bergstroem and Jensen who in their 1998 [76] review of psychosocial and behavioural assessment of chronic pain recommend the use of psychometrically sound instruments, and highlight that the purposes for the use of a measure have to be thoroughly considered in advance. They, and we, also emphasize that 'in clinical practice, each separate measure must be interpreted in a wider context, where clinical findings and judgements are considered as a whole'.

Once one has found a test that might be used, it should be evaluated on clinical utility. This is done by considering the dimensions of the test, including: psychometric properties, suitability for use with head and neck pain patients (where possible norms for this population), ease of use for the patients seen (reading level, clarity of instructions, duration of test taking, etc.) and clinical value for the evaluator (including ease of interpretation, range of information provided, availability of a manual, etc.). When all these dimensions are present one has found a clinically useful tool.

Review articles

A good source for a review of the broad range of psychometric tests available is *Buros' Mental Measurements Yearbook* [77], which is updated every year. As well, the Buros Institute has a website at www.unl.edu/buros at which the reader can search their databanks for tests, reviews and articles. For most general readers, this source offers too many choices.

Bergstroem and Jensen [76] have provided an article that gives clinicians information on basic features to consider when selecting instruments specific to the assessment of chronic benign pain. As well, this article provides a review of some psychosocial and behavioural measurement methods in this area. As with the biopsychosocial considerations delineated above, specific areas of assessment are sometimes difficult to isolate. While the emphasis and specificity of every test differs, most of the assessment tools described below provide a range of information covering a number of different areas that affect our patients' functional capacity. Most of these are generic for all pain patients, as there are few psychological assessment tools specific to head

and neck pain. Where such tools exist, they are highlighted in the discussion.

There are a number of different areas that are assessed in working with a pain population. These include: measures of pain severity, pain behaviour, pain coping strategies, physical functioning, emotional, psychological and cognitive functioning, psychosocial factors at work and home and quality of life [76]. Personality features [78], psychiatric symptoms, reliability of self-report, and self-rated disability are also components of relevance to understanding these patients and have all been included in the discussion which follows.

Turk and colleagues [11,79] have made repeated appeals for comprehensive, integrated, assessment of all chronic pain patients. In their review they advocated for three primary axes in a 'multiaxial' approach. These axes were physical, psychosocial and behavioural functioning. Each axis added to the overall understanding of the chronic pain patient's condition, and no one axis could be considered in isolation. Furthermore, they argued that developing such a multiaxial assessment of pain, or MAP, ought to be incorporated into the IASP taxonomy for chronic pain syndromes.

More recently, Penzien *et al.* [20] in their excellent overview of approaching the assessment of all headache patients proposed a broader multiaxial evaluation. They proposed five axes very similar to, but not identical with, the axes commonly used for DSM diagnoses of psychiatric disorders. The authors proposed that information be collected on:

Axis I   – Physical symptoms of headache and headache diagnosis
Axis II – Psychological/behavioural factors
Axis III – Co-existing physical conditions
Axis IV – Environmental, social, and cultural factors, and
Axis V   – Functional capacity/disability

Healthcare providers in multidisciplinary settings will notice that the accurate diagnosis of the headache syndrome, or of the level of WAD provides the starting point for the complete evaluation. While attention to the co-existing physical conditions (Axis III) and a broad variety of psychological, behavioural, social and cultural factors is essential for a complete understanding of the headache patient, no instruments for this Axis will be reviewed.

What follows is an overview of a range of measurement tools. Some of these, such as the multidimensional pain inventory are broadly used with many kinds of chronic pain patients and also cover a range of psychological domains, while others, such as the cogniphobia scale are more narrowly focused on headache patients, and are also domain-specific, assessing only one variable. The authors have tried to present the best choices available for general clinical usage, but highlight that readers should consider both the specific attributes of each test, as well as the characteristics of the population they work with.

Measuring the pain experience (Axis I)

Martin [14] covers the most important areas of history, pathognomonic signs and the key clinical facets of the person's pain experience. These are incorporated into the Psychological Assessment of Headache Questionnaire (PAHQ). It is structured to permit an easy way of understanding the diagnostic significance of the clinical information collected for making a diagnosis using the International Headache Society [80] nosology for headache syndromes, as well as alerts for referral to a neurologist. Also helpful in establishing a diagnosis is a good clinical interview of the pain patient. Readers are urged to read an excellent overview of structured interviewing provided by Doleys *et al.* [81].

Ancillary information may be needed on pain severity, or other attributes of the pain. A common procedure in evaluation of pain severity is to ask the patient to indicate their pain on a scale of 1 to 10, or to mark such boxes. Such unidimensional measures are not adequate for capturing the character of that person's pain experience. Slightly better is to ask the patient for their usual level of pain in the past week, their maximal level of pain and their minimum level. However, any comprehensive pain evaluation should assess multidimensional aspects of the pain, as well as multiaxial components [11]. The best known multidimensional measure has been the McGill Pain Questionnaire (MPQ.

The McGill Pain Questionnaires [58,82] were developed in order to characterize the

fullness of an individual's experience and responses, which comprise their unique pain experience. The resulting profile of responses would give a complete multidimensional verbal hologram of the person's internal pain experience. It would allow an individual expression of the pain experience, yet it also allowed reliable and objective measurement of the same phenomena repeatedly over time.

The original purpose of the MPQ was to allow an instrument that could demonstrate the effectiveness of different treatment approaches with a variety of pain patients. Whatever the characteristics of a pain patient's pain, the MPQ could quantify it and demonstrate the effectiveness of treatments that ameliorated the pain. Although it is sometimes taken to be conceptually derived from the gate control theory, Melzack's descriptions make it clear that it was actually empirically derived and subsequently shaped into the three components proposed by gate control theory, and by the idea that a scientific measurement tool should seek to quantify the underlying anatomical realities that theory has proposed.

The McGill Pain Questionnaire had its origins in Melzack and Torgerson's [83] review of the clinical literature which yielded 102 adjectives describing the pain experience. They then selected 78 adjectives in 20 subclasses, based on the consideration of balancing parsimony with representing all qualitative properties of the pain experience. However, only the first 16 subclasses of descriptors really follow from the three theoretical components of the model delineated by Melzack and Casey [84]. The last four subclasses are described as 'miscellaneous': but they are not miscellaneous to pain description, only miscellaneous to the theoretical model.

Melzack and Casey [84] made the argument that the final conscious pain experience is derived from the contributions from three components of brain functioning. These three anatomical subsystems are the sensory, motivational and central control determinants. They proposed that sensory inputs to the pain experience include spatial, temporal and magnitude information from the hurt tissue at the periphery. The affective inputs include contributions from the aversive drive system and its corollary experience of negative affects. Finally, they outline that cognitive factors include the meaning of the pain-producing situation, as well as previous experiences including cultural factors, and anxiety and attentional effects.

Interestingly, where the McGill Pain Questionnaire is most inadequate is in evaluating the cognitive component of the pain experience. Although three components are delineated, the third factor is represented by only one set of five adjectives. It certainly cannot be taken as a measure of the cognitive processes that mediate the pain experience. Subsequent factor analytic studies have had difficulty in corroborating the factor structure of the measure, mostly for this reason. On the other hand, the MPQ is excellent in delineating the affective attributes of the pain experience for the person, and norms are available for many pain patient subgroups [85], although headache and whiplash are not among them.

The problems with the MPQ include that it takes a long time to administer (up to 20 minutes), and requires a very good comprehension of English. In addition, the pain information it gives does not help to answer any diagnostic questions. The more recent Short Form [82] overcomes some of the major problems of administering the questionnaire to clinic patients. It takes only 2–5 minutes. But it didn't correct the problem of the underlying factor matrix [86,87]. Overall, the MPQ provides an excellent picture of the unique attributes of the pain experience for that person, but it is susceptible to being easily 'faked' by those simulating whiplash pain [88].

Other alternatives exist but have been less common in pain research. One alternative to the problem of faking is to incorporate psychophysiological recording measures into pain evaluations [89,90], but these are generally more difficult to administer.

Psychological and behavioural factors (Axis II)

Cognition and beliefs

The broad range of cognitive-behavioural measures that are now available to measure chronic pain phenomena will assess pain beliefs, cognitive errors (catastrophizing), self-efficacy and coping strategies. The Multidimensional Pain Inventory (MPI) [91] and the Behavioural Assessment of Pain (BAP) [92] are probably the best single instruments which evaluate a cross-section of this cognitive domain, but if more specific questions require answers, then domain specific measures can be found [93,94]. Neither measure was developed specifically for head and neck pain patients, but the MPI will reference the result obtained with a headache pain norm group. One of the only psychometric tools designed specifically for the headache population is Martin *et al*.'s [95] locus of control scale.

Multidimensional pain inventory

Although few studies have reported item-level factor analyses [94] the West Haven-Yale Multidimensional Pain Inventory (WHYMPI, or MPI) [89] is frequently used in clinical evaluation and research with chronic pain patients. The MPI is a 52-item inventory divided into three parts, each of which contains several subscales. The first part evaluates five dimensions of the pain experience while Part II looks at the responses of significant others to communications of pain. The patients' report of their participation in four categories of common daily activities comprises the third part of the MPI.

As noted by Kerns *et al* [91] the assets of the MPI include its brevity and clarity, its strong psychometric properties, its foundation in psychological theory, and its multidimensional focus. The test is available from the University of Pittsburgh [91].

Behavioural assessment of pain questionnaire

The Behavioural Assessment of Pain Questionnaire (BAP) [92] is a questionnaire which permits the comparison of the patient's answers to a variety of pain related questions, to similar answers provided by a normative sample of similar chronic pain patients who have been experiencing subacute or chronic benign pain. The normative sample was composed of over 600 patients. This assessment provides information on functional level of the patient, pain perception, coping mechanisms as well as providing information on the patient's perceptions of being helped by their doctors. While the BAP provides a lot of clinically useful information we have not found the reliability and validity scales to be particularly useful. We understand that the authors are working to revise the test, to shorten its length and further improve scales.

Fear of pain

One of the main problems with pain patients is that they become very fearful of undertaking activities which could bring on pain. Todd [96] coined the term 'kinesiophobia' for this tendency to avoid activities in order to avoid increased pain. He emphasized that these patients experienced a great deal of anxiety about triggering exacerbations of their pain. This should be distinguished from psychiatric anxiety disorders. Other authors have described the same phenomenon as avoidance learning [97], operant conditioning [6] or activity intolerance [98]. It is definitely one of the most powerful clinical problems which can prevent patients from making their best efforts at rehabilitation [96]. Anxiety has also been implicated in reducing musculoskeletal pain thresholds for normal young adults. Todd also emphasized that the evaluator unfamiliar with pain patients, could mistakenly take the inconsistent efforts of the kinesiophobic patient as an indication of malingering.

Todd designed the Tampa Scale of Kinesiophobia [96,99] to measure its occurrence in chronic pain patients, and is a reliable measure of self-reported fear of movement (re-injury) in this population. This test looks at levels of fear and avoidance of physical movement, but has no response-style scales to assess whether patients exaggerate their responses, and to what degree. Nevertheless, this test should be considered in treatment planning, especially with patients with variable motivation and results.

Other questionnaires seeking to measure the same process include Gross's [100] Pain Anxiety Symptom Scale (PASS), and Waddell *et al.*'s [101] Fear Avoidance Beliefs Questionnaire (FABQ). Gross's PASS scale evaluates four separate factors that make up its anxiety rating: fearful appraisal, cognitive anxiety, physiological anxiety and escape/avoidance. However, none of these tests incorporates a validity scale to assess the patient's response style. Moreover, all three scales were developed for general musculoskeletal chronic pain. Only recently have Todd and colleagues [75,102] developed the Cogniphobia, or C-scale, to specifically measure the impact of

headaches on the individual's activities and beliefs.

Other emotional states in pain

The measurement of emotions is difficult at the best of times. When patients are in pain, they are sometimes not ready to think about other dimensions of their experience, and hence may not attend to the task of providing careful reflection on their experience. For this reason it is often helpful to discuss the reasons why understanding the emotional concomitants of pain can be very helpful for treating the headache. With a thorough discussion of how to use analogue scales, and with some trial-and-error learning on how to convey internal feelings with ratings, visual analogue ratings of depression, anxiety, frustration and anger can be discriminated and included in assessment and monitoring activities.

The Visual Analogue Scales described by Price [103,104] and his colleagues can provide useful insights into the emotions that the person is experiencing. As an alternative to the VAS, one could use the Profile of Mood States [105]. In our experience it is always helpful to use the mood ratings as a basis for further inquiry into the contexts in which the most intense moods were experienced.

The MPQ affective scales can also be helpful in understanding a patient's affective experiences related to their pain. However, very few other scales provide information about mood. The MPI has a subscale called 'affective distress', but this score is the sum of three questions on the level of depression, anxiety and frustration the person has experienced with their pain. The BAP includes a subscale called Kroenig's factor, which represents a mixture of depressive and anxiety symptoms. Neither of these last two scales is focused on emotions. They are closer to measuring psychiatric symptomatology rather than emotional states. These two should not be confused with each other. The examiner using the scales should be clear on the differences between the two before undertaking such assessments.

Behavioural factors

Observation of the patient during a consultation is very important in coming to an understanding about that patient's way of functioning with their pain. As well as paying attention to the elements of the mental status of the patient during the interview, it is also important to observe the way they communicate pain, avoid certain movements or activities and how they persist with their efforts across the period of the consultation [106]. Do they grimace, get out of their chair, etc?

An early effort to conduct such behavioural observations in a more systematic way was Keefe and Block's [107] protocol for evaluating the pain behaviours a patient conveyed in a 10-minute time frame. The patient is asked to proceed through a standardized set of activities for specified periods of time (sitting, standing, walking, reclining), the behaviour is videotaped, and an assessor later scores the number and kind of pain behaviours observed. Pain behaviours of interest included guarding, bracing, rubbing, grimacing and sighing.

Other authors have pointed out that patient behaviour is not always consistent with the degree of pathology noted in physical examination, or that patients can dramatize their pain experiences through their behaviour [108–110]. These behavioural signs, often referred to as Waddell's signs, can be useful in understanding the patient, especially when the examiner is the doctor conducting the physical examination of the patient. The Waddell Equivalency Scale (WES) was designed to elicit non-organic signs of pain. Because the WES comes from a paper-and-pencil test rather than a physical examination, it can be used with patients whose pain locus is other than the back [111].

Self-monitoring of headaches and related behaviour, such as drug use, can be very helpful and informative about the patient's life situation and patterns of headache activity. Martin [14] describes strategies for conducting both time sampling, diaries, as well as event sampling, descriptions of specific events of importance to the patient. These techniques are especially helpful in seeing the broader 24-hour pattern of the patient's life, which otherwise the patient may not be aware of, or not think to discuss with the physician.

Evaluating psychiatric involvement

The most widely used instrument for evaluating pain patients for evidence of psychiatric symptomatology [21] as well as distinctive patterns of pain problems has been the MMPI (now the MMPI-2 [112]. However, it is a test which can only be administered by a psychologist with an appropriate amount of training in working with the scale and with pain patients. Other similar tests in widespread use today are the Millon Health Behaviour Inventory [113] and the Personality Assessment Inventory [114], as full spectrum psychological tests. For assessment of depression one has a choice between The Center for Epidemiologic Studies Depression Scale [71], and the Beck Depression Inventory [115], and for anxiety the State-Trait Anxiety Inventory [116] in focused monosymptomatic assessment. As with the MMPI-2, these are useful, but availability of some may be restricted to psychologists. In addition, there are tests used in different languages, such as the Freiburg Personality Inventory [54] and the Well-Being Questionnaire [54], which may be more appropriate for certain clinical populations, and certain research questions.

Nevertheless, there are other scales that can be used for purposes of screening, or to determine the benefit of referring the patient for a full psychological assessment. Where such a referral is made, it should be borne in mind that not all psychologists have experience in working with pain patients. In addition, on occasion there will be concomitant head injuries and an assessment by a neuropsychologist may be more helpful than a general clinical psychologist.

The Symptom Check List (SCL-90-R)
The SCL-90-R is often used in both clinical work and research with pain patients. It evolved from the Hopkins Symptom Checklist, which had scales for the most commonly presented psychiatric symptomatology, including scales for somatization, obsessive-compulsiveness, interpersonal sensitivity, depression and anxiety [59,117]. Through the addition of scales for hostility, phobic anxiety, paranoid ideation and psychoticism, the SCL-90-R was more able to detect the broader range of psychiatric symptoms that patients most often complain of. The self-report has only 90 questions which makes it ideal for fairly quick administration. It can be hand scored, or sent for computer scoring.

The SCL-90-R was revised in the early 1990s and useful norms exist for whiplash patients

[118]. Although no validity scales are present on the instrument itself, Wallis and Bogduk [119] published the results for university students asked to fake the profile of a whiplash patient. The authors noted that the malingering students' profiles were strikingly different for both the SCL-90-R and the VAS pain ratings. However, pain scores for malingering students could not be distinguished from those of bona fide whiplash patients on the McGill Pain Questionnaire.

The SCL-90-R is available for use by all healthcare providers. It is a very useful tool for screening for the presence of psychiatric symptoms among pain patients. Its brevity is its greatest asset, and it does a good job of alerting the physician to the presence of possible psychiatric symptoms. On the other hand, it does not provide enough information to make specific diagnoses. With elevations above the levels seen among typical head and neck pain patients, referral to a psychologist or psychiatrist is recommended. The test is available from National Computer Systems (NCS) (http://assessments.ncs.com/assessments/tests/scl90r.htm).

Pain patient profile (P-3)

The P-3 inventory was developed by Tollison and Langle [120] to help identify patients who had psychological factors associated with their pain and physical symptoms. It consists of 48 items which load into four subscales: depression, anxiety, somatization and a validity scale assessing whether patients are trying to present themselves in a positive light. It takes 15 minutes to administer, and can be used as an effective screen to determine whether a psychological consultation would be helpful. Norms are available to compare results with both the community population as well as chronic pain patients. No norms are published for whiplash or headache populations specifically. The test is available from Multi-Health Systems (www.mhs.com).

Anxiety after trauma

Mayou and Bryant [39] and Mayou and Radanov [42] have emphasized that post-traumatic stress is often under-reported among the WAD population, and must be considered in early intervention and ongoing management. Recently Jaspers [121] presented evidence that treating only the anxiety caused

by the trauma, resolved the pain symptoms of the patient. This provides compelling evidence that identifying these factors is very important in treating some WAD patients. A number of resources exist which can help the doctor, or multidisciplinary team, to evaluate the existence of these problems among their patient population. Foa and her colleagues [122] published a test of PTSD. In addition, a recent publication by Turner and Lee [123] entitled, *Measures in Post Traumatic Stress Disorder: A Practitioner's Guide*, reviews a number of assessment measures which could be used. However, none of the above measures reviewed contain any validity scales, to evaluate the respondent's response style.

The Trauma Symptom Inventory (TSI) [124] corrects this problem, and provides a range of scales useful to understanding different elements of the presenting symptomatology of these patients. The inventory consists of 100 items designed to evaluate post-traumatic stress and other psychological sequelae of traumatic events. It reports scores for anxious arousal, depression, anger/irritability in addition to the different dimensions of PTSD itself. Ordering the test requires that the healthcare professional has had some training in statistics and test interpretation. The test is available at PAR's website (www.parinc.com/percouns/percouns.html).

Travel anxiety is ubiquitous among whiplash associated disorders [39,55]. Evaluation of travel anxiety has generally been assessed through clinical interview. A search for psychometric tests of travel anxiety did not turn up any tools developed specifically for this purpose.

Environmental, social and cultural factors (Axis IV)

The environment in which the pain patient grew up, and the one he finds himself in currently will both undoubtedly influence his behaviour. This is the 'social' part of the biopsychosocial model. Drummond and Holroyd [125] have discussed how the individual's past experiences, cultural experiences and beliefs about the self, the world and pain all shape the person's actual experience of the pain, and how they go about adapting to it. There are not very many resources available in this area, but two recent additions are worth mention. One focuses on the Asian American population [126], and the other is an edited text entitled *Cultural Issues in the Treatment of Anxiety* [127].

As well as the influence of the past, the way in which those around us respond to us currently will also impact on our level of anxiety, apprehension, confidence and general level of stress. All of those factors in turn will impact on the perception of pain, and more importantly on how we communicate these experiences to those close to us. Determining how the pain patient's current interactions will impact on the patient, most especially with those who they are closest to, is very important. The Multidimensional Pain Inventory includes social scales that provide measures of whether significant others are being overly solicitous, or punishing, in their responses; the Behavioural Assessment of Pain also provides feedback on the person's interactions with others. Finally, the patient should be interviewed for information on how they see others responding to them, whether they feel supported, and whether they evaluate the home environment to be stressful in any respect. Many times the most telling information about social interactions come from the clinical interview with the patient. The astute evaluator will always be asking the patient for examples of interactions, and times when these interactions were most difficult, and most helpful.

Functional abilities and disabilities (Axis V)

Quality of life

The SF-36 [128] is a short, self-administered survey of general health status which has been used a great deal with different groups of headache patients [33,34]. The SF-36 measures patients' functioning across eight dimensions including: physical functioning, role functioning – physical, bodily pain, general health, vitality, social functioning, role functioning – emotional and mental health. While the SF-36 has been referred to as 'the gold standard' [129], we see limitations in its use from a psychological perspective. While it provides a good overview of various areas of health status, it does not account for the personal meaningfulness of these areas from the patient's unique perspective. In the absence of any way of personalizing the ratings of different functions the information obtained is limited to counts of different types of rated data. Setting priorities for treatment requires making further determinations of meaningfulness.

A recent improvement on the SF-36 is the publication of the Treatment Outcomes in Pain Survey, or TOPS [130,131]. It has been designed to provide a reliable way to evaluate response to treatment. The measure consists of scales that evaluate lower and upper body limitations separately, perceived and objective family/social disability, objective work disability, as well as a range of cognitive and social factors important in multidisciplinary pain treatment programmes. The TOPS provides a range of information about the patient's response to treatment, helpful to the clinician and the patient, and sometimes required by third-party payers. Norms are provided for a mixed sample of 947 chronic pain patients. The TOPS had a greater sensitivity to changes seen in treatment than did the SF-36, and would seem to be a very promising tool for use in active multidisciplinary treatment programmes, where treatment needs will dictate treatment provided and response to treatment is periodically re-evaluated, as well as for disability assessments, where a range of information is usually required.

The Ferrans and Powers [132,133] Quality of Life Index provides a solution to this dilemma. This easy to use assessment rates the patients' satisfaction in 34 different areas and then asks the patient to rate the importance of each area for him or herself. The four subscale areas are: health and functioning subscale, socioeconomic subscale, psychological/spiritual subscale and the family subscale. The added dimension of asking the patient to rate the importance each area would appear to be very useful in treatment planning around quality-of-life issues.

Evaluating disability

Conducting impairment and disability evaluations is a very specialized kind of evaluation, which typically carries a great deal of importance to the patient as well as their family, and to all other players involved in providing the health care for that patient [60,74]. Because of its importance for the individual, the possibility that the person could exaggerate their experiences and difficulties must be borne in mind [60]. There are questionnaires that can help the evaluator get the patent's input in these matters, but in all cases other objective measures of pain and disability have to be obtained from a complete assessment.

Such assessments are all conducted by a systematic clinical interview of the patient. As well as history, mechanism of injury, current pain and psychological status, the evaluator must evaluate the factors that are predisposing to disability. Martelli *et al.* [75] have devised what can be considered a prototype of factors to be considered with his Vulnerability to Disability Rating Scale. However, this can only be taken as one consideration, as it has not been validated with any clinical population. Indeed, there is no information available on how reliably the scales can be used by clinicians, and whether they may need revision or adjustment with particular patient populations. Nevertheless, this scale provides a useful starting point for the disability evaluator as well as the clinician interested in heading off problems before they have become overwhelming for the patient. In this context, the work of Radanov and his colleagues, in their longitudinal study of Swiss whiplash patients.

Millard [134] provided a review article on questionnaires for assessing pain-related disability. Millard reviews 14 questionnaires that can be used for assessing pain-related disability and summarizes their comparative attributes. This article organizes the questionnaires into the three groups of: (1) back pain, (2) pain without reference to site, or (3) illness without reference to pain. Each questionnaire is reviewed in terms of background, psychometric findings (reliability and validity) and implementation. Most of the questionnaires included in this review include information about specific activities of daily living, although they vary in terms of structure, content, and intended applications. However, none of those reviewed related specifically to headache or whiplash. The one test in this domain is the Neck Disability Index.

Neck Disability Index

A useful patient questionnaire for use with head and neck pain patients is the Neck Disability Index (NDI) devised by Vernon and Mior [135,136]. This is a 10-question scale which asks the patient to indicate the degree to which their normal activities are interfered with by their head and neck pain. The scale is easy to use and quickly yields the person's estimate of the degree of disability they suffer from (expressed as a percentage). Comparison with physical examination results is essential to understand what this self-report may mean.

Pain Symptom Ratings questionnaire

The Pain Symptom Ratings (PSR) was designed to assess the legitimacy of a pain patient's complaint, by measuring the reliability and validity of pain patients' self-reports of pain and pain related disability. It measures 20 factors including mood, somatization, common and highly unusual symptom endorsement, activity limitation, response consistency, instrumental pain and others. The instrument was standardized on a sample of over 2300 chronic pain patients, males and females, ranging in age between 21 and 65. We have found this test to be particularly helpful when one has to make determinations on the credibility of the patient's self-report, whether it be its reliability or validity.

The PSR extends the methodology which Rogers [137] introduced into assessing malingering among psychiatric patients to the domain of disability assessments involving chronic pain. The scale incorporates a systematic approach to evaluating many dimensions of importance in establishing the reliability and validity of self-reports of subjective phenomena. Most importantly, the PSR has been validated with 98 chronic pain patients in a 'malingering clinical group'. To be included in the criterion group a patient had to have positive results on all three clinical indicators of malingering. The three criteria were (1) invalid protocols on administered psychometric tests, (2) positive results on non-organic signs tests, and (3) elevated results on measured coefficients of variation. Subjects who only manifested two or these three features were not included in the 'malingering' cohort. The PSR also evaluates four psychosocial factors that are sometimes confused with malingering, to understand the interrelationship of many factors that could contribute to a patient's self-reports.

The test has good psychometric properties, consisting of 120 statements that the patient evaluates. It takes about a 30 minutes for most patients to complete. While this test is available to most health professionals it is intended for professionals trained in the diagnosis and treatment of pain conditions, who also have a reasonable understanding of statistics and the appropriate interpretation of psychometrically derived tests. The results of this test, like all tests used in disability determinations, are intended to be used as apart of an interdisciplinary assessment of the legitimacy of a patient's pain and pain-related disability, and must be weighted against other clinical findings of the validity and reliability of patients' self-reports. The test can be obtained from Human Development Consulting (at http://www.hdcus.com) [138].

SUMMARY

The tests described above provide a range of tests that are psychometrically sound and allow formal evaluation of factors shown by research to be important to clinical management of head and neck pain patients. In our view the tests presented provide a useful cross-section of tests assessing different attributes of the pain experience and psychological processes that interact with it. No test answers every question; and every test is subject to any response bias that a given patient may bring with him or her into the testing situation.

Readers interested in reading further in this areas can turn to many sources including the very comprehensive *Handbook of Pain Assessment* [139], as well as numerous reviews and articles [14,81,88,140–142]. Of particular value are two recent reviews of a number of tests assessing cognitive factors in pain including locus of control, coping, extraversion-introversion and perceived optimism [4,78]. Also, readers looking for more testing resources can access the search engine at www.ericae.net, which can locate a broad range of published tests, as well as reviews of them. Also useful in locating material on the Internet is an excellent 'search engine of search engines' (which can be accessed at www.dogpile.com).

Concluding remarks

As well as assessment tools, there are other psychological resources available to help chronic pain patients. Corey [143] has published a self-help guide to help patients with chronic pain to assess and change problematic pain behaviours in a systematic way. This 200-page book provides a comprehensive and multidimensional approach for the pain patient to follow in making a series of changes in behaviour and attitude. Although meant for patients to read and apply, it provides a clear and easy to read understanding of changing psychological factors to manage chronic pain more successfully.

We trust that this chapter has provided a perspective which will help non-psychologists on the multidisciplinary team to understand why they should be open to thinking about psychological aspects of a patient's pain problem, and to be more comfortable in using specific tools to clarify these factors in individual cases. We are sure that efforts made to think psychologically about the patient's situation will make real contributions to more effective treatment. For psychologists who are routinely involved in assessment and treatment of motor-vehicle-accident victims, a very useful resource is the recently published book by Blanchard and Hickling [144] which reviews assessment and treatment issues specific to this general population in great detail.

We have progressed a long way from where Melzack and Wall initiated this journey, bringing psychosocial factors into the arena of pain evaluation. Turk and Rudy extended this perspective by proposing that no evaluation of chronic pain was comprehensive unless it also evaluated the psychosocial and behavioural factors involved. We hope that this chapter has brought the reader closer to integrating this perspective into their clinical practice by providing a range of tools to help in their treatment of head and neck pain complaints. Even so, all who work with head and neck pain patients realize how much further we have yet to go, to provide the range of treatments that meet the range of challenges presented by our patients.

REFERENCES

1. Pargeon KL, Hailey BJ. Barriers to effective cancer pain management: a review of the literature. *J Pain Symp Manag* 1999;**18**:358–368.
2. Turk DC Meichenbaum D, Genest M. *Pain and Behavioral Medicine*. The Guilford Press, 1983.
3. Turk DC. (1996). Biopsychosocial perspective on chronic pain. In *Psychological Approaches in Pain Management* (eds. RJ Gatchel, DC Turk), The Guilford Press, pp 3–32, 1986.
4. Keefe FJ, Bradley L, Main C. Psychological Assessment of the Pain Patient for the General Clinician. In *Pain 1999 – An Updated Review*. Seattle, WA: IASP Press, pp 21–232, 1999.
5. Turk DC, Okifuji A. Evaluating the role of physical, operant, cognitive, and affective factors in the pain behaviors of chronic pain patients. *Behav Mod* 1997;**21**(3);259–280.
6. Melzack R, Wall PD. Pain mechanisms: a new theory. *Science* 1965;**150**:971–979.
7. Melzack R. Pain: past, present and future. *Can J Exp Psychol* 1993;**47**(4):615–629.
8. Melzack R. Pain – An overview. *Acta Anaesth Scand* 1999;**43**:880–884.
9. Turk DC. The role of psychological factors in chronic pain. *Acta Anaesth Scand* 1999;**43**:885–888.
10. Mongini F, Defilippi N, Negro CG, et al. Psychosocial issues: Their importance in predicting disability, response to treatment and search for compensation. *Neurol Clin* 1999;**17**(1):149–166.
11. Turk DC, Rudy TE. Towards a comprehensive assessment of chronic pain patients: A multi-axial model. *Behav Res Therap* 1987; **25**(4):237–249.
12. Price DD. The Dimensions of Pain Experience. In *Psychological Mechanisms of Pain and Analgesia, Progress in Pain Research and Management* 1999;**15**:43–66.
13. Johnson PR. Psychological factors influencing headaches. In *Headache: Diagnosis and Treatment* (eds. CD Tollison, RS Kunkel), Baltimore: Williams & Wilkins, pp. 31–37, 1993.
14. Martin PR. *Psychological Management of Chronic Headaches*. The Guilford Press, 1993.
15. Packard RC. Epidemiology and Pathogenesis of Posttraumatic Headache. *Journal of Head Trauma and Rehabilitation* 1999;**14**:9–20.
16. Drummond PD. Psychological mechanisms of migraine. In *The Headaches* (eds. JP Olesen, P Tfelt-Hansen, KM Welch), 2nd edn, Baltimore: Lippincott Williams & Wilkins, pp. 313–8, 2000.
17. Andrasik F, Passchier J. Psychological mechanisms of tension-type headache. In *The Headaches* (eds. JP Olesen, P Tfelt-Hansen, and KM Welch), 2nd edn, Baltimore: Lippincott Williams & Wilkins, pp. 599–603, 2000.
18. Samuels MA. Headache Syndromes. *Audio-Digest Psychiat* 2000;**29**(1).
19. Passchier J, de Boo M, Quaak HZ, et al. Health-related quality of life of chronic headache patients is predicted by the emotional component of their pain. *Headache* 1996;**36**:556–560.
20. Penzien, D, Jeanetta, C, Holroyd, K. Psychological assessment of the recurrent headache sufferer. In *Headache: Diagnosis and Treatment* (eds C. Tollison and R.S. Kunkel), Baltimore: Williams and Wilkins, pp. 39–49, 1993.
21. American Psychiatric Association. American Psychiatric Association Press. *Diagnostic and Statistical Manual of Mental Disorders*, 4th edn, 1994.
22. Kinder BN, Curtiss G, Kalichman S. Cluster analyses of headache-patient MMPI scores: A cross-validation study. *Psychol Assess: J Consult Clin Psychol* 1991;**3**:226–231.
23. Kinder BN, Curtiss G, Kalichman S. Affective differences among empirically derived subgroups of headache patients. *J Psychol Assess* 1992;**58**:516–524.
24. Ustun TB, Sartorius N (eds.). *Mental Illness in General Health Care: An International Study*, Chichester: John Wiley and Sons, Inc., 1994.
25. Wade JB, Dougherty LM, Hart RP, et al. Patterns of normal personality structure among chronic pain patients. *Pain* 1992;**48**:37–43.
26. Williams DE, Thompson JK, Haber JD, et al. MMPI and headache: A special focus on differential diagnosis, prediction of treatment outcome, and patient-treatment matching. *Pain* 1986;**24**:143–158.
27. Robinson MD, Geisser ME, Dieter JN, et al. The relationship between MMPI cluster membership and diagnostic category in headache patients. *Headache* 1991;**31**:111–115.
28. Kurlman RG, Hursey KG, Mathew NT. Assessment of chronic refractory headache: The role of the MMPI-2. *Headache* 1992;**32**:432–435.
29. Cella DF. Quality of life: Concepts and definition. *J Pain Symp Manage* 1994;**9**:186–192.
30. Skevington SM. Investigating the relationship between pain and discomfort and quality of life, using the WHOQUOL. *Pain* 1998;**76**:395–406.
31. Henriksson CM. Living with continuous muscular pain – patient perspectives:I. Encounters and consequences. *Scand J Caring Sci* 1995;**9**:67–76.
32. Becker N, Thomsen AB, Olsen AK, et al. Pain epidemiology and health related quality of life in chronic non-malignant pain patients referred to a Danish multidisciplinary pain center. *Pain* 1997;**73**:393–400.

33. Solomon GD. Evolution of the measurement of quality of life in migraine. *Neurol* 1997;**48**(Suppl 3):S10–S15.

34. Solomon GD, Skobieranda FG, Gragg LA. Does quality of life differ among headache diagnoses? Analysis using the medical outcomes study instrument. *Headache* 1994;**34**:143–147.

35. Osterhaus JT, Townsend RJ, Gandek B, *et al.* Measuring the functional status and well-being of patients with migraine headache. *Headache* 1994;**34**:337–343.

36. Burckhardt CS, Clark SR, O'Reilly CA, *et al.* Pain-coping strategies of women with fibro-myalgia: Relationship to pain, fatigue, and quality of life. *J Musculoskel Pain* 1997;**5**:5–21.

37. Ward SE, Carlson-Dakes K, Hughes SH, *et al.* The impact of quality of life on patient-related barriers to pain management. *Res Nurs Health* 1998;**21**:405–413.

38. Myers TC, Wittrock DA, Foreman GW. Appraisal of subjective stress in individuals with tension-type headache: The influence of baseline measures. *J Behav Med* 1998; **21**:469–484.

39. Mayou R, Bryant B. Outcome of 'whiplash' neck injury. *Injury* 1996l;**27**:617–623.

40. Gargan M, Bannister G, Main C, *et al.* The behavioural response to whiplash injury. *J Bone Joint Surg* 1997;**79**-B:523–526.

41. Teasell RW, Shapiro AP. Cervical Flexion-Extension/Whiplash Injuries. In *Spine: State of the Art Reviews* (eds. RW Teasell, AP Shapiro), Hanley & Belfus, Inc., p. 7, 1993.

42. Mayou R, Radanov BP. Whiplash neck injury. *J Psychosomat Res* 1996;**40**:461–474.

43. Teasell RW. The Clinical Picture of Whiplash Injuries: An overview. In *Spine: State of the Art Reviews* (eds. RW Teasell, AP Shapiro), Hanley & Belfus, Inc, 1993;**7**:379–383.

44. Kreeft JH. Headache Following Whiplash. In *Spine: State of the Art Reviews* (eds. RW Teasell, AP Shapiro), Hanley & Belfus, Inc. 1993;**7**:391–402.

45. Merskey H. Psychological Consequences of Whiplash. In *Spine: State of the Art Reviews* (eds. RW Teasell, AP Shapiro), Hanley & Belfus, Inc. 1993;**7**:471–840.

46. Teasell RW, Shapiro AP, Mailis A. Medical Management of Whiplash Injuries. In *Spine: State of the Art Reviews* (eds. RW Teasell, AP Shapiro), Hanley & Belfus, Inc. 1993;**7**:481–499.

47. Shapiro AP, Roth RS. The effect of litigation on recovery from whiplash. In *Spine: State of the Art Reviews* (eds. RW Teasell, AP Shapiro), Hanley & Belfus, Inc. 1993;**7**:531–556

48. Bannister G, Gargan M. Prognosis of Whiplash Injuries. In *Spine: State of the Art Reviews* (eds.

RW Teasell, AP Shapiro), Hanley & Belfus, Inc. 1993;**7**:557–569.

49. Spitzer WO, Skovron ML, Salmi LR, *et al.* Scientific monograph of the Quebec Task Force on Whiplash-Associated-Disorders: Redefining 'Whiplash' and its management. *Spine* 1995;**20**:7–73S.

50. Freeman MD, Croft AC, Rossignol AM. 'Whiplash Associated Disorders: Redefining whiplash and its management' by the Quebec Task Force: A critical evaluation. *Spine* 1998;**23**:1043–1049.

51. Radanov BP, Sturzenegger M, Di Stefano G. Long-term outcome after whiplash injury: a 2-years follow-up considering features of accident mechanism, somatic, radiological and psychological findings. *Medicine* 1995;**74**:281–297.

52. Radanov BP, Sturzenegger M. The effect of accident mechanisms and initial findings on the long-term outcome of whiplash injury. *J Musculoskel Pain* 1996;**4**:47–59.

53. Reitav J, McClean K, Cook T, *et al.* Changes in sleep and muscular pain thresholds in college students during examinations. (in press).

54. Radanov BP, Begre S, Sturzenegger M, *et al.* Course of psychological variables in whiplash injury. In *Whiplash Injuries* (eds. R Gunzburg, M Szpalski), Lippincott-Raven, pp.151–159, 1998.

55. Mayou R, Tyndel S, Bryant B. Long-term outcome of motor vehicle accident injury. *Psychosom Med* 1997;**59**:578–584.

56. Wallis BJ, Lord SM, Bogduk N. Resolution of psychological distress of whiplash patients following treatment by radio frequency neuro-tomy:a randomized, double-blind, placebo-controlled trial. *Pain* 1997;**73**:15–22.

57. Lord SM, Barnsley L, Wallis BJ, *et al.* Chronic cervical zygapophysial joint pain after whiplash:a placebo-controlled prevalence study. *Spine* 1996;**21**:1737–1744.

58. Melzack R. The McGill Pain Questionnaire: Major properties and scoring methods. *Pain* 1975;**1**:277–299.

59. Derogatis LR. *Administration, Scoring and Procedures Manual – II. Clinical Psychometric Research*, 1983.

60. Bellamy R. Compensation Neurosis. *Clin Orthop Rel Res* 1997;**336**:94–106.

61. Schrader H, Obelieniene D, Bovim G, *et al.* Natural evolution of late whiplash syndrome outside the medico-legal context. *Lancet* 1996;**347**:1207–1211.

62. Obelieniene D, Bovim G, Schrader H, *et al.* Headache after whiplash: a historical cohort study outside the medico-legal context. *Cephalalgia* 1998;**18**:559–564.

63. Evans RW. Some observations on whiplash injuries. *Neurol Clin* 1992;**10**:975.

64. Freeman MD, Croft AC. The controversy over late whiplash: Are chronic symptoms after whiplash real? In *Whiplash Injuries* (eds. R Gunzburg, M Szpalski), Lippincott-Raven, pp161–162, 1998.

65. Ramadan NM, Keidel M. Chronic posttraumatic headache. In *The Headaches* (eds. J Olesen, P Tfelt-Hansen, KM Welch), 2nd edn, Baltimore: Williams & Wilkins, pp. 771–780, 2000.

66. Radanov BP. Common whiplash – research findings revisited. *J Rheumatol* 1997;**24**:623–625.

67. Ferrari R, Russell AS. The whiplash syndrome – common sense revisited. *J Rheumatol* 1997;**24**:618–623.

68. Editorial Commentary. The rheumatologist and chronic whiplash syndrome. *J Rheumatol* 1997;**24**:618–625.

69. Correspondence. *J Rheumatol* 1998;**25**:1437–1440.

70. Correspondence. *J Rheumatol* 1999;**26**:1205–1120.

71. Cassidy JD, Carroll LJ, Cote P, *et al.* Effect of eliminating compensation for pain and suffering on the outcome of insurance claims for whiplash injury. *N Engl J Med* 2000;**342**:1179–1186.

72. Fordyce WE. On the nature of illness and disability. *Clin Orthop Rel Res* 1997;**333**:47–51.

73. *Guides to the Evaluation of Permanent Impairment*, American Medical Association Press, 1993.

74. Loeser JD, Sullivan M. Doctors, Diagnosis, and Disability. *Clin Orthop Rel Res* 1997;**336**:61–66.

75. Martelli MF, Grayson RL, Zasler ND. Posttraumatic Headaches: Neuropsychological and psychological effects and treatment implications. *J Head Trauma Rehab* 1999;**14**:49–69.

76. Bergstroem G, Jensen IB. Psychosocial and behavioural assessment of chronic pain: recommendations for clinicians and researchers. *Scand J Behav Ther* 1998;**27**:114–123.

77. Buros Institute of Mental Measurements. In *Thirteenth Mental Measurements* (eds. JC Impara, BS Plake), Yearbook, Mental Measurements Press, 1998.

78. Gatchel RJ ,Weisberg JN, eds. *Personality Characteristics of Pain Patients*, American Psychological Association Press, 1999.

79. Turk DC, Okifuji A. Assessment of patients' reporting of pain: An integrated perspective. *Lancet* 1999;**353**:1784–1788.

80. International Headache Society. Classification and diagnostic criteria for headache disorders, cranial neuralgias and facial pain. *Cephalgia* 1988;**8**:1–96.

81. Doleys D, Murray J, Klapow J, *et al.* Psychological assessment of the pain patient. In *The Management of Pain* (eds. MA Ashburn, LJ Rice), Edinburgh: Churchill Livingstone, pp.27–49, 1997.

82. Melzack R. The short-form McGill Pain Questionnaire. *Pain* 1987;**30**:191–197.

83. Melzack R, Torgerson WS. On the language of pain. *Anesthesiol* 1971;**34**:50–59.

84. Melzack R, Casey KL. Sensory, motivational and central control determinants of pain: a new conceptual model. In *The Skin Senses* (ed. D Kenshalo), Springfield, IL: Thomas, 1968.

85. Wilkie DJ, Savedra MC, Holzemer WL, *et al.* Use of the McGill Pain Questionnaire to measure pain: a meta-analysis. *Nurs Res* 1990:36–41.

86. Turk DC, Rudy TE, Salovey P. The McGill Pain Questionnaire reconsidered: confirming the factor structure and examining appropriate uses. *Pain* 1985;**21**:385–397.

87. Holroyd K, Holm A, Keefe F, *et al.* A multicenter evaluation of the McGill Pain Questionnaire: results from more than 1700 chronic pain patients. *Pain* 1992;**48**:301–311.

88. White P. Pain measurement. In *Principles and Practice of Pain Management* (ed. CA Warfield), McGraw-Hill, pp. 27–42, 1993.

89. Flor H, Miltner W, Birbaumer N. Psychophysiological recording methods. In *Handbook of Pain Assessment* (eds. DC Turk, R Melzack), The Guilford Press, pp. 169–192, 1992.

90. Price DD, Harkins SW. Psychophysiological approaches to pain measurement and assessment. In *Handbook of Pain Assessment* (eds. DC Turk, R Melzack), The Guilford Press, pp. 111–134, 1992.

91. Kerns RD, Turk DC, Rudy TE. The West Haven-Yale Multidimensional Pain Inventory (WHYMPI). *Pain* 1985;**23**:345–356. (Available from the University of Pittsburgh, Pain Evaluation and Treatment Institute, 4601 Baum Boulevard, Pittsburgh, PA, 15213–1217 USA.)

92. Lewandowski MJ, Tearnan BH. Behavioural Assessment of Pain Questionnaire. Pendrake, Inc. (Available by e-mailing publisher at: editor@pendrake.com)

93. DeGood DE, Shutty MS Jr. Assessment of pain beliefs, coping, and self-efficacy. In *Handbook of Pain Assessment* (eds. DC Turk, R Melzack), The Guilford Press, pp. 214–234, 1992.

94. Riley JL, Zawacki TM, Robinson ME, *et al.* Empirical test of the factor structure of the West Haven-Yale Multidimensional Pain Inventory. *Clin J Pain* 1999;**15**:24–30.

95. Martin N, Holroyd KA, Penzien DB. The headache-specific locus of control scale:adaptation to recurrent headaches. *Headache* 1990;**30**:729–734.

96. Todd D. Kinesiophobia:the relationship between chronic pain and fear-induced disability. *Forens Exam* 1998;**7**:14–20.

97. Fordyce WE. *Behavioral Methods for Chronic Pain and Illness*, St Louis: Mosby-Year Book, 1976.

98. Fordyce WE (ed.). *Back Pain in the Workplace: Management of Disability in Nonspecific Conditions, Task Force Report.* Seattle, WA: International Association for the Study of Pain, 1995.

99. Vlaeyen JW, Kole-Snijders AM, Boeren RG, *et al.* Fear of movement/(re)injury in chronic low back pain and its relation to behavioral performance. *Pain* 1995;**62**:363–372.

100. McCracken LM, *et al.* Pain Anxiety Symptom Scale (PASS): Development and validation of a scale to measure fear of pain. *Pain* 1992;**50**:67–73.

101. Waddell G, Newton M, Henderson I, *et al.* A Fear-Avoidance Beliefs Questionnaire (FABQ) and the role of fear-avoidance beliefs in chronic low back pain and disability. *Pain* 1993;**52**:157–168.

102. Todd DD, Martelli MF, Grayson RL. The Cogniphobia Scale (C-Scale): A measure of headache impact. 1998. (Available from Dr Martelli (see reference 75)).

103. Price DD, McGrath PA, Rafii A, *et al.* The validation of visual analogue scales as ratio scale measures for chronic and experimental pain. *Pain* 1983;**17**:45–56.

104. Wade JB, Price DD, Hamer RM, *et al.* An emotional component analysis of chronic pain. *Pain* 1990; **40**:303–310.

105. McNair DM, Lorr M. Profile of Mood States – Bipolar Form (POMS-Bi). Educational and Industrial Testing Service, 1982.

106. Keefe FJ, Williams DA. Assessment of Pain Behaviors. In *Handbook of Pain Assessment* (eds. DC Turk, R Melzack), The Guilford Press, pp. 275–288, 1992.

107. Keefe FJ, Block AR. Development of an observation method for assessing pain behavior in chronic low back pain patients. *Behav Ther* 1982;**13**:363–375.

108. Waddell G, McCulloch JA, Kummel E, *et al.* Nonorganic physical signs in low back pain. *Spine* 1980;**5**:111.

109. Waddell G, Bircher M, Finlayson D, *et al.* Symptoms and signs: Physical disease or illness behaviour? *BMJ* 1984;**289**:739–741.

110. Main C, Waddell G. Spine update: Behavioural responses to examination:a re-examination; a reappraisal of the interpretation of 'nonorganic' signs. *Spine* 1998;**23**:2367–2371.

111. Dirks JF, Wunder J, Reynolds J, *et al.* A scale for predicting nonphysiological contributions to pain. *Psychother Psychosom* 1996;**65**:153–157

112. Butcher JN, Dahlstom WG, Graham JR, *et al. MMPI-2: Manual of administration and scoring*, University of Minnesota Press, 1989.

113. Millon T, Green CJ, Meagher RB. *Millon Behavioral Health Inventory*, 3rd edn, Interpretive Scoring System, 1982.

114. Morey LC. *An Interpretive Guide to the Personality Assessment Inventory (PAI)*, Psychological Assessment Resources, 1996.

115. Beck AT. *Beck Depression Inventory*, Philadelphia Center for Cognitive Therapy, 1978.

116. Spielberger CD, Gorsuch R, Lushene R. *State-Trait Anxiety Inventory*, Consulting Psychologist Press, 1970.

117. Derogatis LR. Rickels K, Rock A. The SCL-90 and the MMPI: a step in the validation of a new self-report scale. *Br J Psychiatr* 1976;**128**:280–289.

118. Wallis BJ, Lord SM, Barnsley L, *et al.* Pain and psychological symptoms of Australian patients with whiplash. *Spine* 1996;**21**:804–810.

119. Wallis BJ, Bogduk N. Faking a profile: can naive subjects simulate whiplash responses? *Pain* 1996;**66**:223–227.

120. Tollison DC, Langley . The Post-Traumatic Personality Profile. *Br J Clin Psychol* 1990;**29**:383–394.

121. Jaspers JP. Whiplash and post-traumatic stress disorder. *Disab Rehab* 1998;**20**:397–404.

122. Foa EB, Riggs DS, Dancu CV, *et al.* Reliability and validity of a brief instrument for assessing post-traumatic stress disorder. *J Traum Stress* 1993;**6**:459–473.

123. Turner S, Lee D. *Measures in Post-Traumatic Stress Disorder: A Practitioner's Guide*, Nfer-Nelson, 1998.

124. Briere J. *Psychological Assessment of Adult Post-traumatic States.* American Psychological Association Press, 1997.

125. Drummond PD, Holroyd KA. Psychological modulation of pain. In *The Headaches* (eds. J Olesen, P Tfelt-Hansen, KM Welch), 2nd edn, Baltimore: Williams & Wilkins, pp 217–221, 2000.

126. Lee E (ed.). *Working with Asian Americans*, The Guilford Press, 1997.

127. Friedman S (ed.). *Cultural Issues in the Treatment of Anxiety*, The Guilford Press, 1997.

128. McHorney CA, Ware JE, Raczek AK. The MOS 36–item short form health survey (SF-36): II Psychometric and clinical tests of validity in measuring physical and mental health constructs. *Med Care* 1993;**31**:247–263.

129. Wilson T. Applications of the SF-36 Health Survey. *J Rehab Outcomes Meas* 1997;**1**:26–34.

130. Rogers WH, Wittink HM, Wagner A, *et al.* Assessing individual outcomes during outpatient multidisciplinary chronic pain treatment by means of an augmented SF-36. *Pain Med* 2000;**1**:44–54.

131. Rogers WH, Wittink HM, Ashburn MA, *et al.* Using the 'TOPS,' an outcomes instrument for multidisciplinary outpatient pain treatment. *Pain Med* 2000;**1**:55–67.

132. Ferrans C, Powers, M. Quality of Life Index: Development and psychometric properties. *Adv Nurs Sci* 1985;**8**:15–24.

133. Ferrans C, Powers M. Psychometric assessment of the Quality of Life Index. *Res Nurs Health* 1992;**15**:29–38.

134. Millard RW. A critical review of questionnaires for assessing pain-related disability. *J Occup Rehab* 1991;**1**:289–302.

135. Vernon H, Mior S. The Neck Disability Index: a study of reliability and validity. *J Manip Physiol Ther* 1991;**14**:409–415.

136. Vernon H. The Neck Disability Index: Patient assessment and outcome monitoring in whiplash. *J Musculoskel Pain* 1996; **4**:95–104.

137. Rogers R. *The Clinical Assessment of Malingering and Deception.* The Guilford Press, 1988.

138. Human Development Consulting. Pain Symptom Ratings questionnaire, 1998 (available at: http://216.223.91.98).

139. Turk DC, Melzack R. *Handbook of Pain Assessment*, The Guilford Press, 1992.

140. Hebben N. Toward the assessment of clinical pain in adults. In *Evaluation and Treatment of Chronic Pain* (ed. GM Aronoff), Baltimore: Williams & Wilkins, pp. 384–393, 1992.

141. Ott BD. The use of psychological testing with the chronic pain patient. In *Evaluation and Treatment of Chronic Pain* (ed. GM Aronoff), Baltimore: Williams & Wilkins, pp. 475–483, 1992.

142. Hinnant DW. Psychological evaluation and testing. In *Handbook of Pain Management* (ed. CD Tollison), Baltimore: Williams & Wilkins, pp. 18–35, 1994

143. Corey D. *Pain: Learning to Live Without It.* McMillan Press, 1993 (available by e-mailing author at: group@healthrecovery.on.ca)

144. Blanchard EB, Hickling EJ. *After the Crash: Assessment and Treatment of Motor Vehicle Accident Survivors.* Washington, DC: American Psychological Association Press, 1997.

Chapter 11

Whiplash injury and the upper cervical spine

Robert W. Teasell and Allan P. Shapiro

INTRODUCTION

The Quebec Task Force [1] adopted the following definition of whiplash:

> 'Whiplash is an acceleration-deceleration mechanism of energy transfer to the neck. It may result from rear-end or side-impact motor vehicle collisions, but can also occur during diving or other mishaps. The impact may result in bony or soft tissue injuries (whiplash injuries), which in turn may lead to a variety of clinical manifestations (Whiplash-Associated Disorders).'

The incidence of whiplash claims is about 1 per 1000 population per year [2]; however, most victims of a motor vehicle accident do not develop symptoms and most symptomatic patients do not become chronic [3]. After an acute whiplash injury approximately 80% are asymptomatic by 12 months [4]. After 12 months, only between 15% and 20% of patients remain symptomatic and about 5% are severely affected [3].

PATHOPHYSIOLOGY OF WHIPLASH INJURIES

Typically the injured individual is the occupant of a stationary vehicle which is struck from behind [5–11] although injury frequently occurs following side-on and head-on collisions [6]. The Quebec Task Force [1] noted,

'Apart from anatomic studies, much of the scientific understanding of soft tissue injury and healing is derived from animal models, and there is little information on the normal recuperation period. In the animal model of soft tissue healing, there is a brief period (less than 72 hours) of acute inflammation and reaction, followed by a period of repair and regeneration (approximately 72 hours to up to 6 weeks), and finally by a period of remodeling and rematuration that can last up to 1 year.'

These limited animal data and the fact most whiplash injuries resolve quickly have led to the misconception that all whiplash injuries should heal.

The assumption that all whiplash injuries recover has been challenged with research evidence that points to an organic origin for whiplash pain. Experimental research involving animals or human cadavers have demonstrated that a variety of musculoskeletal injuries can occur, ranging from muscle and ligament tears to fractures of the cervical vertebrae [2,3]. However, fractures on radiographic studies are uncommon [12].

Bogduk and Teasell [3] have noted that during the early phases of a rear-end impact, the body's trunk is forced upwards causing the cervical spine to undergo a sigmoid deformation. About 100 ms following a collision the lower cervical vertebrae extends causing the anterior aspects of the vertebrae to separate while the posterior zygapophysial joints are crushed [13]. Such a movement would be expected to result in tears of the anterior anulus fibrosus and sprains of the zygapophysial joints. In fact, autopsy studies of individuals killed in motor vehicle accidents, when compared with control non-trauma autopsy subjects, show these very lesions [14,15].

Supporting research has shown that supporting structures around facet joints may suffer cartilaginous damage or fracture [16–18]. This research demonstrated in a carefully controlled trial of diagnostic local anaesthetic blocks that chronic whiplash pain can be relieved. In these blinded studies, 50 and 68 consecutively referred patients with chronic neck pain following whiplash injury were studied by means of controlled diagnostic blocks of cervical zygapophyseal joints [16,18]. Each joint was separately injected with a short-acting (lignocaine) and a long-acting (bupivacaine) local anaesthetic. In the latter study [18], normal saline blocks were also used. Well over half the patients obtained pain relief with injection concordant with the expected duration of the anaesthetic, thereby dealing with the placebo effect. Gibson *et al.* [19] note that cervical zygapophysial joint pain accounts for 80% of cases following high speed accidents. In a recent randomized controlled trial, the same investigators clearly demonstrated statistically and clinically significant relief for cervical zygapophyseal joint pain for periods in excess of 6 months with radiofrequency neurotomy of the dorsal cervical rami [20]. It is notable that this treatment study was a randomized, double-blind trial incorporating a sham surgical control procedure in patients with a median pain duration of 34 months. The cervical facet joints most commonly affected are C5–6 and C2–3.

THE CLINICAL PICTURE OF WHIPLASH INJURIES

The clinical syndrome

The clinical syndrome of whiplash is dominated by head, neck and upper thoracic pain and often is associated with a variety of poorly explained symptoms such as dizziness,

tinnitus and blurred vision. The symptom complex is remarkably consistent from patient to patient and is frequently complicated by psychological sequelae such as anger, anxiety, depression and concerns over litigation or compensation. In their cohort study, the Quebec Task Force [1] found the highest incidence of whiplash claims among the 20–24-year age group.

A delay in onset of symptoms of several hours following impact is characteristic of whiplash injuries [21–23]. Most patients feel little or no pain for the first few minutes following injury, after which symptoms gradually intensify over the next few days. In the first few hours, findings on examination are generally minimal [24]. After several hours, limitation of neck motion, tightness, muscle spasm and/or swelling and tenderness of both anterior and posterior cervical structures become apparent [24,25]. This delay is probably due to the time required for traumatic oedema and haemorrhage to occur in injured soft tissues [26,27].

Neck pain

Patients with whiplash injuries invariably complain of an achy discomfort in the posterior cervical region radiating out over the trapezius muscles and shoulders, down to the interscapular region, up into the occiput, and/or down the arms. This deep aching discomfort is often associated with burning and stiffness with the latter typically being most apparent in the morning. Initially, there is marked restricted range of motion of the cervical spine which may be associated with palpable muscle spasm and localized paraspinal tenderness. When the C2–3 region is involved, patients tend to have more difficulty with forward flexion.

Headaches

Headache is a common symptom following whiplash injury and the characteristic clinical sequelae of a C2–3 facet-joint injury. Within 24 hours of the accident, many patients complain of diffuse neck and head pain. The headache may be limited to the occipital area or may spread to the vertex, temporal-frontal and retro-orbital areas [28]. The pain may be a dull pressure or a squeezing sensation and include pounding and throbbing (migrainous) components [28,29]. Muscle contraction and vascular headaches often are present simultaneously (post-traumatic mixed headache). Patients may experience concomitant nausea, vomiting and photophobia. The frequency of these various forms of headache in whiplash is not known. However, the incidence of unspecified headache in a retrospective analysis of 320 cases referred for medico-legal assessment was 55% [30]. Lord *et al.* [31] note that of patients with chronic headache as the dominant complaint, 53% of cases can have their pain traced to the C2–3 zygapophysial joints.

Visual disturbances, dizziness and tinnitus

Whiplash patients may complain of intermittent blurring of vision [9,11,32]. Blurring of vision by itself is not believed to have diagnostic significance unless associated with damage to the cervical sympathetic trunk, which is regarded as rare. Complaints of dizziness or vertigo-like symptoms are common following whiplash injuries [33]. Several theories have been postulated to explain these features including vertebral artery insufficiency, inner ear damage, injury to the cervical sympathetic chain and an impaired neck righting reflex [5,34]. The 'reflex' or 'neuromuscular' theory proposes that interference with normal signals coming from the upper cervical joints, muscles or nerves to the inner ear produces a feeling of ataxia [11,35]. The entire concept of chronic vertigo arising from the cervical region has been questioned because of the relatively small cervical afferent input to the vestibular nuclei and the capacity of the system for making adjustments [23,36].

Tinnitus or difficulties with auditory acuity are frequently reported in association with whiplash injuries [11,27,37]. Tinnitus may theoretically be due to vertebral artery insufficiency, injury to the cervical sympathetic chain or inner ear damage [5,38]. Tinnitus alone does not appear to have prognostic significance [11] although anecdotally we have noted it to be common with more severe injuries. Additional auditory complaints include decreased hearing and loudness recruitment [27,39].

NATURAL HISTORY OF WHIPLASH INJURIES

It is difficult to be definitive regarding the natural history of whiplash as there continues to be a paucity of longitudinal studies in anything but selected populations, e.g., individuals who attend a specialist's office or who seek attention in a local emergency room. Only two studies, the Quebec Task Force (QTF) Study [1] and the Lithuanian study [40], have attempted to study a more representative cohort of patients.

The QTF cohort study [1] retrospectively determined that 87% and 97% of insurance claimants recover at 6 and 12 months respectively; however, the criterion for recovery was that the claimant was no longer receiving insurance payments and patients who suffered 'recurrences' were excluded from the dataset. Using this outcome criterion, it is unclear how many subjects actually recovered compared with those who remained both symptomatic and disabled but had their benefits discontinued for lack of a demonstrable organic basis (as is the case for all soft-tissue pain) for their symptoms. The criterion of discontinuance of insurance benefits significantly overestimates actual 'recovery' in soft-tissue injuries. Teasell and Merskey [41] estimate the actual recovery rate of 1 year in the QTF cohort as less than 90% when 'recurrences' are returned to the dataset.

Schrader and colleagues [40] used police accident records from a city in Lithuania to identify 202 individuals whose cars were hit from behind in automobile collisions 1–3 years earlier. They compared these subjects with a non-accident control group selected randomly from the population register and found no statistically significant differences between groups in the incidence of neck/back pain, headache or memory/concentration difficulties. They concluded that 'the late whiplash syndrome has little validity' and argued that reports of chronic whiplash in other countries are probably due to the existence of a medico-legal context which compensates whiplash injury – in Lithuania few drivers are covered by car insurance. However, the sex ratio in the Lithuanian accident group was four males to one female, whereas most studies on chronic whiplash report a higher ratio of females to males. A review of the scientific literature on sex variation and pain concluded that women are more likely than men to experience a variety of recurrent pains and report more severe levels of pain, more frequent pains and pain of longer duration [42]. Likewise, relative to men, women report higher rates of disability for cervical pain [43] and headache [44]. Accordingly, the sex bias in the Lithuanian study probably resulted in a significantly lower incidence of chronic pain and disability.

Only 31 of the 202 accident subjects in the Lithuanian study actually reported any acute injury and of these, only nine reported that their pain lasted a week or more. A prospective study of acute whiplash injury from Switzerland [45] of subjects who had pain at initial intake which was, on average, 1 week post-injury found that 24% continued to report symptoms at the 2-year follow-up. Based on this research we would expect that of the nine Lithuanian accident victims whose pain lasted more than a week, 24% or two subjects would continue to report symptoms at 1 year. Indeed, the Lithuanian study reported that three more subjects in the accident group reported chronic neck pain relative to the non-accident group, a difference, which given the small sample could not have reached (and did not reach) statistical significance. The study lacks power and would need about 1000 accidents before it could reliably come to the conclusion it did.

The study of Radanov *et al.* [45] is widely regarded as the best study of whiplash. They looked at whiplash patients solicited from family doctors and were insured under a typical 'no-fault' insurance plan with no compensation for 'non-economic' loss, i.e., pain and suffering. One hundred and sixty-four consecutive patients were referred, of whom 27 did not meet study criteria and 20 dropped out at 6 months. One hundred and seventeen subjects (74 women, 43 men) completed the study at 1 year. Within 10 days of injury, patients underwent a thorough physical and psychosocial assessment. Recovery at 3-, 6- and 12-month follow-up was 56%, 69% and 76% respectively. No difference between symptomatic and asymptomatic patients on baseline personality inventories was noted. The authors concluded that psychological and cognitive problems were the result of somatic symptoms. Persistence of symptoms at 1 year was predicted by physical aspects of

Table 11.1 Cohort studies on whiplash patients: percentage of acute patients who 'recover'

Time since MVA	QTF*	Radanov**
3 months	70%	56%
6 months	87%	69%
1 year	97%	76%

* Retrospective, all claims in jurisdiction and recovery defined as claim no longer compensated [1].
** Prospective, representative cases from family doctors and recovery defined as asymptomatic [45].

the injury including initial intensity of neck pain and headache, rotated or inclined head position at impact, unpreparedness at the time of impact and the car being stationary when hit.

Prospective studies without selection bias utilizing objective measures of recovery are lacking. The trial of Radanov *et al.* [45] comes the closest to avoiding the selection bias which besets most prospective studies. There are other studies looking at selected populations, either attending an emergency room or a specialty clinic, which have demonstrated failure to recover in 62% [46] and 58% [47] of whiplash patients respectively. However, as is evident from Table 11.1, the majority of individuals who recover do so within the first 3–6 months.

MANAGEMENT OF WHIPLASH INJURIES

Radiological investigations

Radiological studies of the cervical spine taken at the time of the accident are generally unremarkable or reveal evidence of pre-existing degenerative changes. The most commonly reported abnormal X-ray finding is straightening of the normal cervical lordotic curve [8]] However, Hohl [48] noted that straightening of the cervical spine was not necessarily indicative of a pathological condition [8,49,50] and can be regarded as a normal variant. Rarely, X-rays may reveal evidence of bony injury such as posterior joint crush fractures or minimal subluxation [11]. Radiological investigations are of limited value in the diagnosis and prognosis of whiplash injuries and their main use is in ruling out surgically correctable anatomical injuries. CT scanning and MRI imaging should be reserved for cases where cervical disc protrusion or spinal cord injury are suspected. Radionucleotide bone scanning is warranted only when there is significant clinical suspicion of an undiagnosed fracture [48].

Quebec Task Force review of interventions and treatment guidelines

The Quebec Task Force (QTF) [1] reviewed the research literature on treatment interventions for whiplash patients. For almost every treatment, the QTF found either no studies or a lack of independent studies, i.e., the specific intervention was only included as a part of a multi-intervention treatment or in conditions other than whiplash. Only facet joint injections, pulsed electromagnetic treatment and magnetic necklace were not found to be of benefit in acceptable clinical trials and even these conclusions were based on only one study for each treatment. Based on the QTF review the most common conclusion for the efficacy of treatments was 'no studies.' Therefore, based on the Quebec Task Force review one cannot definitively conclude whether these interventions are effective or ineffective, just that they have not been studied in isolation. However, for many of these treatments, multimodal interventions did not suggest they would be effective.

Manual and manipulative therapy

Aker *et al.* [51] conducted a systematic overview and meta-analysis of conservative management of mechanical neck pain, some of it secondary to whiplash injuries. They found studies with nine randomized assignment to either treatment or control groups utilizing various forms of manual treatments (including manipulation, mobilization and massage) met

their methodological eligibility criteria. For manual treatments alone there were two studies. Both compared manipulation with mobilization. The best study, Cassidy *et al.* [52], showed no significant difference between treatments while Vernon *et al.* [53] reported a significant improvement in the manipulation group.

Seven studies compared manual treatment in combination with other forms of treatment with a control. Control groups were relatively similar, consisting of rest, education, and use of analgesics with or without the use of exercise, cold packs or cervical collars. The case mix included acute whiplash [54,55], acute [56] or subacute and chronic mechanical disorders [58] and chronic cervical headache [59]. All conformed to the definition of a mechanical neck disorder although the duration of the complaint (acute and chronic) and the methodological quality varied between studies. All the studies assessed outcomes, shortly after treatment, between 1 and 4 weeks. Aker *et al.* [51] concluded that there was moderate evidence to support the use of manual treatments in combination with other treatments for short-term pain relief in patients with mechanical neck pain. There was limited evidence that manual treatments were no better than mobilizations [51]. One must be careful in extrapolating these data to whiplash injuries alone.

Exercise therapy

Aker *et al.* [51] reported on two randomized controlled trials utilizing exercise therapy for mechanical neck pain. Goldie *et al.* [60] compared exercise in combination with drug treatment and advice to a control group and reported no significant difference. Levoska *et al.* [61] compared active exercises to a combination treatment of stretching, heat and massage and reported a significant difference ($P<0.01$) favouring active exercise. Pennie and Agambar [62] published a prospective, non-randomized treatment study where 135 whiplash patients who presented to two emergency rooms in England were subsequently referred to a research clinic. Seventy-four patients received a collar with advice about mobilization while 61 had traction and exercises; 128 patients subsequently underwent the full review. No benefit was noted with active treatment over a neck collar and advice. In contrast, a randomized controlled study by Mealy *et al.* [56] reported that patients receiving Maitland mobilization techniques had more short-term relief of pain and better range of motion than did patients prescribed rest and a soft cervical collar.

In a study [54] of 247 consecutive patients attending an Irish hospital within 72 hours of an acute whiplash injury, patients were randomly assigned to one of three treatment groups: (1) general advice about mobilization after an initial rest period of 10–14 days; (2) active physiotherapy exercises combined with other physical modalities (local heat and cold, short-wave diathermy, hydrotherapy); or (3) a 30-minute session of advice on mobilization of the neck by a physiotherapist. Of the 247 patients who entered into the study, 77 failed to attend for 1- and 2-month review, but dropouts were evenly distributed among the three groups. Neck range of motion and pain severity improved significantly at 1 and 2 months in both the active and advice groups but did not do so until 2 months for the rest group. Neck range of motion and pain severity were not statistically different between the active treatment and advice groups. However, both treatment groups improved significantly more than the rest group.

Borchgrevink *et al.* [63] studied 201 patients, 81 men (40%) and 120 women (60%), with neck sprain injuries following a car accident who presented to an emergency room of a Norwegian hospital. These patients were randomly assigned to two treatment groups. An 'act-as-usual' group was instructed to act as usual and received no sick leave or collar. Patients in the 'immobilized' group received sick leave and were immobilized in a soft neck collar for 14 days. They were instructed to alternate use of the soft collar during the day with 2 hours on and 2 hours off and to use it continuously during the night. Patients were examined at intake and at 2-week, 6-week and 6-month follow-up. Only 138 patients completed all the questionnaires. There was a statistically significant reduction of symptoms from the time of intake to 24 weeks after treatment in both groups. Relative to the immobilized group, the 'act-as-usual' group demonstrated greater improvement on measures of pain localization, pain during daily activities, neck stiffness, memory and concentration and visual analogue scale measurements of neck pain and headache. Although this difference was 'statistically significant', the clinical significance was limited.

Jordan *et al.* [64] randomly assigned 119 consecutive patients with neck pain (not necessarily whiplash) of at least 3-months 'duration into one of three groups: (1) intensive exercise training of the neck and shoulder musculature; (2) individual physiotherapy treatment; and (3) high-velocity, low-amplitude spinal manipulation performed by a chiropractor. All three groups experienced considerable reduction in pain (approximately 50%) on completion of treatment and at 4- and 12-month follow-up. However, there were no significant differences between groups.

In summary, there is evidence that advice to remain active, active physiotherapy and manipulation exercises result in a better outcome early after whiplash injury when compared with rest and a cervical collar. These interventions were not substantially different in terms of clinical outcomes.

Other physical modalities

There are a variety of physical modalities which are listed in Table 11.2. Most of these therapeutic modalities have not been adequately studied in the acute or chronic phase of whiplash injuries. The lack of efficacy of the cervical collar when compared to advice to remain active and exercise therapy was noted above. Some information is available on high frequency pulsed electromagnetic therapy, a cervical collar and cervical traction. Overall, there is little evidence supporting the use of these physical modalities in whiplash injuries.

Table 11.2 Physical modalities used in whiplash injuries

- Cervical collar
- Physical modalities
- TENS (transcutaneous electrical nerve stimulation)
- Cervical traction
- Massage therapy
- Acupuncture
- Magnetic therapy

High frequency pulsed electromagnetic therapy (PEMT)

Foley-Nolan *et al.* [65] assigned 40 patients with whiplash presenting to a Dublin hospital emergency room within 72 hours of the accident either to an active treatment (magnetic collar) or a sham control group (non-magnetic collar). Treatment involved wearing the collar 8 hours/day for 12 weeks. Patients in both groups also received an individualized physiotherapy programme. The magnetic collar reported significantly less ($P<0.05$) pain at the 2- and 4-week assessments but the groups did not differ at 12 weeks. Movement scores were significantly better ($P<0.05$) in the magnetic collar group at 12 weeks only. Analgesic use decreased significantly in both groups over 12 weeks but was significantly less at 4 and 12 weeks in the treatment group. Overall, PEMT treatment resulted in a statistically significant greater improvement [65].

Traction

Aker *et al.* [51] identified three randomized controlled trials investigating the use of traction in neck pain. Goldie *et al.* [60] compared traction with a control treatment of analgesics, muscle relaxants and postural advice. There was no significant difference between the two groups. Pennie and Agambar [62] compared traction, exercise and patient education with collar and exercise. No significant difference was noted between the groups. Loy [66] compared traction and short-wave diathermy with electro-acupuncture. The latter was reported to improve symptoms significantly better than traction and diathermy. From these three trials it does not appear traction is superior to other treatments.

Medications

Aker *et al.* [51] reviewed two placebo controlled trials [67,68] using muscle relaxants (cyclobenzaprine) for neck and low back pain. Both reported significant improvement. Tricyclic antidepressants have been shown to have some benefit in the treatment of neuropathic pain and even fibromyalgia. The evidence with regards to low back pain has been mixed. There are no randomized controlled trials of tricyclic antidepressants and opioids specifically in whiplash injuries.

Cervical facet joint injections and surgical techniques

Barnsley *et al.* [69] conducted a randomized controlled trial of corticosteroid injections with chronic whiplash patients who demonstrated clear cervical facet joint involvement on diagnostic (anaesthetic blocks) testing. No significant benefit was noted when compared to placebo corticosteroid injections. Lord *et al.* [20] using radiofrequency neurotomy of the dorsal cervical rami, achieved virtually complete relief of chronic whiplash pain in patients with a median pain duration of 34 months. In this randomized, double-blind clinical trial, seven of 12 patients receiving the active treatment obtained complete pain relief in excess of 6 months. Only one of the 12 patients in the sham surgical placebo control group was rendered pain free. Patients in the active treatment group obtained complete pain relief of their primary pain complaint for a median duration of 263 days compared with 8 days in the placebo group. More recent work has demonstrated that if the first procedure is successful in providing greater than 90 days of complete relief, then subsequent repeat procedures have an 82% success rate [70].

Multimodal rehabilitation

Provinciali *et al.* [71], in an Italian study, recently studied the efficacy of a multimodal rehabilitation approach to whiplash injuries. Sixty patients with whiplash injuries were recruited within 2 months of injury (average 30 days). Patients were randomly assigned to one of two treatments: a multimodal treatment consisting of postural training, manual therapies and psychological intervention (primarily 10 sessions of relaxation training); or a control group using several physical modalities only (TENS, pulsed electromagnetic therapy, ultrasound and calcic iontophoresis). Both groups improved, but the multimodal therapy group showed statistically more improvement on measures of pain reduction, self-assessment of recovery and return to work at 6 months. Neck range of motion was not statistically different between the two groups. Full recovery occurred in six patients receiving the multimodal treatment but none of the comparison group. The authors argued that multiple factors may influence the late whiplash syndrome and, in particular, speculated that psychological support (primarily relaxation training) may have reduced the emotional influence on muscle tone and increased pain tolerance.

SUMMARY

The natural history of acute whiplash is that most patients will improve or recover relatively quickly. In carefully controlled diagnostic blocks of cervical facet joints the two most commonly affected joints are C5–6 and C2–3. Higher cervical injuries involving C2–3 facet joint injuries typically experience headaches as a sequelae. Supportive education and a progressive exercise programme involving stretching of the involved region and an aerobic component are the mainstays of medical management. Other physical treatments (physical modalities, manipulation, TENS) and pharmacological treatments provide short-term pain reduction at best and should not be used in isolation. Injections and surgical interventions are rarely useful in uncomplicated whiplash. The one exception is percutaneous facet-joint denervation, which appears effective for patients with demonstrable (via diagnostic blocks) facet-joint involvement. Psychosocial interventions, including vocational counselling, are becoming more popular as we recognize the importance of treating the person with a whiplash injury and not just the injury itself. However, psychosocial interventions remain unproved.

REFERENCES

1. Spitzer WO, Skovron ML, Salmi LR, *et al.* Quebec Task Force on Whiplash-Associated Disorders. *Spine* 1995;**20**(85):1S-73S.
2. Barnsley L, Lord S, Bogduk N. The pathophysiology of whiplash. In *Cervical Flexion-Extension/Whiplash Injuries. Spine: State of the Art Reviews* (ed. G.A. Malanga), Philadelphia: Hanley & Belfus 1998;**12**:209–242.
3. Bogduk N, Teasell R. Whiplash: The evidence for an organic etiology. *Arch Neurology* (in press).
4. Radanov BP, Sturzenegger M, DiStefano G. Long-term outcome after whiplash injury: a 2-year follow-up considering features of injury mechanism and somatic, radiologic, and psychosocial findings. *Medicine* 1995;**74**:281–297.
5. Bogduk N. The anatomy and pathophysiology of whiplash. *Clin Biomech* 1986;**1**:92–101.
6. Deans GT. Incidence and duration of neck pain among patients injured in car accidents. *BMJ* 1986;**292**:94–95.
7. Frankel VH. Pathomechanics of whiplash injuries to the neck. In *Current Controversies in Neurosurgery* (ed. TP Morley), Philadelphia: WB Saunders, pp. 39–50, 1976.
8. Hohl M. Soft tissue injuries of the neck in automobile accidents: Factors influencing prognosis. *J Bone Joint Surg* 1974;**56A**:1675–1682.
9. LaRocca H. Acceleration injuries of the neck. *Clin Neurosurg* 1978;**25**:205–217.
10. Macnab I. Acceleration injuries of the cervical spine. *J Bone Joint Surg (Am)* 1964;**46**:1797–1799.
11. Macnab I. Acceleration extension injuries of the cervical spine. In *The Spine* (eds. RH Rothman, FA Simeone), 2nd edn, Philadelphia: WB Saunders, pp. 647–660, 1982.
12. Hoffman JR, Schriger DL, Mower W, Luo JC, Zucker M. Low-risk criteria for cervical-spine radiography in blunt trauma: a prospective study. *Ann Emerg Med* 1992;**21**:1454–1460.
13. Kaneoka K, Ono K, Inami S, Hayashi K. Motion analysis of cervical vertebrae during whiplash loading. *Spine* (in press).
14. Jonsson H, Bring G, Ranschning W, Sahlstedt B. Hidden cervical spine injuries in traffic accident victims with skull fractures. *J Spinal Disorders* 1991;**4**:251–263.
15. Taylor JR, Twomey LT. Acute injuries to cervical joints. *Spine* 1993;**18**(9):1115–1122.
16. Barnsley L, Lord SM, Wallis BJ, Bogduk N. The prevalence of chronic cervical zygapophysial joint pain after whiplash. *Spine* 1995;**20**:20–25.
17. Lord S, Barnsley L, Bogduk N. Cervical zygapophyseal joint pain in whiplash. In *Spine: State of the Art Reviews* (eds. RW Teasell, AP Shapiro), 1993;**7**(3):355–372.
18. Lord SM, Barnsley L, Wallis BJ, Bogduk N. Chronic cervical zygapophysial joint pain after whiplash. A placebo-controlled prevalence study. *Spine* 1996;**21**(5):1737–1745(a).

19. Gibson T, Bogduk N, Macpherson J, McIntosh A. The accident characteristics of whiplash associated chronic neck pain. *J Musculoskeletal Pain* (in press).

20. Lord SM, Barnsley L, Wallis BJ, McDonald GJ, Bogduk N. Percutaneous radio-frequency neurotomy for chronic cervical zygapophyseal joint pain. *N Engl J Med* 1996;**335**:1721–1726(b).

21. Deans GT, McGailliard JN, Kerr M, Rutherford WH. Neck pain – a major cause of disability following car accidents. *Injury* 1987;**18**:10–12.

22. Dunsker SB. Hyperextension and hyperflexion injuries of the cervical spine. In *Neurological Surgery* (ed. JR Youmans), 2nd edn, Philadelphia: WB Saunders, pp. 2332–2343, 1982.

23. Evans, RW. Some observations on whiplash injuries. In *The Neurology of Trauma. Neurologic Clinics* (ed. RW Evans), 1992; **10**(4):975–995.

24. Hohl M. Soft tissue injuries of the neck. *Clin Orthop* 1975;**109**:42–49.

25. Wickstrom JK, LaRocca H. Management of patients with cervical spine and head injuries from acceleration forces. *Curr Pract Orthop Surg* 1975;**6**:83.

26. Jeffreys E. *Disorders of the Cervical Spine.* London: Butterworths, 1980.

27. Lieberman JS. Cervical soft tissue injuries and cervical disc disease. In *Principles of Physical Medicine and Rehabilitation in the Musculoskeletal Diseases*, Grune & Stratton, New York, pp. 263–286, 1986.

28. Speed WG. Psychiatric aspects of post-traumatic headaches. In *Psychiatric Aspects of Headache* (eds. CS Adler *et al.*), Baltimore: Williams & Wilkins, pp. 210–216, 1987.

29. Balla JI, Moraitis S. Knights in armour. A follow-up study of injuries after legal settlement. *Med J Aust* 1970;**2**:355–361.

30. Wiley AM, Lloyd J, Evans JG, Stewart BM, Sanchez J. Musculoskeletal sequelae of whiplash injuries. *Advocates Quarterly* 1986;**7**:65–73.

31. Lord SM, Barnsley L, Wallis BJ, *et al.* Third occipital headache: a prevalence study. *J Neurol Neurosurg Psychiatry* 1994;**57**:1187–1190.

32. Horwich H, Kasner D. The effect of whiplash injuries on ocular functions. *South Med J* 1962;**55**:69–71.

33. Oosterveld WJ, Kortschot HW, Kingma GG, *et al.* Electronystagmographic findings following cervical whiplash injuries. *Acta Otolaryngol (Stockh)* 1991;**111**:201–205.

34. Toglia JV. Acute flexion-extension injury of the neck. Electronystagmographic study of 309 patients. *Neurology* 1976;**26**:808–814.

35. DeJong PTVM, DeJong JMBV, Cohen B, Jongkees LBW. Ataxia and nystagmus induced by injection of local anaesthetics in the neck. *Ann Neurol* 1977;**1**:240–246.

36. Balch RW. *Dizziness, Hearing Loss and Tinnitus, the Essentials of Neurology.* Philadelphia: FA Davis, 1984, p. 152, discussed in Evans (1992).

37. Chrisman OD, Gervais RF. Otologic manifestations of the cervical syndrome. *Clin Orthop* 1962;**24**:34–39.

38. *Medical News.* Animals riding in carts show effects of 'whiplash' injury. *JAMA* 1965;**194**:40–41.

39. Gibson JW. Cervical syndromes: Use of comfortable cervical collar as an adjunct in their management. *South Med J* 1974;**67**:205–208.

40. Schrader H, Obelieniene D, Bovim G, *et al.* Natural evolution of the late whiplash syndrome outside the medical legal context. *Lancet* 1996;**347**:1207–11.

41. Teasell R, Merskey H. The Quebec Task Force on Whiplash Associated Disorders and the British Columbia Whiplash Initiative: A study in insurance industry initiatives into the natural history and management of whiplash injuries. *J Pain Research and Management* (in press).

42. Unreh AM. Gender variations in clinical pain experience. *Pain* 1996;**65**:123–167.

43. Hasvold T, Johnsen R. Headache and neck as shoulder pain-frequent and disabling complaints in the general population. *Scand J Primary Health Care* 1993;**11**:219–224.

44. Taylor H, Curran NM. *The Nuprin Pain Report*, New York: Louis Havris and Associates Inc., 1985.

45. Radanov BP, Sturzenegger M, DeStefano G, Schnidrig A. Relationship between early somatic, radiological, cognitive and psychosocial findings and outcome during a one-year follow-up in 117 patients suffering from common whiplash. *Br J Rheumatol* 1994;**33**:442–448.

46. Gargan MF, Bannister GC. The rate of recovery following whiplash injury. *Eur Spin* 1994;**J3**:162–164.

47. Hildingsson C, Toolanen G. Outcome after soft tissue injury of the cervical spine: A prospective study of 93 car-accident victims. *Acta Orthop Scand* 1990;**61**:357–359.

48. Hohl M. Soft tissue neck injuries. In *The Cervical Spine* (eds. The Cervical Spine Research Society Editorial Committee), 2nd edn, Philadelphia: JB Lippincott Co., pp. 436–441, 1989.

49. Borden AGB, Rechtman AM, Gershom-Cohen J. The normal cervical lordosis. *Radiology* 1960;**74**:806.

50. Rachtman AM, Borden AGB, Gershon-Cohen J. The lordotic curve of the cervical spine. *Clin Orthop* 1961;20:208.

51. Aker PD, Gross AR, Goldsmith CH, Peloso P. Conservative management of mechanical neck pain: systematic overview and meta-analysis. *BMJ* 1996;**313**:1291–1296.

52. Cassidy JD, Lopes AA, Yong-Hing K. The immediate effect of manipulation versus mobilization of pain and range of motion in the cervical spine: a randomized controlled trial. *J Manipulative Physiol Ther* 1992;**15**:570–587. Correction in: *J Manipulative Physiol Ther* 1993;**16**:279–280.

53. Vernon HT, Aker P, Burns S, Viljakaanen S, *et al*. Pressure pain threshold evaluation of the effect of spinal manipulation in the treatment of chronic neck pain: a pilot study. *J Manipulative Physiol Ther* 1990;**13**:13–16.

54. McKinney LA, Dornan JO, Ryan M. The role of physiotherapy in the management of acute neck sprain following road traffic accidents. *Arch Emerg Med* 1989;**6**:27–33.

55. McKinney LA. Early mobilization and outcomes in acute sprains of the neck. *BMJ* 1989;**299**:1006–1008.

56. Mealey K, Brennan H, Fenelon GCC. Early mobilization of acute whiplash injuries. *BMJ* 1986;292:656–657.

57. Nordemar R, Thorner C. Treatment of acute cervical pain – a comparative group study. *Pain* 1981;**10**:93–101.

58. Koes BW, Bouter LM, van Mameren H, Esser AH, *et al*. Randomized clinical trial of manipulative therapy and physiotherapy for persistent back and neck complaints: results of one-year follow-up. *BMJ* 1992;**304**:601–605.

59. Jensen OK, Nielsen FF, Vosmar L. An open study comparing manual therapy with the use of cold packs in the treatment of post-traumatic headache. *Cephalgia* 1990;**10**:242–250.

60. Goldie I, Landquist A. Evaluation of the effects of different forms of physiotherapy in cervical pain. *Scand J Rehab Med* 1970;**2–3**:117–121.

61. Levoska S, Keinanen-Kiukaanneimi S. Active or passive physiotherapy for occupational cervicobrachial disorders? A comparison of two treatment methods with a 1-year follow-up. *Arch Phys Med Rehabil* 1993;**74**:425–430.

62. Pennie BH, Agambar LJ. Whiplash injuries. A trial of early management. *Bone and Joint Surgery* 1990;**78B**(2):277–279.

63. Borchgrevink GE, Kaasa A, McDonagh D, Stiles TC, *et al*. Acute treatment of whiplash neck sprain injuries. *Spine* 1998;**23**(1):25–31.

64. Jordan A, Bendix T, Nielsen H, Rolsted Hansen F, *et al*. Intensive training, physiotherapy, or manipulation for patients with chronic neck pain. *Spine* 1998;**23**(3):311–319.

65. Foley-Nolan D, Moore M, Codd M, Barry C, *et al*. Low energy high frequency pulsed electromagnetic therapy for acute whiplash injuries. A double-blind randomized controlled study. *Scand J Rehab Med* 1992;**24**:51–59.

66. Loy TT. Treatment of cervical spondylosis. Electroacupuncture versus physiotherapy. *Med J Aust* 1983;**2**:32–34.

67. Bercel NA. Cyclobenzaprine in the treatment of skeletal muscle spasm in osteoarthritis of the cervical and lumbar spine. *Curr Ther Res* 1977;**22**:462–465.

68. Basmajian JV. Cyclobenzaprine hydrochloride effect on skeletal muscle spasm in the lumbar region and neck: Two double-blind controlled clinical and laboratory studies. *Arch Phys Med Rehabil* 1978;**59**:58–63.

69. Barnsley L, Lord SM, Wallis BJ, Bogduk N. Lack of effect of intra-articular corticosteroids for chronic cervical zygapophysial joint pain. *N Engl J Med* 1994;**330**:1047–1050.

70. McDonald G, Lord SM, Bogduk N. Long-term follow-up of cervical radiofrequency neurotomy for chronic neck pain. *Neurosurg* (in press).

71. Provinciali L, Baroni M, Illuminati L, Ceravolo MG. Multi-modal treatment to prevent the late whiplash syndrome. *Scand J Rehab Med* 1996;**28**:105–111.

Chapter 12

Manual therapy in children: with special emphasis on the upper cervical spine

Heiner Biedermann

INTRODUCTION: PRINCIPLES OF MANUAL THERAPY IN CHILDREN

The essence of manual medicine is the restoration of impaired function, albeit in the framework of a pre-existing form. This 'form' has two components:

1. The morphology, individually expressed on the basis of our genetic patterns and their interaction with the environment during growth.
2. The cybernetic patterns which are morphologically fixed on a microhistological level in the central nervous system and as important a base for (mal)function as the macromorphology.

In an adult, the balance between function and form tends towards the latter. In adolescents, children and, especially in babies and newborns, the reverse is true. Here, function (and malfunction) determines the developing form in the two facets mentioned above. This is the essential difference. Manual therapy in children (MTC) bears only scant resemblance to the much less dramatic and currently well-known effects we see in adults. There, we are only too aware that we often 'repair' without being able to heal; thus condemning therapist and patient to repeat this exercise sooner or later. In schoolchildren and babies, one adjustment can stop incessant week-long crying, can turn a 'hyperactive little nerve-wracker' into the darling of the family, can

relieve a schoolchild of disabling headaches – and permanently so. Not all of these problem children benefit from MTC, but many more than the average paediatrician or general practitioner might concede do so spontaneously.

MTC is *not* a scaled-down version of the procedure for adults. It is quite understandable for somebody only busy treating adults to regard any non-adult as 'a child' and, thus, belonging to a group mainly defined by this one quality of not yet having reached the status of a grown-up. Like most conceptual assumptions this lofty idea withers upon close scrutiny. Since the idea of 'punctured equilibria' was introduced into evolution by Gould [1] we have a better insight into the dynamics of phylogenetic development. On the ontogenetic level the same principles apply. Relatively stable periods alternate with rather short transition phases which are inevitably more sensitive to disturbances than the rest periods. Disequilibration of a given level of organisation to attain a higher complexity implies a dangerous period of vulnerability – but a unique chance for far-reaching therapeutic effects too.

The development of a child is not a continuous process of accretion of body mass. As every parent knows, growth happens in leaps and bounds. The beloved offspring can wear the same shoes for several months over the winter but by the following spring, the parents have to buy a new pair of jeans every third week because they are quicker outgrown than paid for. This variable growth rate is but the most basic and easiest to notice of these discontinuities. Other phenomena are less easily isolated, but the results are the same. Everybody just *knows* that 'she was just a baby last year and now she's a little girl' – or 'how quickly he changed from a carefree kindergarten kid to the serious schoolboy he is now'.

We are best aware of changes after they have happened; and we can categorize the 'before and after' more or less precisely only with hindsight. Thus, the transition itself is elusive. These changes are important with regard to our way of interacting with the young and, therefore, the average adult knows about them. But the complexity of the process observed, i.e., the transition from one stage in their development to the next, prevents us from using clear-cut and measurable criteria. This creates a frustrating situation for all those who want to find sharp and enforceable boundaries for our therapeutic activities. They are not easily submitted to a rigid quality control.

A multidimensional process

Something as simple as a light ray needs several models of explanation (wave *and* photon) to come to grips with the results of experiments. From the viewpoint of the physicist, it is almost endearing to see how the biomedical sciences struggle to get their field into line with a 'structured and well-designed protocol'. Reductionism still seems to reign supreme but 'the ability to reduce everything to simple fundamental laws does not imply the ability to start from those laws and reconstruct the universe' [2].

As the developing child chooses (mostly unconsciously) its individual path out of the myriad of possibilities offered by its genetics, environment and education, there is such a thing as a 'butterfly effect' wherein a minor stumbling block at the wayside may alter the entire biography. But the sheer complexity of the web of influences makes it impossible to attribute simple and straight interconnections to this process. Expelled from 'the paradise of linear equations' [3], we have lost the comfort of a world where every possible development

can be mechanically predicted if one knows the initial constellation well enough [4].

The new qualities emerging when complex structures are assembled from simpler basic blocks, and which are the essential ingredients for any form of life, prevent the application of rigid boundaries once one comes sufficiently close to the subject of observation. This knowledge gives us the basis to live happily with fuzzy edges wherever we deal with a quickly changing and ever more complex situation. The emergence of new qualities is the essence of growing up. As much as the phylogenetic restraints of gene and culture define a 'corridor of possibilities', our individual use of them depends on a series of accidents in the true sense of the word; and if these happen at a crucial point in time, their influence on the later development can hardly be overestimated.

There are two ways to present MTC to those without prior knowledge: at first look, one might concentrate on the usual phalanx of statistics, preferably with a diagnostic score and a 'significant' outcome study best done double-blinded. One might thus avoid many points of friction; but this would not do justice to this incredibly exciting topic and would only reproduce a methodological bias far too often applied to manual medicine in general; thus treating it as a mere technique. But, as Lewit put it, 'it is not enough to master the various techniques which are effective in orthopaedic medicine; it is as important to understand dysfunction' [5]. So I shall try to describe the *gestalt* of MTC or manual medicine in children. Whenever statistics are useful, they will be presented, but more as means to an end. One cannot grasp the beauty of a painting by listing the colours it contains. This 'open' approach is meant as a foundation for discussion. There is a great deal we have learned about the possibilities of manual therapy in small children during the past 20 years and the broad lines presented here have proved themselves during the examination and treatment of thousands of babies.

Determining the stages

The developmental steps of childhood are usually defined according to the viewpoint of the examiner. An endocrinologist will look for different transition points than someone dealing with the pulmonary system or, as in our case, researchers and/or therapists interested in the process of sensorimotor development. From our viewpoint, anything which changes the way in which we interact with the world is of interest and has to be examined with this question in mind: 'is there a fundamentally different situation *before and after*?'

Fortunately, the limitations of space exert a welcome pressure to stay concise; so we shall concentrate on three transitions that have a profound impact on the individual development:

A Birth
B Verticalisation
C Cessation of growth

At first sight, one might consider birth as an exactly localisable point in time. But even this first and indispensable prerequisite of all the following events is not that easy to define. Is it the appearance of the head, the first breath or the cutting of the umbilical cord? As always, in complex situations, it helps to step back and choose a slightly coarser unit of measurement: the hour of birth or even the birthday.

The second item in the list needs further clarification. What does verticalisation mean? We mean here the conquest of the third dimension; the step from being fixed in a basically two-dimensional area to a three-dimensional space. Normally, this happens during a few weeks. The toddler pulls himself up and is amazed by the experience of standing on his own feet; shortly afterwards the first steps can be observed. Here, too, we have to choose the right unit of measurement to get meaningful information: whereas it is most certainly meaningless to be precise to a day, we can in most cases fix the month of verticalisation for girls, between the 10th and the 13th month, for boys, 1–3 months later, but still considered normal till the 18th month [6,7].

The third item – cessation of growth – is even less precisely located in time, and mostly only afterwards: 'She stopped growing at 15' is in most cases the best level of precision available and sufficient for all practical uses.

These three steps are of vital interest for those busy with MTC; the first as one main origin of traumatic lesions of the spinal poles, the second and third as important points in time where changes in the function of the spine have wide-ranging consequences for the way we can interact therapeutically.

THE TRAUMA OF BIRTH

'The birth channel is one of the most dangerous passages we have to traverse in our whole life'. This quote is attributed to various authors, mostly obstetricians. We tend to forget how dangerous these few centimetres are. General anaesthesia and modern pharmacology provide us with powerful tools to overcome most of the problems mother and child can face during birth. But one should not forget that the older obstetric literature was filled with gruesome procedures to dismember the fetus in utero if the normal birth had not succeeded.

The use and abuse of caesarean sections is controversially discussed. There is no need to reiterate the arguments here; suffice it to say that from our viewpoint as specialists of functional disorders of the vertebral spine, the advantages of a broad indication for a caesarean seem obvious. In all our studies, babies born by caesarean section are underrepresented, and even more so if one excludes the oblique position from this group.

Phylogenetically, there are two main problems regarding the delivery mechanism of the fetus. Firstly, the bipedal gait necessitates a profound alteration of the pelvis. Its function in quadrupeds implies an open and oval construction, connecting the hind member with the vertebral spine at an angle of about 90°; this leaves ample space for the delivery of the fetus. With the upright posture of the trunk in humans, the pelvis had to be closed as much as possible to carry the intra-abdominal structures and the ilium had to be bent outwards to make room for the gluteal muscle group. These muscles have a different working angle once the trunk sits on top of the hindlegs and not in front of them [8–10]. The birth channel is in direct contradiction to these constructive principles as the fetus has to pass through this now much smaller aperture. This is one of the reasons why the sexual dimorphism of the pelvis is bigger in humans than in any other mammal group [11].

Another constructive problem adds to this dilemma: the acquisition of the upright posture, as a consequence, means that the femoro-spinal angle of roughly 90° has to be enlarged to almost 180° and beyond. This is achieved by redesigning the lumbo-sacral junction, and it leads to the almost angular sacral promontory, [12] which is a uniquely human achievement and another obstacle for the fetus. No other region of the human musculo-skeletal system has such a large inter-individual variability as the sacrum and its neighbouring structures [13]. Obstetricians were among the first to analyse the pelvic architecture and its consequences for, for example, low back pain [14].

The redesign of the pelvis to suit it for its role in bipedal posture is one problem aggravating the situation of the fetus on its entry into the world. The second aspect is almost as important and in some ways similar to the constructive dilemma at the caudal pole of the vertebral spine. In quadrupeds the orientation of the skull, i.e., visual axis, is, grosso modo, an extension of the vertebral axis. The vertical positioning of the trunk makes it necessary to align the visual axis with the horizon. In most animals that assume a vertical position only for a limited period (e.g., bears, prairie dogs, etc. [11]), this is achieved by a lordosis of the cervical spine and no further adaptation of the cranial structures ensues.

The evolution of humans took a different path. Here, the realignment of the visual field with the horizon was accomplished by an angulation between the upper cervical spine and the craniofacial region. The result of this complicated development was a wider base for the neocranium and an angle of ±90° between the orientation of the vertebral spine and the visual axis. One of the side-effects of this new relationship between head and spine was the change of the birth mechanism: whereas in most mammals the facial part of the skull is delivered first, in humans the dome of the skull is the first structure to go through the birth canal [15].

The main diameter of the head lies in the sagittal plane; that of the trunk in a frontal orientation. The two redesigns of the vertebral poles interact to produce a complicated birth mechanism. The construction of the lower pelvis leads to a semicircular trajectory for the fetus. As the main diameters of head and trunk have to be aligned during delivery, a 90° angle between the two is established while traversing the lower pelvis. This leads to a necessarily asymmetrical positioning of the occipito cervical junction which cannot be reversed during the entire delivery.

MRI studies of the intracranial structures of apparently healthy newborns have shown a high percentage of signs of microtrauma of brainstem tissues in the periventricular areas [16]. It seems probable that the exposed structures of the occipito-cervical (OC) junction suffer at least as much as the cranium [17]. Wischnik *et al.* [18] have shown this in experimental studies of the biomechanics of delivery (see also Govaert *et al.*[19]). Injury of the intracranial and subcranial structures is, thus, the rule, not the exception. The ability of most newborns to overcome and repair these lesions shows the enormous capacity of the not yet fully developed brain to cope with trauma at this stage.

Taking into account that the optimal development of the brain, which lasts at least until the 12th year [20], depends on consistent sensory inputs, the importance of proprioceptive dysbalances for the efficient repair of cerebral lesions becomes evident.

Verticalisation

All movement, and therefore all sensorimotor development, interacts with and works against gravity. The importance of this transition from the mainly two-dimensional '*way of life*' into the third dimension is still widely underestimated. We have to consider this transition as an important expansion of the possibilities of the developing child; alas, in connection with all the instabilities which accompany any newly acquired degree of freedom. Before these new options can be put to use, the child has to master the instability of keeping the spine upright. To a major extent, this means that the function of the spine has to be reinvented, as its habitual position in most mammals is horizontal.

The contour of the spine is the result of the intrinsic phylogenetic programme [21] and its interaction with these external factors. These latter forces play a much bigger part than previously assumed. Meyer observed that the unilateral torsion of the lying baby turns into a bilateral scoliotic posture after verticalisation [22]. 'After the child starts walking, the muscular reaction changes completely and we find scoliosis, lumbar hyperlordosis and hyperkyphosis of the dorsal spine (*M. Scheuermann*)'. Like many successful practitioners, Meyer did not publish his results systematically and we have only a few anecdotal sources [23]. But even in this limited material we find many of the observations on the determinative influence of early irritations of the cervical spine on the form and function of the adult spine.

It is very important to be aware of the different patterns of reaction before and after verticalisation in order to interpret the possibilities of corrective measures. As very often seen in developmental physiology, a certain fixation of the already acquired abilities precedes the new phase. Consequently, it is easier and more efficient to treat postural imbalances before verticalisation occurs than afterwards. In an analysis of the effectiveness of MTC, we were able to show that the incidence of readjustments depends on whether the first treatment was applied before or after verticalization [24].

It is important to keep this in mind when communicating the possibilities of manual therapy to paediatricians. Before the first birthday, the success rate of the initial treatment is between 80% and 90% with only about one third of these babies needing further physiotherapy [25]. After the 12th to 14th month, most of the children have to be seen at least twice by an MTC specialist and about half of them need re-education in the form of physiotherapy or ergotherapy. These numbers reflect the situation of central Europe and the work-sharing arrangements we have here. I suppose that the different structure of health care in North America shifts the percentage of the professions involved considerably, albeit without changing the underlying qualitative aspect.

Cessation of growth

Similar considerations apply to this transition phase, but to a lesser extent. After the growth of the bones is completed, the adaptation of the musculoskeletal apparatus continues at a much slower pace and often in creating changes which are classified as 'degenerative', i.e., negatively connoted.

It is obvious that we have more possibilities to influence the postural patterns of a 10- or 11-year-old than of somebody who is already 16. At the age of 10, we are still able to use the last growth periods to alter the course of development; the treatment of scoliosis is a good and well-documented example. Later on, the acquired morphological and cybernetic form establishes the limits of our therapeutic efforts. Having said that, one has to add immediately that these limits are by no means fixed; but the closer we get to the adult stage, the more we have to accept the individual situation as being more or less stable. We can correct functional problems, but we have to accept that the underlying morphological and/or cybernetic structures will make a reappearance of similar complaints likely.

The dividing line between the treatment regime applicable to an adult is quite similar to that of an adolescent of 12 or 13 years of age. Their individual complaints are similar, too. The main difference lies in the fact that an adolescent (at least before the last big growth periods of 11–13 years) has the possibility to alter the physical structure and thus the functional base after an adjustment.

These considerations influence more the way we inform about the long-term perspectives than the actual treatment procedures. This is the main reason why this article concentrates on the examination and treatment of small children.

Torticollis neonatorum

Asymmetry in newborn babies is a well-known problem and is often considered benign and spontaneously remitting if left alone long enough. It is certainly true that we have to be patient in the first days and weeks. After passing through the birth channel, a realignment of the asymmetrical cranial bones and a resorption of soft-tissue oedema and/or haematomas take time. An initially asymmetrical posture should be noted and observed, not more or less (see Figures 12.1 and 12.2).

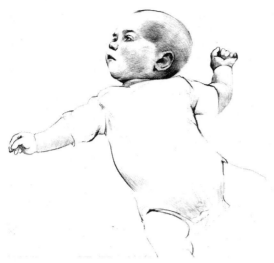

Figure 12.1 *A typical KISS baby (Type I). This baby is unable to move spontaneously from this position. The head was fixed in a right-rotated and left-tilt position.*

If this asymmetry persists after 3–4 weeks, or additional symptoms appear, it is advisable to check if the range of movement of the head is impaired. This restricted movement is, in most cases, a sign of a protective immobilisation of the upper cervical spine. For a long time this was linked to a malfunction of the sternocleidomastoid muscle, leading to the common diagnosis of 'muscular torticollis' [26–31]. The most visible symptom was thought to be the cause. At least in the early phases, the shortened and thick sternocleidomastoid muscle is so prominent that it is regarded as the 'natural' culprit. Late cases of infantile torticollis often show a fibrosis of the sternocleidomastoid [32,33]. The two facts were then easily combined: early haematoma results in later fibrosis.

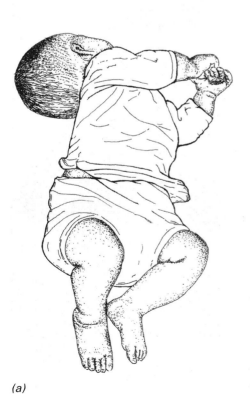

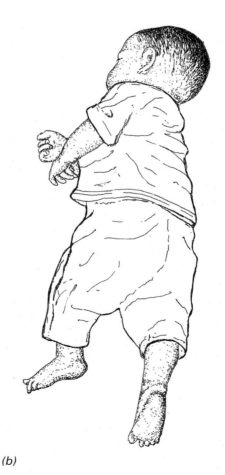

(a)   *(b)*

Figure 12.2 *Child sleeping in a fixed retroflexion (KISS type II). (a) before treatment; (b) 4 weeks later. Drawings based on photos taken by the father.*

Our experience has led to different conclusions. There is no direct and linear connection between the initial haematoma and a late fibrosis. Children with an initial haematoma do not have a greater chance of developing a late fibrosis than newborns without a palpable tumour of the sternocleidomastoid. The connection between the two phenomena is much more intricate than such a linear concept suggests. The sternocleidomastoid is a co-victim of the underlying trauma to the articular structures of the cervical spine and, as such, it is not a good starting point for therapy or analysis. It is far better used as an indicator of the improvement brought about by other therapeutic measures, as a correct therapy of the suboccipital joints results in an alignment of the muscular tonus of the sternocleidomastoid.

There is controversy about how to react to a fixed or asymmetric posture in newborn babies. Some consider this a 'physiological scoliosis' and think it wears off without treatment [34,35]. More recent papers stress the importance of asymmetries in perception and posture for the development of more severe consequences later on [36]. Buchmann has remarked 'the existence of an asymmetrical range of tilt in the suboccipital region of a child is no big deal. Only if additional signs accompany this, an immediate treatment might be necessary' [37]. Asymmetry is frequently found in testing newborns [38,39] and its clinical significance has to be carefully examined. Seifert published data of unselected groups of newborn babies where she found that more than 10% of them showed signs of asymmetry of the functioning of the upper cervical spine [40].

No one advocates a treatment schedule where all these initially asymmetrical babies have to be treated routinely; but these babies should be re-examined later on and treated if the functional deficit has not subsided spontaneously after 4–6 weeks. We would propose to take a large margin, especially as MTC is a low-risk procedure, quite uncomplicated and has not to be repeated more than once or twice. Keessen *et al.* show that the accuracy of the proprioception of the upper limb is reduced in cases with idiopathic scoliosis and spinal asymmetry [36]. As we know that the proprioception of the arms depends heavily on a functioning SO region [39], functional deficits in this region should be corrected as soon as possible.

As is often seen in the history of medical knowledge, our frame of reference changes over time. In 1727 Nicolas Andry, who coined the word 'orthopaedics', had already mentioned the treatment of the torticollis as one important field of this new discipline [40]. In going back to these roots, we understand that good posture in children was at the forefront of orthopaedic diagnostics and treatment. 'Ortho-Paedics –

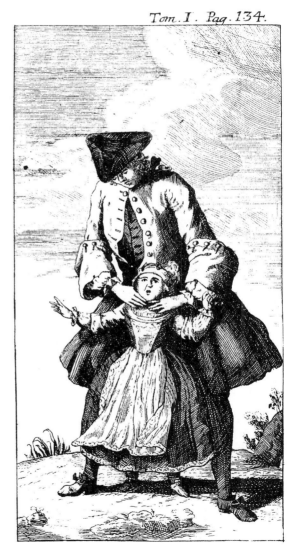

Tom. I . Pag. 134.

Figure 12.3 *An illustration from Andry's book, demonstrating a treatment we would easily identify as a manipulation today.*

straightening the young' was so important for Andry that he used this concept as the definition of the medical procedures he published in his book. This fundamental underpinning of the new discipline was lost in later centuries and Andry's eminently functional approach had to make way for the mechanistic paradigms which have dominated orthopaedics in the last decades (see Figure 12.3).

The effects of a fixed posture of the head in newborns have great breadth and depth, the former evaluated in the presentation of the KISS syndrome, the latter being compiled as KIDD (see below).

Colic

Infants in Western societies cry more in the first 3 months than in any other period of their lives [43]. This phenomenon has its peak at 6 weeks and declines rapidly thereafter [44]. It is very difficult to assess the dividing line between 'normal' and 'abnormal' crying. Several definitions have been proposed to define this crying as pathological. Wessel's definition 'more than 3 hours per day, more than 3 days per week for more than three weeks' [45] is widely used in publications but is at least a little unrealistic, as it asks a stoicism of the parents which may not be found very often nowadays. 'I am still too impressed by the parental feelings of hopelessness and helplessness, their anger and anxiety, their feeling that something is really wrong with their child, to leave them alone with this, in nature, self-limiting problem' says Lucassen [43]; and one might add that, although infantile colic is known to subside spontaneously, there are reasons enough to try to shorten this period:

• It is very stressful for the parents and may sometimes lead to aggressive and violent behaviour of parents and/or baby-sitters.*
• It may result in lasting communication problems between parents and the baby [46,47] in the years to come.
• Many functional disorders of the school-age period and even later can be traced back to these early signs.[48]

* Think of the recent well-publicised trials of several au-pair girls in the USA.

A recent publication by a team of colic specialists is entitled 'The enigma of infantile colic' [49]. Discussing the possible origins of this problem, the authors mention that 'more than half of the babies concerned showed slight to medium deficits in functional neurological tests ... the quality of spontaneous motor patterns was not normal'. As with many other authors, this team also did not find convincing evidence of the feeding pattern on the incidence of colic [50–52].

Can persistent crying in the first months be considered a 'benign condition' [53]? The first contacts with the effect of manual therapy on colic babies came through serendipity. Quite a few newborns who were presented because of their fixed posture recovered from colic, too, after the treatment administered for the C-scoliosis or the fixed retroflexion. At that time there were only very few observations of functional factors contributing to colic; most authors were looking for clues related to nutrition or mother-child interaction; even something as elusive as 'the temperament' [54] of the baby was considered relevant; alas, difficult to influence therapeutically, one might hasten to add.

We had already known for a long time about the intricate connections between the oro-facial muscles and the upper cervical spine [55–57]. The next step was to look for factors in the individual case history that might enable us to screen babies with colic for those who might benefit most from the use of manual therapy. The results of this inquiry were twofold. In the group of successfully treated cases of colic, we found mostly babies with a fixed retroflexion of the head and trunk (see Figure 12.2a) and feeding problems. This led to a cooperation pattern with paediatricians concerning referral of babies with incessant crying. The paediatricians check for other concerns, e.g., infections or pylorospasm, and then for signs of an involvement of functional vertebrogenic factors. This includes the screening of the case history, checking the flexion of the head and the local irritability of the neck as well as neurological tests [58,59] for asymmetry. If they, thus, have reason to believe that a functional problem of the upper cervical spine contributes to the problem of colic, the babies are referred to a specialist in MTC.

The qualitative evaluation of the effectiveness of MTC in these cases still has to be demonstrated conclusively, but there its very success is the biggest obstacle: paediatricians and parents who are aware of the enormous efficiency of MTC in these cases (see Table 12.1) resolutely refuse to allow control groups.

The KISS syndrome

Having treated newborns and small children with postural problems for many years, a pattern began to emerge which directed our attention beyond the purely positional dimension. In a monograph published in 1984 [60] one chapter was dedicated to the treatment of babies and small children. At that time we did not yet have a clear idea about the full impact of the pathology we were about to discuss. We simply did not have the large number of cases needed to recognise the underlying patterns. In the 1970s, Gutmann treated one or two children every month; in 1999 we see between 50 and 100 small children every week. This increase is reflected in the much clearer clinical picture we were able to develop. Not all of the symptoms listed below can be found in every single case; most of the time some symptoms are dominant and others may be completely absent. But as a whole this list has been quite useful in the evaluation.

In 1992 we proposed the KISS syndrome for the first time to the Anglo-American public [61]: Kinematic Imbalances due to Suboccipital Stress (1991 in German [62]). The reason for this 'new' syndrome is that its definition gives us a taxonomic frame to accommodate the pathogenetic base (irritation of the suboccipital structures of the cervical spine) and the clinically dominant item, i.e., the asymmetry.

Strictly speaking, nobody is symmetrical; but symmetry is nevertheless perceived as ideal in art and nature [63], and might even convey evolutionary advantages to its bearer [64,65]. A comprehensive treatment of symmetry and its evolutionary role can be found in Møller and Swaddle [66].*

Blickhorn [67] summed up a recent publication [68]: '... fluctuating asymmetry could account for almost all heritable sources of variability in IQ'. This is but one hint to the

importance of symmetry as a marker and/or cause of other more fundamental problems. The impairment of sensorimotor development in KISS children seems to point to the same conclusions. Complete symmetry is empty, dead [69]. A person or object needs a certain amount of symmetry to be considered beautiful, but the addition of a little bit of asymmetry can really make us like what we see [70]. Strong asymmetry on the other hand is seen as 'sick' [71]. Between these two extremes the ideal has to be found by intuition – or trial and error.

For structures connected to sensory input, symmetry is more than an embellishment: most of the information has to be related to a three-dimensional analysis of its origin and, here, symmetry of the supporting structure simplifies processing. Strong asymmetry necessitates a higher level of 'input-correction' and is therefore of evolutionary disadvantage.

Asymmetry of posture is normal immediately after birth. The forces exerted on the newborn during delivery routinely lead to a temporary tilt posture in at least one third of all cases [72]. Most of these babies recover spontaneously and if re-examined 4–6 weeks later only about 6% of all newborn still show signs of an impairment of the motion range of the head. In these cases further evaluation should be done to establish other symptoms and eventually treat these.

In the recent neuropaediatric literature, more and more importance is attributed to symmetrical posture and movement patterns. The search for asymmetry is a basic part of the diagnostics of all major examination schemes [6,58,73,74]. As neurologists, these authors attribute the origin of these asymmetrical patterns to a malfunctioning of the central nervous system, and extensive literature exists searching – mostly in vain – for a visualizable correlate in MRI or PET scans. Specialists of manual medicine will need even more successfully treated children to convince the other medical professionals of the role of faulty proprioception in the suboccipital vertebral structures in these cases; but 'function (physiology) is as real as is anatomy (pathology)' [5].

Any fixed posture of the head of a small child exerts a strong influence on the sensorimotor development. In the beginning it is hard to differentiate between any underlying pattern; the more so as most children display

---

* The authors put additional material on their website www.oup.co.uk/MS-asymmetry

mixed symptoms. As there exists a different pattern of complaints and a slightly different long-term development pattern it is worthwhile to note the main forms. We distinguish between two types of KISS (see Figure 12.2a and b):

- Type I: fixed lateroflexion of head and trunk
- Type II: fixed retroflexion of the head with hyperextension of the thoraco and/or lumbar spine.

These two forms share many symptoms, and a pain-avoiding protective immobilisation of the traumatically irritated suboccipital structures is at the base of both. This trauma may have been caused by an intrauterine irritation through fixed oblique positioning of the fetus and/or a direct birth trauma.

Ongoing research seems to indicate that type II facilitates the development of symptoms of colic and incessant crying whereas in babies with Type I we tend to find more cases of unilateral retardation of the development of the hip joints.

The items mentioned in Table 12.1 show that in many cases the two types of KISS overlap. One has to take into account that it is easier for a paediatrician to recognise the laterally fixed posture as pathological. The fixed retroflexion more often than not has to be actively searched for. Often it is best seen in the sleeping position of the children (see Figure 12.2 a and b). Initially we did not pay much attention to it and it was only after the parents reported spontaneously that their children slept much more calmly and in a markedly more relaxed position that we

became aware of the diagnostic importance of a fixed retroflexion of the head.

Through these observations of the parents, the idea developed to check systematically if and how much we were able to relieve the sufferings of 'cry-babies' (i.e. colic) and their families. Initially quite a few of these small children were referred to us for the treatment of postural asymmetries and the accompanying colic was not mentioned by the parents during our interviews. In the questionnaire we asked the parents to send back to us 6 weeks after their visit, they mentioned that the babies were much calmer and slept better.

In a simple descriptive pilot study, we found that up to 55% of those who said that incessant crying was one of the main reasons their child was presented in our consultation registered an improvement of more than two-thirds in the week after treatment (see Tables 12.1 and 12.2). A prospective study is ongoing.

The basic trigger which makes paediatricians send the babies to a specialist in manual therapy is the hypersensitivity of the neck region in combination with a restricted range of movement of the head. Those who already observed the success of manual therapy in cases of colic or feeding problems are looking actively for these signs to help them decide if it is advisable to present these babies at a specialist. Others find it easier to first look for signs of asymmetry before they take into account manual therapy as a treatment option. In both cases it helps to have the pattern of typical KISS complaints present, even if not all symptoms can be found in an individual case.

KIDD: KISS-Induced Dyspraxy and Dysgnosy

Since the 1980s, the awareness of the long-ranging consequences of pre-birth conditioning has risen considerably. British cardiologists were the first to note that children born in poor families with a high incidence of malnutrition suffer from a higher rate of heart failure decades later [75]. Similar results came from epidemiological studies in the Netherlands and in Finland [76]. It seems probable that our organism is assigned an 'operating mode' early in life according to the environmental condi-

Table 12.1

Spontaneous complaints reported by the parents (n = 263) [25]

Torticollis	89.3%
Reduced range of head movements	84.7%
Cervical hypersensitivity	76.0%
Cranial asymmetry	40.1%
Opisthotonos	27.9%
Restlessness	23.7%
Forced sleeping posture	14.5%
Unable to control head movements	9.5%
Uses one arm much less	7.6%

Table 12.2 Results of treatment (interviews with parents) [25]

Symptom	(Very) good result after				Improved	No change	Total
	1 day	1 week	2 weeks	3 weeks			
Torticollis	78	28	33	19	40	25	223
Opisthotonos	10	6	5	7	12	5	45
Restless/crying	26	5	6	2	6	7	52
Fixed sleeping posture	16	3	3	6	4	1	33

tions reigning during pregnancy and the first months after birth.

Learning about these results made it easier to come forward with observations we made with schoolchildren and young adults. In many cases (72% [77]) where we had to treat patients for headaches, postural problems or coordination malfunctions, we were able to establish KISS-related problems in the first year of life. In order to find this connection one can rely on the checklists which are filled out regularly during the predetermined visits at the paediatrician (see Table 12.4). Another valuable source of information is the photograph collection of the first year (see Figure 12.4). Very often one finds the baby again and again in the same posture as it grows into a kindergarten kid. When asked about other signs we associate with a dysfunction of the occipitocervical junction, we often got affirmative answers. Because of the 'fuzziness' of these symptoms it is difficult to put this in a tight diagnostic frame.

Forthcoming research aims at establishing the effectiveness of MTC treating school problems. Before this prospective study, which we have undertaken in collaboration with the paediatric department of the University of Cologne, a sample of schoolchildren in Hagen (Germany) were examined and treated. This group of children between 6 and 10 years of age came from a school specialised in pupils with learning difficulties. These children were evaluated by their teachers and an initial interview to document the case history was conducted. Two X-rays of the cervical spine were obtained and at a second session the documentation was checked, the X-ray pictures analysed and a manipulation of the cervical spine performed. Four and 8 weeks later the parents and teachers were asked to evaluate the development of the children.

Table 12.3

	KISS points	Score before treatment	Score after treatment
Group I	17	17	9
Group II	8	15	14

The results are summarized in Table 12.3. Of the pupils taking part in the pilot phase, we assembled two groups. Group I were those children where the case history contained items which fit a KISS-Syndrome; Group II were the other half (6/6 children; for the points see Table 12.3). For the evaluation of the individual cases, we relied on the internal system of the school before and after treatment that is mainly based on the SIPT [78]. A detailed report is due to be published in 2000 [79].

These findings reflect our previous experience well; if it is possible to establish a case history typical of KISS children in a pupil with learning difficulties, it is worthwhile to examine and treat such a child with MTC. To prove the influence of functional vertebrogenic disorders on a given sensorimotor problem, it is often most effective to simply perform a test treatment and evaluate the results, as Lewit and Janda remarked already more than 30 years ago [80]. In order not to be overwhelmed by desperate parents, a prescreening by a paediatrician who is able to filter out the most promising cases is helpful. Once confronted with an individual case it is almost always better to treat one too many than to let a possible improvement slip away. It is fair to say that there is no risk involved if one limits the treatment to a single manipulation. As we were able to show in an analysis

Table 12.4 Questionnaire for children

Birth	
mother's age	
first/second/third . . . delivery	
duration of delivery (<1 hour ; 1–3 hours; 3–6 hours; >6 hours)	x
birth weight	
birth length	
oblique presentation	x
twin	x
forceps	
vacuum	x
caesarean	x
The first months:	
bad sleeper during first months – 6–12 months – later	x
did/does the child often wake up at night	x
crying at night – how often	x
fixed sleeping pattern	x
problems with breastfeeding on one side	x
signs of colic	x
orofacial hypotonus	x
hypersensitivity of the neck region	x
General health:	
bronchopulmonary infections	
headaches	x
neurological disorders	
mouth is often open	x
Sensorimotor development slower than expected:	
posture and movement	x
language	x
concentration	x
social integration	x
Asymmetry:	
visible immediately after birth	x
only later (when?)	x
obstetrician/midwife saw it	
parents observed A. first	
localisation	
arm	
trunk	
head	
baby looks only to one side	x
moves only one arm/leg	
face is smaller on one side	x
occiput flat on one side	x
has a bald spot on the occiput	x

of fatal complications after manual therapy almost all these cases occurred at the second of third intervention and/or using rotational manipulation [81].

During the first year, the most important direct sign of functional problems of the occipito-cervical junction is asymmetry. The closer the child gets towards verticalization the less

pronounced these signs become. The additional information furnished by the third dimension obviously helps the child to compensate for the faulty proprioceptive patterns of C0/C2. Similar to the 3-month-old who stops crying spontaneously the problem of asymmetry seems to disappear if only we have the patience to wait long enough. In the second and third year

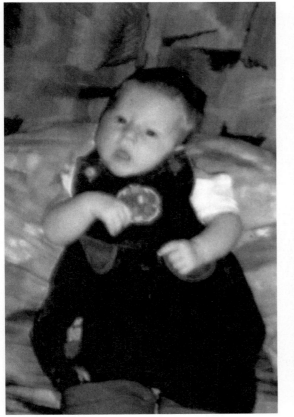

(a)

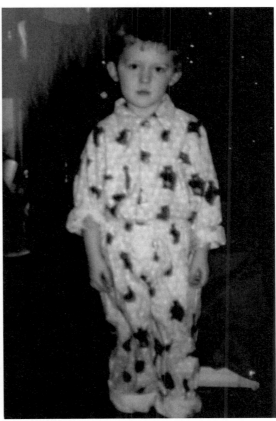

(b)

Figure 12.4 *Two pictures of the same boy who came to our consultation because of his headaches. The parents' photo collection showed how the fixed position of the head could be traced back The parents had not noticed anything abnormal regarding the posture until we started to talk about it.*

children enter a phase where they show little or no signs of any functional or motor disorder.

Later on, when children are between 4 and 6 years old, other symptoms appear. These children are reported as being 'clumsy' or 'slow'; parents tell that they have difficulties learning to bike or to roller-skate. 'We were so astonished that she still cannot ride a bike as she was walking at 8 months already' is a remark we often hear. This is the situation where you have to inquire further: how was the delivery, how were the first months? The relevant questions are compiled in Table 12.4. Those items marked with an 'x' contribute to a 'KISS score' which we use to improve the accuracy of the prognosis. The definite form of this score is not yet fixed and the discussion in

the EWMM* should lead to a usable standard in the near future, which shall be made publicly available via our website.

These questions – translated into a non-medical language – form the base of our interviews with the parents. If used judiciously, this list helps to avoid being overeager when examining potential cases. As already mentioned, it does little harm to treat one child too many – but on the other hand it's not helpful to claim to be able to treat all and anything with the same method. Once we have found the typical pattern of KISS in the case history we have to ascertain that the problems

* European Workgroup for Manual Medicine (see www.manmed.org).

which brought the children to our consultation are consistent with the 'KISS pattern'.

Differential diagnosis

Asymmetry, at least temporarily, is very often present during the child's development. If it was the only diagnostic criterion to filter out functional problems of the vertebral spine we would be in a difficult situation. Luckily we have an entire assortment of clues to rely on for a reasonably precise diagnosis. Nevertheless, it is only after evaluating the eventual result of a manipulation that the relevance of the functional disorders of the SO region for a given problem can be assessed. The threshold for intervention is relatively low as there are no known risks as long as the proper procedure is followed.

One of the most important diagnostic problems is the detection of spinal tumours. The severity of these cases and the need for timely intervention attributes much more importance to their detection than the rarity of their occurrence might suggest (5/100 000, of these, 10%-20% in children [82]). Some of the signs are quite specific, e.g., a protrusion of the papilla of the optic nerve or impairment of the pyramidal tract. Others are far less specific and can easily be confounded with functional problems. Even specialists note that a wrong initial diagnosis is the rule and not the exception [83].

Quite often the first symptoms which attract the attention are secondary problems due to functional disorders, i.e., a torticollis [84–86]. These symptoms are identical to those caused by primary vertebrogenic causes and may even improve at first. Gutmann published such a case of a young boy he treated initially successfully for headaches and neck pain [87]. After a complete remission the problems reappeared, seemingly after a minor trauma, as happens quite frequently. When the boy came back a third time, again after some minor knock on the head, Gutmann, nevertheless, insisted on an MRI, which resulted in the diagnosis of a tumour.

One caveat is a crescendo of symptoms. Most functional disorders show a flat curve of development and are often traceable back to an initial trauma. If the pain pattern or the

amount of dysfunction shows a rapid increase, further diagnostic measures are necessary. As much as conventional X-ray plates of the cervical spine are essential for the evaluation of functional disorders of the spine, they do not furnish the necessary information to diagnose intramedullary tumours. MRI scans are by far the best method. As soon as details in the case history or in the clinical examination are discovered which point toward an origin of the problems beyond the functional level, a neuropaediatrician should be consulted.

In a recent publication we summarised the items necessitating further diagnostics as follows [88]:

- inadequate trauma
- late onset of symptoms
- multiple treatments before first presentation
- crescendo of complaints
- 'wrong' palpatory findings.

This last item is by far the most important and in those cases where I had to diagnose a tumour it was this 'wrong' feeling which alerted me. This impression is difficult to describe; one has to examine many necks to calibrate one's hands finely enough in order to filter out these cases. In two of them the main area of pain sensitivity was unusually low; in another case, the sensitivity was so extreme that even after trying to palpate gently and for a long time, the hyperaesthesia persisted. These three children were referred to a neuropaediatrician and the preoperative diagnosis was mainly based on MRI.

In 1997–8 we asked for MRI scans in 12 cases (of a total of 2316 children examined). In two cases a tumour was found (one haemangioma, one astrocytoma). It has to be added that most of the children we see have already been examined by a paediatrician and the normal waiting period for an appointment is 2–4 weeks. This filters out all those cases where the rapid deterioration necessitates immediate action.

In our aim to find the few cases with a serious background we cannot rely on an initial trauma as an exclusion criterion against tumour. In several of these cases where we had to diagnose a tumour in the end, an 'appropriate' trauma was reported. The young girl whose cervical spine is shown in Figure 12.5 complained first about pain in the neck and

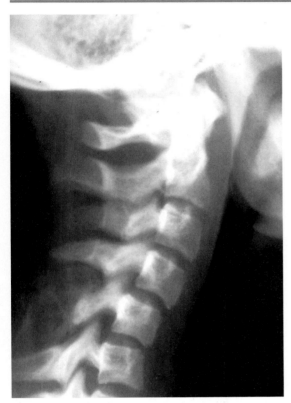

Figure 12.5 *This young girl aged 12 years came because of neck pain after jumping into a swimming pool. Note the rarefication of the osseous structure of proc. spin. C5; haemangioma.*

arm after a dive into a pool, allegedly having touched bottom. In the end we found a haemangioma of the spinous process of C6; this was one of the rare cases where a conventional X-ray plate showed enough to alert the examiner.

Clinical examination

The basis of the clinical examination can be 'borrowed' from neuropaediatric manuals, e.g., [6,89,90]. The evaluation of those findings varies between a purely neurological approach and one which includes the vertebral function. Asymmetry of posture and movement are the first warning signs that the suboccipital structures should be closely checked. Hypersensitivity and restricted range of movement in this area ideally triggers a referral to a specialist.

Once the child has arrived in our consultation we routinely repeat the paediatric test scheme based on Vojta's proposals [59]. These tests are complemented by a segmental examination of the entire spine and a test of the passive range of movements of the joints of the extremities, thereby comparing the two sides (see Figures 12.6 and 12.7).

For older children the situation becomes much more complex. Here, the basic pattern of complaints directs the examination towards different focal points. To test the sensorimotor development one scheme frequently used is the Sensory Integration and Praxis Tests (SIPT, Ayres; see Fisher *et al* [78]). For the functional analysis of the spine a few coordination tests suffice: one-leg stand on the floor or on a soft support, walking on a line, finger-nose test (with open and closed eyes), tiptoeing and walking on the heels are our standard tests, optionally complemented by additional procedures. In most cases these rather simple tests supply a solid base of the functional evaluation.

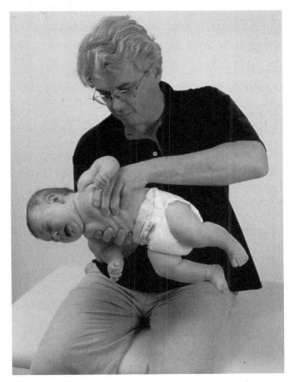

Figure 12.6 *Examining the babies: during examination special emphasis is given to the functioning of the upper cervical spine.*

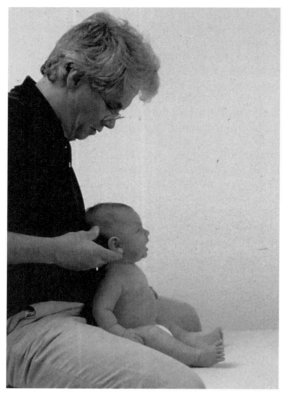
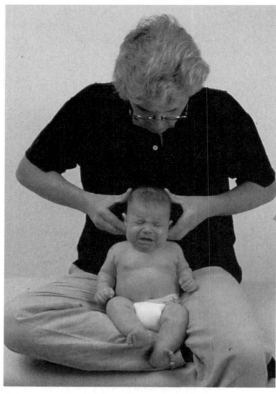

(a)   *(b)*

Figure 12.7 *Examining the babies: during examination special emphasis is given to the functioning of the upper cervical spine.*

All of these tests are important and a base for the evaluation. But at least as important as these tests is a sensitivity for the surrounding details: How does the child react, how tense are they, how is the base of communication, etc? These 'non-classifiable' items have to be taken into account and they finally form the bedrock on which we have to rely to grasp the *gestalt* of a clinical problem.

Radiological examination

There are different opinions about the need to take X-rays before treating the cervical spine, to put it euphemistically. Many therapists active in the field reckon it is safe and sufficient to rely on the palpatory findings and the clinical interview. They consider the classic two-plane radiography a superfluous exercise. Anybody

with daily experience of the difficulties one encounters in trying to convince our little patients to cooperate is only too willing to accept any excuse to get rid of this time-consuming part of the examination. But the information obtained by the functional and morphological analysis of these pictures renders the effort worthwhile. An in-depth analysis of the functional radiology of the cervical spine would cover more space than the entire book provides, let alone one chapter. So we have to content ourselves with a few examples of the interaction between functional and morphological analysis of the 'classic' X-ray plates of the cervical spine (see Figure 12.8a and b).

The X-ray picture complements and verifies the clinical findings. If the de-symmetrization of the occipito-cervical junction follows the established pattern (see Figure 12.9) the direction of the impulse is confirmed. This is the case in more than 80% of the newborn and

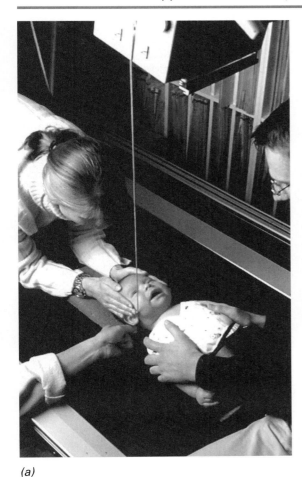

(a)

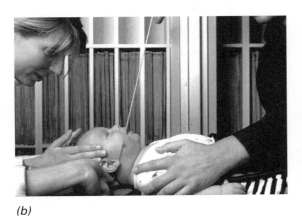

(b)

Figure 12.8 *The difficult picture. We ask the parents to fixate the baby for the exposure. This tests the patience of all concerned. The rope shows the slightly tilted orientation of the X-ray to avoid superposition of the scull base and the cranio-cervical junction.*

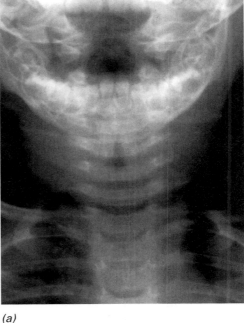

(a)

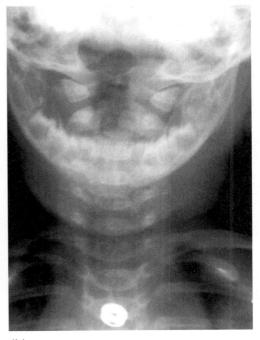

(b)

Figure 12.9 *A typical X-ray picture. The linea intercondylaris, the lateral massae of the atlas and the rudimentary dens should be easily distinguishable on a correctly taken picture.*

small children [24,77]. In these cases there would be no difference between what happens with and without radiography.

But it is the other 20% that interest us. We have not yet been able to find conclusive tests that might enable us to sort out the one-fifth of our patients who need to have X-ray plates before actually having examined them. If that was possible we might indeed first test for these criteria and take X-ray pictures only in those cases that fulfil these, non-existing, criteria. But as long as we do not have them at our disposal it is by far the lesser evil to screen systematically.

The risk of the use of ionising radiation often triggers highly emotional arguments. Quite frequently a nebulous 'cancer risk' is quoted to justify avoiding a standard radiological examination. 'It is true that fetuses and children are about twice as radiosensitive as adults, but not much more than that' [91]. 'It is time to scientifically challenge the old tenet stating that

cancer risk is always proportional to dose, no matter how small' [92]. If we add to that the fact that the energy density used for plates of the cervical spine of small children is one of the lowest dosages used in conventional radiology it should be obvious that a risk-benefit analysis clearly favours the standard procedure of taking X-ray plates before *any* treatment of the cervical spine regardless of the age of the patient.

Just the morphological findings of the conventional X-ray studies of the cervical spine in children would easily fill a book. Wackenheim's monograph (albeit focusing on adults) is still the most comprehensive account [93]. By far the most common finding is the fusion of two vertebrae. Its relevance depends mostly on the levels involved and if the symmetry is preserved. A fusion of, for example, C3/C4 is much less relevant for the individual biography than a fusion of C2/C3 which impairs the anteflexion of the head considerably.

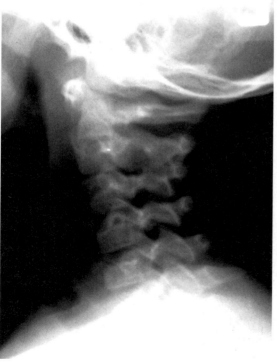

(a)

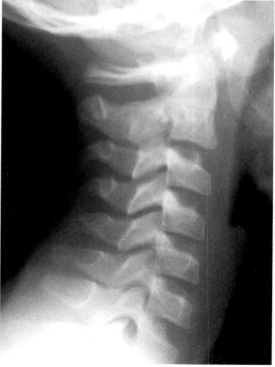

(b)

Figure 12.10 *Open arcus dorsalis C1 and strong rotation below C2. The arcus dorsalis is hypoplastic and the double contour at its end clearly visible. The proc. articularis inferior from C2 on is clearly double projected, whereas the head is not rotated. After the treatment the rotation is gone, the morphology persists.*

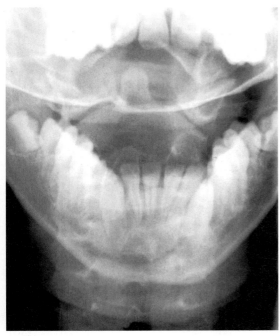

A second quite frequent finding is a hypoplasia of the dorsal arc of C1. As this structure does not have a direct static role, these variants often remain unnoticed. Statistical evaluation of our material indicates a strong correlation between a hypoplastic arcus dorsalis C1 and asymmetries of the lumbosacral region on one hand and unilateral hypoplasia of one hip joint.

Once a non-standard form of the atlas is noticed it seems at least advisable to check for clinical signs of asymmetry of the pelvic girdle and functional deficits of one of the hip joints. If there are signs of asymmetry found there one can continue the examination with conventional X-ray plates or CT scans.

The plates presented in Figures 12.10–12.12 show some of these aspects. Once one has learned to overcome the difficulties of obtaining correct projections, it is astonishing how much detailed information can be extracted. But it takes time and constant training to get to a satisfactory quality level.

Figure 12.11 *Dysplastic C2 the abnormal articulation and the differences between the two joint facets C1/C2 shows a strong morphological component in this case.*

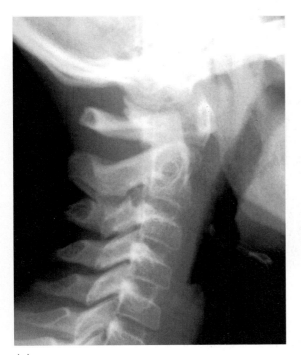

(a)

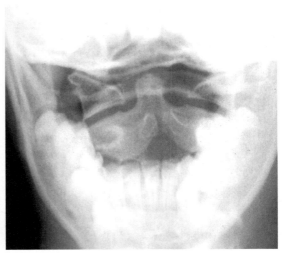

(b)

Figure 12.12 *Dysplastic C2 + insufficiency of the lig. transversum atlantis.*

Manipulative techniques

Manual therapy is one of the oldest forms of healing we know. It is a craft; an interpersonal action involving direct bodily contact. Whenever we try to put this into a conceptual frame we have to concentrate on one or a few of the many dimensions involved in such a complex interaction. It is absolutely legitimate and necessary to do, for example, experimental studies focussing on the amount of force used in the treatment of children and adults [94], but in discussing these findings, we have to keep in mind that it needs more than the right amount of force to make a manipulation successful.

This is one reason why it is next to impossible to separate the effect of a given method from the person who applies the treatment. We can teach the anatomical basics and the pathophysiological processes involved and the state of the art regarding the techniques applicable. But we cannot turn an eminently personal interaction between two individuals into an industrial product. Publications like this one are as good and as bad as a cookbook. If one knows something about the topic at hand, the lecture of such a book may be of advantage. For the non-initiated it provides frustrating reading or it provokes plain refusal.

After everything said until now, it should be evident that the main point is to recognise the pattern and intervene in a timely manner. The choice of the optimal method depends to a large degree on constitutional factors of the therapist. In treating children and adolescents, the age of the little patient is at least as important. As soon as we reach the age range of schoolchildren, the techniques used are more and more similar to these of adults. Clinically, too, we find comparable patterns of complaints as in adults, but with a special 'tilt'.

In most cases the direction of the manipulation is determined by the radiological findings (85%). In the other cases the orientation of the restricted movement, the palpation of segmental dysfunction or the local pain reaction help to find the best approach [95]. The manipulation itself consists of a short thrust of the proximal phalanx of the medial edge of the second finger (see Figure 12.13). It is mostly lateral; in some cases the rotational

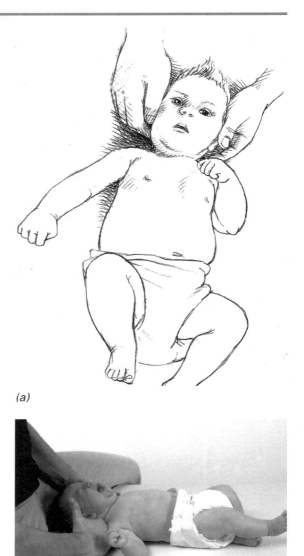

(a)

(b)

Figure 12.13 *The treatment.*

component can be taken into account but in small children this is the exception. In cases where KISS type II is pre-eminent and the fixed retroflexion is the main component, the manipulation can be applied via the transverse process of C1 in a sagittal direction.

We believe that the selection of the specific technique without functional analysis of the radiography of the cervical spine lessens the effectiveness of this treatment. Apart from the improved treatment technique, a correct analysis reveals morphological problems in 6–8% of the cases [85,88,96]. Standard X-rays – during the first 18 months an A/P plate of the cervical spine including the SO region suffices – have to be of optimal quality and no manipulation in the SO region should be done without them.

The technique itself needs subtlety and long years of experience in the manual treatment of the upper cervical spine of adults and school-children. In the hands of the experienced practitioner the risk is minimal; we have not yet encountered any serious complications (see also Meyer [22]). The forces used during the manipulation were tested with a calibrated pressure gauge; they do not exceed the force used to push a bell-button energetically [94]. Most children cry for a moment, but stop as soon as they are in their mothers' arms. In five cases (of approx. 8000 infants) the children vomited after the treatment; this had no negative effect on the outcome, and there were at least as many babies vomiting already during the test routine to determine their neurological status.

Outlook: the fourth dimension

The most fascinating thing about MTC is its far reach. It determines many different details of a baby's wellbeing on one hand and the development of such an individual on the other. This long-distance influence into a fourth dimension (time) distinguishes functional disorders of this biographical period from those encountered later on. The importance of early trauma for the individual development in adult life was already mentioned more than 100 years ago by Palmer and Still, alas without defining exactly which signs to look for.

Such a general conjecture renders this statement almost useless, as everybody encounters more or less violent accidents while growing up. Only when we are able to look for specific signs in the case history will it be possible to advance our understanding of the impact of the birth trauma on the clinical pattern of complaints of our patients.

The concept of KISS and KIDD should be seen as a tool to come to grips with *one* aspect of this wonderfully multidimensional endeavour the readers of these lines mastered already: growing up. Which is why I dedicate this article to our children and grandchildren. Let's hope MTC can remove a few stones from their rocky road to adulthood.

REFERENCES

1. Gould SJ. *Ever since Darwin: Reflections in Natural History*. Nortan, 1977.
2. Waldrop MM. *Complexity*. New York: Simon & Schuster, 1992.
3. Parisi G. Cacciati dal paradiso delle equitazione lineari. In *Gli ordini del chaos*. Rome, pp. 73–79, 1991.
4. Bak P. *How nature works. The science of self-organised criticality*. New York: Copernicus/Springer, 1996.
5. Lewit K. The functional approach. *J Orthop Med* 1994;**16**:73–74.
6. Ambühl-Stamm D, *Früherkennung von Bewegungsstörungen beim Säugling*. Munich: Urban & Fischer, 1999.
7. Largo RH. Verhaltens- und Entwicklungsauf-fälligkeiten: Störungen oder Normvarianten? *Monatsschr Kinderheilk* 1993;**141**:698–703.
8. Gracovetsky SA. *The Spinal Engine*. Vienna, New York: Springer, 1988.
9. Preuschoft H. Body posture and mode of locomotion in Early Pleistocene Hominids. *Folia Primat* 1971;**14**:209–240.
10. Preuschoft H. Zur Evolution der menschlichen Becken- und Rumpfform. In *Manualtherapie bei Kindern* (ed. H Biedermann), Stuttgart: Enke, pp. 77–88, 1999.
11. Starck D. *Vergleichende Anatomie der Wirbeltiere*. Berlin: Springer, Vol. 2, 1979.
12. Fick R. *Handbuch der Anatomie und Mechanik der Gelenke*. Jena: Fischer, 1911.
13. Gutmann G, Biedermann H. *Funktionelle Röntgenanalyse der Lenden – Becken- Hüftre-gion*. Stuttgart: Fischer,1990.
14. Martius H. *Der Kreuzschmerz der Frau*. Stuttgart: G. Thieme, 1947.
15. Wiltschke-Schrotta K. Zur Evolution der Geburt. In *Manualtherapie bei Kindern* (ed. H Biedermann), Stuttgart: Enke, pp. 89–98, 1999.
16. Valk J, *et al.* The role of imaging modalities in the diagnosis of posthypoxic-ischaemic and haemorrhagic conditions of infants. *Klin Neuro-radiol* 1991;**2**:83–140.
17. Lierse W. Das Becken. In *Praktische Anatomie* (ed. VL Wachsmuth), New York: Springer, 1984.
18. Wischnik A, Nalepa E, Lehmann KJ. Zur Prävention des menschlichen Geburtstraumas I. Mitteilung: Die computergestützte Simulation

des Geburtsvorganges mit Hilfe der Kernspintomographie und der Finiten-Element-Analyse. *Geburtshilfe Frauenheilkunde* 1993;**53**:35–41.

19. Govaert P, Vanhaesebrouck P, de-Praeter C. Traumatic neonatal intracranial bleeding and stroke. *Arch Dis Child* 1992;**67**:840–845.

20. Giedd JN, Blumenthal J. Jeffries NO, *et al.* Brain development during childhood and adolescence: a longitudinal MRI study. *Nat Neurosci* 1999;**2**(10):861–863.

21. Kolár P. The sensorimotor nature of postural functions. Its fundamental role in rehabilitation of the motor system. *J Orthop Med* 1999;**21**(2):40–45.

22. Meyer T. Das KISS-Syndrom. (Kommentar). *Man Med* 1994;**31**:30.

23. Meyer T. *Methodiek van Manuele Therapie.* Rotterdam, p. 37, 1991.

24. Biedermann H, Pathogenese und Therapie frühkindlicher Symmetriestörungen (Teil 1 & 2). *hautnah paediatrie*, 1995;**7**:4–14, 84–98.

25. Biedermann H. KISS-Kinder: eine katamnestische Untersuchung. In *Manualtherapie bei Kindern* (ed. H Biedermann), Enke: Stuttgart, pp. 27–42, 1999.

26. Binder H, Gaiser JF, Koch B. Congenital muscular torticollis: results of conservative management with long-term follow-up in 85 cases. *Arch Phys Med Rehabil* 1987; **68**:222–225.

27. Entel RJ, Carolan FJ. Congenital muscular torticollis: magnetic resonance imaging and ultrasound diagnosis. *J Neuroimag* 1997; **7**(2):128–130.

28. Porter SB, Blount BW. Pseudotumor of infancy and congenital muscular torticollis. *Am Fam Phys* 1995;**52**(6):1731–1736.

29. Robin NH. Congenital muscular torticollis. *Pediatr Rev* 1996;**17**(10):374–5.

30. Tom LW, Handler SD, Wetmore RF, *et al.* The sternocleidomastoid tumor of infancy. *Int J Pediatr Otorhinolaryngol* 1987;**13**:245–255.

31. Vojta V, Aufschnaiter DV, Wassermeyer D. Der geburtstraumatische Torticollis myogenes und seine krankengymnastische Behandlung nach Vojta. *Krankengymnastik* 1983;**35**:191–197.

32. Kraus R, Han BK. Babcock DS, *et al.* Sonography of neck masses in children. *Am J Roentgenol* 1986;**146**:609–613.

33. Ljung JGBM, Guerry T, Schoenrock LD. Congenital torticollis: evaluation by fine-needle aspiration biopsy. *Laryngoscope* 1989; **99**:651–654.

34. Bratt HD, Menelaus MB. Benign paroxysmal torticollis of infancy. *J Bone Joint Surg* 1992;**74**-**B**:449–451.

35. Kamieth H. Die chiropraktische Kopfgelenksdiagnostik 'unter funktionellen Gesichtspunkten' nach Palmer-Sandberg-Gutmann aus schul- medizinisch-radiologischer Sicht. *Z Orthop* 1988;**126**:108–116.

36. Keesen W, Crow A, Hearn M. Proprioceptive accuracy in idiopathic scoliosis. *Spine* 1993;**17**:149–155.

37. Buchmann J, Bülow B, Pohlmann B. Asymmetrien der Kopfgelenksbeweglichkeit von Kindern. *Man Med* 1992;**30**:93–95.

38. Groot L.D Posture and motility in preterm infants. In *Fac Bewegingswetenschappen.* Frije Universiteit: Amsterdam, The Netherlands, p. 155, 1993.

39. Rönnqvist L. A critical examination of the Moro response in newborn infants-symmetry, state relation, underlying mechanisms. *Neuropsychologia* 1995;**33**:713–726.

40. Seifert I. Kopfgelenksblockierung bei Neugeborenen. *Rehabilitacia Prag (Supp)* 1975;**10**:53–57.

41. Hassenstein B. *Verhaltensbiologie des Kindes.* München: Piper, 1997.

42. Andry de Boisregard N, *L'orthopédie ou l'art de prévenir et de corriger dans les enfants les difformités du corps.* Paris: Vv Alix, 1741.

43. Lucassen P. Infantile Colic in Primary Care. In *Faculteit Geneeskunde.* Amsterdam: Vrije Universiteit, p. 135, 1999.

44. Spock B. Etiological factors in the hypertrophic stenosis and infantile colic. *Psychosom Med* 1944;**6**:162.

45. Wessel MA, *et al.* Paroxysmal fussing in infancy, sometimes called 'coli'. *Pediatrica* 1954; **14**:421–434.

46. Papousek M, von Hofacker N. Persistent crying in early infancy: a non-trivial condition of risk for the developing mother-infant relationship. *Child Care Health Dev* 1998;**24**(5):395–424.

47. Rautava P, Lehtonen L, Helenius H, *et al.* Infantile colic: child and family three years later. *Pediatrics* 1995;**96**:43–47.

48. Kühnen H. Erfahrungen mit der Manualmedizin in der neuropädiatrischen Landpraxis. In *Manualtherapie bei Kindern* (ed. H Biedermann), Stuttgart: Enke, pp. 187–198, 1999.

49. Hofacker Nv, *et al.* Rätsel der Säuglingskoliken. *Monatschr Kinderheilk* 1999;**147**:244–253.

50. American Academy of Paediatrics, Committee on Nutrition: Hypoallergenic Formulas. *Pediatrics* 1989;**83**:1069–1086.

51. Brazelton BT. Crying in infancy. *Pediatrics* 1962;**29**:579–588.

52. St James-Roberts I, Halil T Infant crying patterns in the first year: normal community and clinical findings. *J Child Psychol Psychiatry* 1991;**32**(6):951–968.

53. Miller AR, Barr RG. Infantile colic: Is it a gut issue? *Pediatr Clinics N Am* 1991;**38**:1407–1423.

54. Lehtonen L, Korhohnen T, Korvenranta H. Temperament and sleeping patterns in colicky

infants during the first year of life. *J Dev Behav Pediatr* 1994;**15**:416–420.

55. Biedermann F. *Fundamentals of Chiropractic from the Standpoint of a Medical Doctor*. (ed. LCJ Iekeler), ICRC, 1959.

56. Gutmann G, HWS, *Krankheiten HNO*, Arzt HNO. 1968;**10**:289–298.

57. Hülse M, Neuhuber WL, Wolff UD (eds.) *Der Kranio- zervikale Übergang*. Berlin: Springer, pp. 176, 1998.

58. Bobath B. *Abnorme Haltungsreflexe bei Gehirn-schäden*. Stuttgart: Thieme, 1976.

59. Vojta V, Peters A. *Das Vojta-Prinzip*. Berlin: Springer, 1992.

60. Gutmann G, Biedermann H, (eds.). *Die Halswirbelsäule. Teil 2: Allgemeine funktionelle Pathologie und klinische Syndrome*. Stuttgart: Fischer Verlag, 1984.

61. Biedermann H. Kinematic imbalances due to suboccipital strain. *J Man Med* 1992;**6**:151–156.

62. Biedermann H. Kopfgelenk-induzierte Symmetriestörungen bei Kleinkindern. *Kinderarzt* 1991;**22**:1475–1482.

63. Enquist M, Arak A. Symmetry, beauty and evolution. *Nature* 1994;**372**:169–172.

64. Shackelford TK, Larsen RJ. Facial asymmetry as an indicator of psychological, emotional, and physiological distress. *J Pers Soc Psychol* 1997;**72**(2):456–466.

65. Thornhill R, Gangestad SW. Human facial beauty: averageness, symmetry and parasitic resistance. *Hum Nat* 1993;**4**:237–269.

66. Møller AP, Swaddle JP. *Asymmetry, Developmental Stability and Evolution*. Oxford: Oxford University Press, 1997.

67. Blickhorn S. Symmetry as destiny-taking a balanced view on IQ. *Nature* 1997;**387**:849–850.

68. Furlow FB, Armijo-Prewitt T, Gangestad SW, *et al.* Fluctuating asymmetry and psychometric intelligence. *Proc R Soc Lond B Biol Sci* 1997;**264**:823–829.

69. Landau T. *About Faces*, New York: Doubleday, 1989.

70. Swaddle JP, Cuthill IC. Asymmetry and human facial attractiveness: symmetry may not always be beautiful. *Proc R Soc Lond (B)* 1995;**261**:111–116.

71. Parson PA. Fluctuation asymmetry: an epigenetic measure of stress. *Biol Rev* 1990;**65**:131–145.

72. Buchmann J, Bülow B. Asymmetrische frühkindliche *Kopfgelenksbeweglichkeit*. Berlin: Springer, 1989.

73. Flehmig I. *Normale Entwicklung des Säuglings und ihre Abweichungen*. Stuttgart: Thieme, 1979.

74. Vojta V. *Der zerebralen Bewegungsstörungen im Säuglingsalter*. Stuttgart: Enke, 1988.

75. Barker DJ. Intrauterine programming of adult disease. *Mol Med Today* 1995;**1**(9):418–423.

76. Nathanlielsz PW. *Life in the Womb: The Origin of Health and Disease*. Promethan Press, 1999.

77. Biedermann H. Primary and Secondary Cranial Asymmetry in KISS-Children. In *Clinical management of the cranio-cervical and cranio-facial pain and dysfunction* (eds. H v Piekartz, L Brydon), Oxford: Butterworth-Heinemann, 1999.

78. Fisher AG, Murray EA, Bundy AC. *Sensory Integration*. Philadelphia: FA Davis, 1991.

79. Biedermann H. Manualtherapie bei Teilleistungsstörungen: eine Pilotstudie. *Manuelle Medizin* 2000 (in press).

80. Lewit K, Janda V. Die Entwicklung von Gefügestörungen der Wirbelsäule im Kindesalter und die Grundlagen einer Prävention vertebragener Beschwerden. In *Neurologie der Wirbelsäule und des Rückenmarkes im Kindesalter*. (ed. D Müller), Jena: Fischer, pp. 371–389, 1964.

81. Gutmann G. Die funktionsanalytische Röntgendiagnostik der Halswirbelsäule. Funktionelle Pathologie und Klinik der Wirbelsäule. (eds. G Gutmann, H Biedermann), Vol. 1/2. Fischer, 1983.

82. Obel A, Jurik AG. Alternating scoliosis as a symptom of spinal tumor. *Fortschr Rö* 1991;**155**:91–92.

83. Matson DD, Tachdjinan MO. Intraspinal tumors in infants and children. *Postgrad Med* 1963;**34**:279–285.

84. Bussieres A, Cassidy D, Dzus A. Spinal cord astrocytoma presenting as torticollis and scoliosis. *J Manip Physiol Therap* 1994;**17**:113–118.

85. Shafrir Y, Kaufman BA. Quadriplegia after chiropractic manipulation in an infant with congenital torticollis caused by a spinal cord astrocytoma. *J Pediatr* 1992;**120**:266–269.

86. Visudhiphan P, Chiemachanya S, Somburanasin R, *et al.* Torticollis as the presenting sign in cervical spine infection and tumor. *Clin Pediatr* 1982;**21**:71–76.

87. Gutmann G. Hirntumor Atlasverschiebung und Liquordynamik. *Man Med* 1987;**25**:60–63.

88. Biedermann H, Koch L. Zur Differentialdiagnose des KISS-Syndroms. *Man Med* 1996;**34**:73–81.

89. Lietz R. Klinische-neurologische Untersuchung im Kindesalter. *Deutscher Ärzteverlag*, 1993.

90. Prechtl HFR. *The neurological examination of the full-term newborn infant*. London: Heinemann, 1977.

91. National Research Council. *Health effects of exposure to low levels of ionizing radiation*. Washington, 1990.

92. Goldman M. Cancer risk of low-level exposure. *Science* 1996;**271**:472.

93. Wackenheim A. *Roentgen Diagnosis of the Cranio-Vertebral Region.* Berlin: Springer, 1975.

94. Koch LE, Girnus U. Kraftmessung bei Anwendung der Impulstechnik in der Chirotherapie. *Man Med* 1998;**36**(1):21–26.

95. Biedermann H. Manual therapy in newborns and infants. *J Orthop Med* 1995;**17**:2–9.

96. Biedermann H. Biomechanische Besonderheiten des occipito- vervicalen Überganges. In *Manualtherapie bei Kindern.* (ed. H Biedermann), Enke: Stuttgart, p. 19–28, 1999.

Chapter 13

Cervicogenic vertigo: with special emphasis on whiplash-associated disorder

Carsten Tjell

INTRODUCTION

In the search for an explanation of how whiplash-associated disorders (WAD) develop and why these conditions do not heal like a distorted ankle or a tennis elbow, it might be fruitful to focus on the symptom patterns of most patients. All patients with WAD have pain in the neck, and many patients experience some kind of dizziness or disturbed vision, which fluctuates in intensity from day to day. Most patients agree that they feel quite comfortable after a longer period of rest and inactivity; however, every time they start to raise their activity they experience a considerable increase in pain and, often, in dizziness, as well as in cognitive dysfunction. By focusing on these entities – neck pain, dizziness, the chronicity of the disorder, despite the probable healing of any connective tissue lesions, and the pattern of symptom fluctuation in relation to physical activity level – it might be possible to propose a tentative explanation of the development of WAD, and why the condition often continues without adequate improvement.

Neck pain

All patients with WAD have neck pain. Studies have shown a close relation between muscle spindles and chronic inflammation in painful muscle disorders. The muscle spindles are small sensory organs in muscles parallel with the muscle fibres. Their main tasks are to register movements and positions, to be involved in muscle coordination and to regulate reflex-mediated muscle stiffness. During muscle contraction, various substances like lactic acid and potassium ions as well as substances associated with inflammation (i.e., arachidonic acid, bradykinin and serotonin) are produced in the muscles [1,2]. These substances stimulate chemoreceptors in the muscles. Signals from these are transmitted to cells of the spinal medulla, which activate the muscle spindle system and primary and secondary muscle spindle afferents. Primary spindle discharge increases reflex-mediated muscle stiffness. Under certain circumstances, such as prolonged static muscular effort, metabolites collect in the tissues, and a vicious circle can be established (Figure 13.1). These substances also cause pain. The vicious circle may be reinforced by an additional circuit. The secondary muscle-spindle afferents stimulate a positive feedback circuit to the cells, which control the muscle spindles [1–3].

The deepest neck muscles, especially the more delicate ones, have numerous muscle spindles. The spinal joints seem to contain the same proprioceptors as the knee joints. Therefore, it seems possible that the ligaments and capsules of the spinal joints act as sensors which, via the muscle-spindle system, could be important as a source of sensory feedback [1]. Moreover, Hu *et al.* [4] showed that 'stimulation of cervical paraspinal tissues by an inflammatory irritant results in an inflammatory

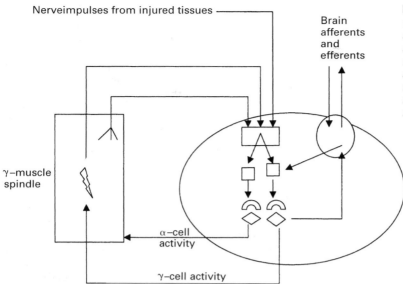

Nerveimpulses from injured tissues

Brain afferents and efferents

γ–muscle spindle

α–cell activity

γ–cell activity

Figure 13.1 *Basal scheme of the γ-muscle spindle system (see text). α-cell activity stimulates ordinary muscle contraction. γ-cell activity is involved in muscle coordination, and regulates the nervous reflex-mediated muscle stiffness.*

response in the paraspinal tissues and in a sustained and reversible activation of both jaw and neck muscles. This activation is especially prominent in the deep neck muscles'.

It is considered that there is an increased risk for a pathological development if the muscle-spindle system is simultaneously afflicted in different ways: by concentrating metabolites and inflammatory substances due to static muscle work, by stretching of ligaments, by joint and muscle inflammatory states and by CNS-originated influence on the muscle spindle system. Since dizziness is a common symptom of patients with WAD, the hypothesis is proposed that a disturbance of the balance system may influence, via efferent signals from the CNS, the muscle spindle system in a pathological direction. Also, it is supposed that the balance function of patients with WAD is affected by abnormal proprioceptive activity of the injured neck. The theoretical basis of the potential link between neck pain and disturbances of the balance system manifesting as cervicogenic vertigo will now briefly be surveyed.

The postural system

Equilibrium is ensured by a steady input of signals of vestibular, visual and proprioceptive origin to the brain. The vestibular system tells the brain of the movements and positions in space of the head, the visual systems brings information of the surroundings, the proprioceptors of the neck transmit information regarding the position of the head in relation to the rest of the body. Finally, the proprioceptors of the rest of the body give information concerning its position and velocity. This sensory input forms 'sensory pictures' which are integrated and stored in a 'bank of memory pictures' [5] which is supposed to be located in the parapontine reticular formation of the brainstem. (Figure 13.2). Every moment, 'sensory pictures' concerning the position and movement of the body are presented for the 'bank of memory pictures'; if the incoming 'sensory pictures' are recognized, the signals pass through at a subconscious level. Efferent activity from this postural control centre is transmitted for adjustment to the muscles of the neck and the rest of the body. This creates a feedback system with a series of new 'sensory pictures'. If inexperienced 'sensory pictures' caused by overstimulation or disease are transmitted to the 'memory bank', they will not be recognized. This will lead to neural activity at a conscious level. Vertigo and dizziness result from an abnormality of the 'sensory picture' or from a disturbance in the complex perceptive system containing interacting and integrating

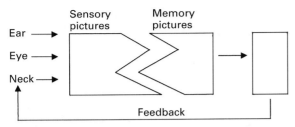

Figure 13.2 *The main principles of the equilibrium (see text). Ear: vestibular input; Eye: visual input; Neck: proprioceptive input. Feedback represents the adjustment of muscle tension in the neck, extremities and torso.*

signals of vestibular, visual and proprioceptive origin.

The complexity of dizziness might be more 'digestible' by the following example. It is well known that the feeling of dizziness can occur when sitting in a stopped train at a railway station and the neighbouring train starts moving. It can be explained as follows: Our eyes register that the 'whole world' (the window) is moving, which is interpreted as we are moving; however, the vestibulum organs of the ear tell the brain that we are not in motion. The brain (i.e., parapontine reticular formation and mid-cerebellum) cannot accept the conflicting information (i.e., the 'sensory picture') that we simultaneously are and are not in motion. Since we do not have such contradicting memory pictures, we will experience dizziness. As soon as we look in the opposite direction the dizziness immediately disappears because both the eyes and the ears give the same information that the train still is stationary.

The vestibular system

The vestibular system constitutes one of the phylogenetically oldest CNS functions, which in all species acts to achieve stability, although in higher animal forms, it is especially developed to maintain posture and locomotion on land, sea or in the air (for a review see Gacek [6] and Schwarz and Tomlinson [7]). The purpose of the reflex from the labyrinth to the eye muscles, the vestibulo-ocular reflex (VOR) is to stabilize images on the retina during head movements. The reader can immediately verify how critically important this reflex is by attempting to read this text while shaking the book through a small angle a few times per second. Reading will become impossible because the visual tracking reflexes are far too slow to manage sufficient visual stability, when the visual target is moving at such frequencies. If, on the contrary, the book is kept still, and the head is correspondingly shaken, reading will be easy, since the relative movements between the visual target and the head are compensated by the VOR. The reflexes to the eye muscles and the trunk and limb muscles are developed to meet the needs of these functions. The vestibular part of the labyrinth, with its three semicircular canals, and the otolith systems of the inner ear are located in the temporal bone. These receptor organs are stimulated by angular and linear acceleration and deceleration, respectively.

· The signals from the labyrinth are conveyed through the vestibular nerve. The vestibular nerve continues as a component of the central part of the VOR, described by Lorente de No [8]. An outline of the VOR is shown in Figure 13.3. The main route is from the labyrinth to the vestibular nuclei (VN) and further to the oculomotor muscle system which is responsible for the eye movements. Both are situated in the brainstem. The first-order vestibular neurons of the vestibular nerve terminate in the vestibular nuclei and also directly in the mid-cerebellum. The second-order vestibular neurons are the efferent projection pathways of the VN complex: (1) to the oculomotor muscle system (III, IV, VI); (2) to the mid-cerebellum; (3) to the paramedian pontine reticular formation (PPRF); (4) to the opposite located vestibular nuclei; (5) to the neck via the medial vestibulo-spinal tract; and (6) to the trunk and neck via the lateral vestibulo-spinal tract.

The vestibulo-cerebellar connection is an important projection between the vestibular nuclei and the mid-cerebellum where the primary visual-vestibular interaction occurs [9] (Figures 13.3 and 13.4). This is the system used when a moving target is followed by an individual in motion, e.g., to see sharply the face of a meeting person when both are walking.

The vestibulo-reticular projections (VRP) are integrated in a circuit (Figure 13.3) with the paramedian pontine reticular formation

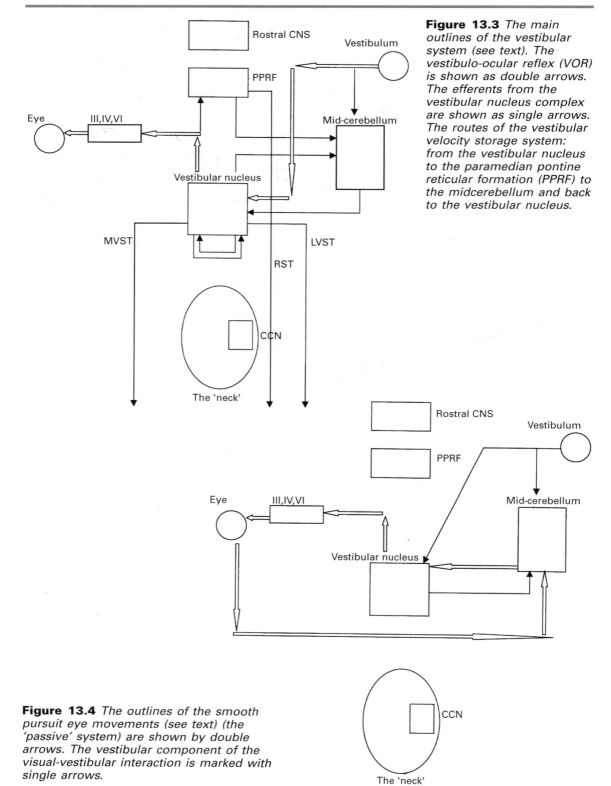

Figure 13.3 *The main outlines of the vestibular system (see text). The vestibulo-ocular reflex (VOR) is shown as double arrows. The efferents from the vestibular nucleus complex are shown as single arrows. The routes of the vestibular velocity storage system: from the vestibular nucleus to the paramedian pontine reticular formation (PPRF) to the midcerebellum and back to the vestibular nucleus.*

Figure 13.4 *The outlines of the smooth pursuit eye movements (see text) (the 'passive' system) are shown by double arrows. The vestibular component of the visual-vestibular interaction is marked with single arrows.*

(PPRF) and the mid-cerebellum [10]. This circuit probably constitutes a vestibular velocity storage system, which further has a smoothing function on the eye movements and the body tonus via the mid-cerebellum [11]. The PPRF is probably one of the major locations for comparison of 'sensory and memory pictures'.

Visual-postural systems

As the VOR helps the animal to keep a stationary target on the fovea, i.e., the hunting animal sees the stationary prey sharply during its advance, the visual systems assist in the opposite situation. The function of the smooth pursuit eye movement (SP) system is to stabilize images of smoothly moving foveal targets, like following a bird in the sky. There are three eye-movement systems with which the VOR must interact. The smooth pursuit (SP) system functions to stabilize images of smooth moving foveal targets [12]. The optokinetic (OK) system stabilizes images whenever the entire visual world moves. The saccadic system is used to move a target from the peripheral retina onto the fovea.

The smooth pursuit eye movement system

A dual system of 'active' and 'passive' visuoocular reflexes has been suggested by Yee *et al.*[13]. The 'active' system involves the fovea of retina and the calcarine cortex, while the 'passive' originates in the peripheral retina and terminates in the mid-cerebellum, without cerebral cortical participation, for adjustment of the eye motor signals during coordination of visual and vestibular signals (i.e., the visual-vestibular interaction) [11] (Figure 13.4).

The optokinetic system

The entire visual field is moving when an animal moves slowly along a curved track in a forest, or we are walking alongside the shelves in warehouses. The optokinetic stimulus, alternating vertical black-and-white zebra stripes, is similar to the visual impression one gets in the forest. The transmission of optokinetic signals involves both the optokinetic and the SP

systems. When changes in the angular velocity are less than 0.1 Hz, the VOR is not activated and blurred vision results. This is due to inertia in the kinetic sensory organ of the inner ears. Consequently, the information they supply concerning changes in head velocity is accurate only at frequencies above 0.1 Hz. The brain deals with this problem by utilizing information from the visual system to supply the VOR with the perceptive inputs about low-frequency movements [14] (Figure 13.5). All VN neurons with angular stimulation can also be activated by an optokinetic stimulus in the appropriate plane (the first-order neurons). The function of this optokinetic input to VN neurons is to compensate for the weak low-frequency reaction of the canals. The optokinetic signal is derived from the same specialized peripheral retinal ganglion cells as the SPs and is also passed to the mid-cerebellum.

The saccadic system

Targets located more than 20 degrees from the line of sight are acquired with a stereotyped combined eye and head movement called 'gaze saccade' [15]. In the evolution of vertebrates this system has proved to be of great value to both the prey as well as to the hunter. It gives them a chance to react immediately. If they detect any movement at the visual periphery they can see the target at once. This they achieve by a firing of excitatory and inhibitory burst neurons in the PPRF, which supply the saccadic pulse (Figure 13.6). Such burst cells are under the influence of visual signals at the retinal periphery and vestibular input during head movement [16]. Nystagmus is rhythmical oscillations of the eyeballs, either pendular or jerky. In jerky nystagmus there is a slow drift of the eyes in one direction, followed by a rapid recovery movement, always described in the direction of the recovery movement. It usually arises from labyrinthine or neurological lesions or stimuli, whether caloric or optokinetic. The slow drift is caused either by a lesion or by stimulation, whereas the rapid eye movement is a non-voluntary saccade generated in the PPRF. The teleological purpose of nystagmus lies in stabilizing a visual target. Saccades are influenced by the flocculus of the mid-cerebellum, which seems to integrate various sensory modalities, the

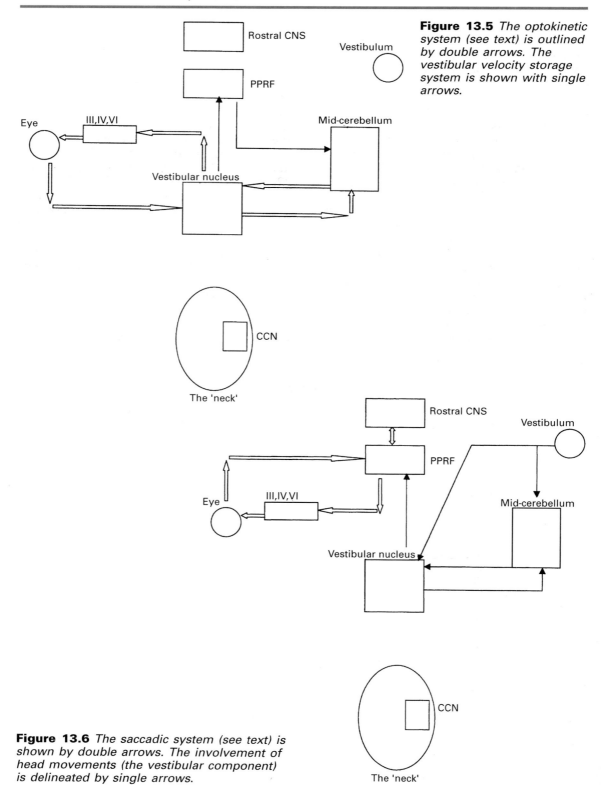

Rostral CNS

Vestibulum

PPRF

Eye

III,IV,VI

Mid-cerebellum

Vestibular nucleus

CCN

The 'neck'

Figure 13.5 *The optokinetic system (see text) is outlined by double arrows. The vestibular velocity storage system is shown with single arrows.*

Rostral CNS

Vestibulum

PPRF

Eye

III,IV,VI

Mid-cerebellum

Vestibular nucleus

CCN

The 'neck'

Figure 13.6 *The saccadic system (see text) is shown by double arrows. The involvement of head movements (the vestibular component) is delineated by single arrows.*

vestibular, the visual and the proprioceptive [17]. Thus, in concert with voluntary eye movements the mid-cerebellum seems to exert control over both head and eye movements.

Proprioceptive postural system

The third component of the 'sensory picture' of postural information presented to the 'memory bank' is the proprioceptive activity of the neck and the rest of the body . The muscles of the neck are distributed in three layers (for a review, see Karlberg [18]); the most superficial being long and extending from the occiput to the shoulder girdle. The middle layer stabilizes the skull to the cervical spine. The deepest layer interlinks the cervical vertebrae [19]. The neck muscles, especially the deepest finer ones, are well supplied with muscle spindles of the same density as the muscles of the hand (Figure 13.1). Muscle spindles, but not joint receptors, seem to be the main generators of cervical proprioception and kinaesthesia according to Dutia [20]. However, the mechanoreceptors are normally found in the facet joints of the human cervical spine according to McLain [21]. The proprioceptive reflexes of the neck are the cervico-collic reflexes (CCR) [22] and the cervico-ocular reflex (COR) [23] (Figure 13.7). The CCR and the COR have different functions; indeed, their effects tend to counteract or compete with each other. The CCR tends to stabilize the neck and protect it against over-rotation [24,25] and it counteracts the VOR [26]. The COR, on the contrary, normally a weak reflex, seems to be a 'helper' reflex if the labyrinth has been damaged [27]. The CCR is probably generated from the muscle spindles of the deepest neck muscles [28]. Their projections terminate at the central cervical nucleus (CCN) in the upper spinal cord [29,30] with its axons crossing the midline and entering the mid-cerebellum [31]. According to Pyykkö *et al.* [17] and Wilson *et al.* [32], the mid-cerebellum is an unique integrator of vestibular,

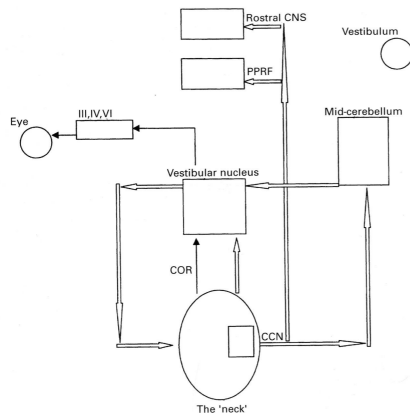

Figure 13.7 *The proprioceptive postural system (see text). The cervico-collic reflex (CCR) is outlined with double arrows. The cervico-ocular reflex (COR) is shown with single arrows.*

smooth pursuit and saccadic eye movements, as well as proprioceptive information. Moreover, the CCN neurons respond to electric stimulation of the contralateral vestibular nerve and to the single fibres of semicircular canals [29]. Thus, the CCN seems to be of importance for vestibular and proprioceptive integration concerning dynamic and static aspects of head movements [33]. A CCR derived vestibulo-proprioceptive interaction occurs in the PPRF [34], as well as in the cerebral cortex [35].

The COR is a reflex of less importance to man than the VOR and CCR [36,37]. Its function seems to provide information about the position of the neck and to cooperate with the VOR for clear vision during motion. The COR originates in proprioceptors in the neck muscles and in the cervical joints of the upper cervical spine [21]. According to Hikosaka and Maeda [23], these ascending signals cross at the midline to terminate in the contralateral vestibular nuclei. At this level, there is an interaction of the COR and VOR leading to modulated activity in the connection to the oculomotor nuclei. The effect of COR can be registered by rotation of the torso when the head is held still. The eyes move to the opposite side of the direction of head rotation, e.g., the torso moves to the left which turns the head relatively to the right, stimulating, the eyes to the left via the COR. At this moment – from a teleological viewpoint – in order to look forward, the saccadic system intervenes with involuntary horizontal saccades, which move the eyes to the midpoint. Again the COR drives the eyes to the left, etc. In this way, a rightwardly directed cervical nystagmus is induced [38–43]. This cervical nystagmus can be elicited in some people with increased proprioceptive neck activity and in people with unilateral vestibular dysfunction [27,44].

Some evidence has been presented that the SP system might be influenced by abnormal proprioceptive activity. For instance, various authors have shown that 'artificial' neck proprioceptive stimulation by muscle vibration affects the perceived location of a visual target [45–47]. The increased proprioceptive activity in patients with WAD has been shown by Tjell and Rosenhall [48] by the smooth pursuit neck torsion (SPNT) test. The CCR and COR reflexes are assumed to form the

basis for the SPNT test. This test is a conventional smooth pursuit eye movement test, performed in three head positions – one in neutral position and the others with the head stationary, turned to the right and the left in relation to the torso, after active turning. Patients should not feel any increase in pain during the test. The velocity gain (i.e., the eye velocity/stimulus velocity relationship) in each head position and direction of the eye movements is recorded. The test parameter chosen to represent the SPNT test was called the SPNT (diff) and is defined according to the formula:

SPNT (diff) = (neutral position (gain R ± gain L)/2) – (right turn (gain R ± gain L) ± left turn (gain R ± gain L)/4)

where gain R represents the velocity gain of smooth pursuits, tracking a target, which moves to the right, and gain L represents the corresponding gain to the left. In that study it was documented that vertigo and dizziness of cervical, but not of vestibular or CNS origin did influence the SPNT test [48]. A new study on patients without head or neck trauma with diagnoses like cervical spondylosis, fibromyalgia and maxillo-facial pain had demonstrated only a slight influence on the test results [49]. This difference in test response is interpreted as an effect of the acceleration-deceleration on the neck and the proprioceptors. It is feasible that this G-impact has lead to an hypersensibility of the proprioceptors.

The vestibulo-spinal tract

The final component in the postural model – after the 'sensory picture' has been compared with the 'memory picture' – is the 'feedback system' constituted by the vestibulo-spinal reflexes (VSR). These are the reflexes that save us from falling after a carousel ride. They transmit the feedback signals so as to establish an appropriate tone of the neck and body muscles for the purpose of balance. However, the effect of the VSR is not as well defined as the VOR because the influence of the vestibulo-spinal tract is only one of the many inputs into a complex multisensory orientational control system. Reflexes to the trunk and limbs are mediated via the lateral vestibulo-spinal tract (LVST) which originates primarily in the lateral vestibular nucleus [50] and via the reticulo-spinal tract from the bulbar reticular formation (Figure 13.3). These long tract reflexes are, in fact, open loops without a directly negative feedback [51].

The medial vestibulo-spinal tract (MVST) is not so extensive as the LVST. It projects to the cervical and upper thoracic cord levels [52]. Most MVST neurons are second-order vestibular cells, which are monosynaptically activated by semicircular canal afferents [50] (i.e., the vestibulo-collic reflex [53]). The sensory input from the neck to the MVST neurons in the VN probably occurs via the CCR. Thus, torsion of the neck stimulates the semicircular canals and their vestibular neurons activate the adjacent MVST neurons, which influence the tonus of the neck muscle. This arrangement serves as a protection against over-rotation.

HYPOTHESIS OF HOW WAD DEVELOPS

After this synopsis of the muscle spindle system and the postural system, a hypothesis is proposed of how neck pain and often dizziness are developed and fluctuate in parallel with one's level of physical activity. The hypothesis is presented in Figure 13.8. The trauma with the supposed impact on ligaments, capsules and muscles is the take-off. Impulses from injured soft tissues evoke cell activity in the spinal medulla, which leads to muscle contraction. An increased muscle tension – due to several days of elevated impulse activity from damaged spine-supporting tissues – releases arachidonic acid, bradykinin, serotonin, etc., which are important generators of pain. These substances stimulate chemoreceptors that also stimulate spinal cells. Hence, the circuit is closed and a vicious circle has been created even without considerable new input from the primary injured tissues.

This mechanism probably provides an explanation of many harmless conditions like neck-strain or temporary muscular low-back pain. However, patients with WAD seem to have permanent pain often accompanied by dizziness, always following increased physical activity. The spinal-cell activity is not only conveyed to the neck muscles but also to the central cervical nucleus (CCN). Signals are transferred from the CCN to the mid-cerebellum, the vestibular nuclei and the PPRF. These most important central postural 'control centres' are involved in the comparison of 'sensory and memory pictures', and the stabilizing feedback is performed via the vestibulo-collic reflex. Because of the increased cell activity to the CCN the 'sensory picture' is contradictory. The message of the proprioceptors is that the head is moving, and the vestibular organ and the eyes give the opposite information. Therefore, there is no corresponding 'memory picture', and dizziness often is experienced. Moreover, the level of feedback activity (i.e., via the vestibulo-collic reflex) is raised, which leads to increased neck muscle tension and further release of pain-evoking inflammatory substances. By this mechanism, the muscle spindle vicious circle is ratcheted up. From Figure 13.4 it can be deduced that besides the latter, a postural vicious circle is also established, and they both are integrated in and reinforce each other.

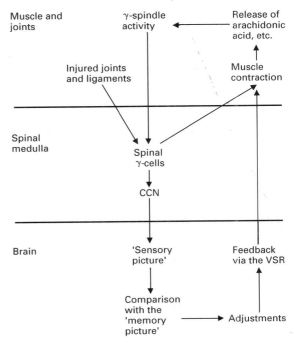

Figure 13.8 *The hypothesis of the development of WAD (see text).*

Clinical aspects of cervicogenic vertigo

The vertigo or dizziness of the patient with WAD is frequently described as a diffuse nautic unstable sensation or a feeling of unreality during a few seconds up to several hours or days. The dizziness often fluctuates with the neck pain, and the dizziness normally does not have the characteristics of the vestibular or visual systems. Therefore, their symptoms, not unusually, are declared as of psychogenic origin. However, in the former it has been shown that all postural systems involve the mid-cerebellum, which receives 'showers' of proprioceptive activity via the cervico-collic reflex over the central cervical nucleus. These proprioceptive signals act as 'noise-signals' on the mid-cerebellum. All interactions, integrations and fine adjustments are affected. Patients declare that the eyes are 'left back' when turning the head; this is due to a disturbed vestibular velocity storage system (i.e., the timing of the PPRF and the mid-cerebellum). Reading or watching TV implicate smooth pursuit and saccadic eye movements that involve the mid-cerebellum. Visiting shopping centres – which often is terrible for the victims – activates visual-vestibular interaction, which is necessary for having a clear vision of the moving people in one's surrounding. When walking along the shelves of a shop the optokinetic system is activated. In all these daily-life situations the mid-cerebellum is involved. Every time this happens the brain experiences an uneven comparison of 'sensory and memory pictures' which leads to compensatory muscular adjustments via the vestibulo-collic reflex, and once more the vicious circles are stimulated.

Suggestions for treatment of cervicogenic vertigo

What happens with a seasick sailor? After a few days he will improve, he will get accustomed to the sea. In fact, his paramedian pontine reticular formation acts as a network computer, and it is 'updated' as it gets new 'memory-pictures', i.e., his brain is learning that it is normal that the sea is moving. As soon as a new order is established, the vertigo and sickness will disappear, and so also the increased muscular feedback activity. This is the basic principle (habituation) in treatment of balance disorders [54,55]. Normally, patients are encouraged to take very intensive training with the positive effect of fast improvement. During the training these patients have an intense increase in the muscular feedback system; however, this is not serious for an otherwise healthy person.

A patient with WAD also needs to be 'updated', i.e., to get new 'memory pictures'. However, activation of the muscular feedback system is deleterious. Therefore, the principle of the proposed treatment is a very delicate balance training (habituation), which should be guided by the following day's neck pain, and every training 'round' should be finished by muscle relaxation with the aim of minimizing the muscular feedback activity. In practice, patients simply do balance exercises (gaze- and walk-gaze training) until they have felt dizziness for about 15 seconds, and then repeat this after a minute followed by a new rest and the next exercise. A training 'round' takes about 15 minutes and is finished with 20 minutes of relaxation with any kind of warmth under the neck. The training is done once or twice a day. The starting level of exercises is 'titrated' by the following day's neck pain, i.e., balance training is not allowed to increase pain. Each week the training burden is cautiously increased according to the principle that after 1 week the 'memory picture' has approximated the 'sensory picture' a little. This will implicate a lesser need for muscular feedback activity and so a lesser need for muscle-spindle activity and consistently the pain. This process has to be very slow. After 3 months of a very smooth increase in balance training the patient may evaluate if she had improved in pain and dizziness and also in cognitive functions, which probably are influenced by the proprioceptors [56–58]. After 6 months many have experienced a consistent improvement. According to the hypothesis presented every kind of treatment that is based on balance training and relaxation has the opportunity to be of benefit.

Finally, there may be a role for manual therapy in the management of cervicogenic vertigo. The role of upper cervical joint dysfunction has been proposed by numerous authors [59–62]. Spinal manipulation [63–66] and mobilization [67,68] have been reported in uncontrolled studies to provide symptomatic relief and to produce normalized ENG testing in a majority of subjects with cervicogenic vertigo. Jurk and Becker [69] reported a randomized clinical trial of manual traction therapy in 120 cases with 80% of subjects relieved in the treated group and 30% in the control group. A recent case report proposes that manual therapy be combined with postural retraining in order to optimize results [70].

List of abbreviations:

CCN, central cervical nucleus; CCR, cervico-collic reflex; CNS, central nervous system; COR, cervico-ocular reflex; LVST, lateral vestibulo-spinal tract; MVST, medial vestibulo-spinal tract; PPRF, paramedian pontine reticular formation; RST, reticulo-spinal tract; SP, smooth pursuit eye movement; SPNT, smooth pursuit neck torsion; VOR, vestibulo-ocular reflex; VSR, vestibulo-spinal reflexes; WAD, whiplash-associated disorders.

REFERENCES

1. Johansson H, Sjölander P. The neurophysiology of joints. In *Mechanics of Joints: Physiology, Pathophysiology, and Treatment*. (eds. V Wright, EL Radin), New York: Marcel Dekker, pp. 243–290, 1993.
2. Djubsjöbacka M, Johannson H, Bergenheim M. Influences on the gamma muscle-spindle system from muscle afferents stimulated by increased intramuscular concentrations of arachidonic acid. *Brain Res* 1994;**663**:293–302.
3. Johansson H, Sojka P. Pathophysiologic mechanisms involved in genesis and spread of muscular tension in occupational muscle pain and in chronic musculoskeletal pain syndromes. A hypothesis. *Med Hypoth* 1991;**35**:196–203.
4. Hu JW, Yu X-M, Vernon H, *et al.* Excitatory effects on neck and jaw muscle activity of inflammatory irritant applied to cervical paraspinal tissues. *Pain* 1993;**55**:243–250
5. Roberts TDM. *Neurophysiology of Postural Mechanisms*. New York: Plenum Press, 1967.
6. Gacek RR. Anatomy of the central vestibular system. In *Neurotology*. (eds. RK Jackler, DE Brackmann), St Louis: Mosby, pp. 41–58, 1994.
7. Schwarz DWF, Tomlinson RD. Physiology of the vestibular system. In *Neurotology*. (eds. RK Jackler, DE Brackmann), St Louis: Mosby, pp. 59–98, 1994.
8. Lorente de No R. Vestibulo-ocular reflex arc. *Arch Neurol Psychiatr* 1933;**30**:245–291.
9. Ito M. The vestibulo-cerebellar relationship: Vestibulo-ocular reflex arc and flocculus. In *The Vestibular System*. (ed. RF Naunton), New York: Academic Press, 1975.
10. Ladpli R, Brodal A. Experimental studies of commisural and reticular formation projections from the vestibular nuclei of the cat. *Brain Res* 1968;**8**:65–96.
11. Ito M. *The cerebellum and motor control*. New York: Raven Press, 1984.
12. Westheimer G. Eye movements responses to horizontally moving visual stimulus. *Arch Ophthalmol* 1954;**52**:932–941.
13. Yee RD, Baloh RW, Honrubia V, *et al.* Pathophysiology of optokinetic nystagmus. In *Nystagmus and Vertigo. Clinical Approaches to the Patient with Dizziness*. (eds. V Honrubia, M Brazier), New York: Academic Press, pp. 251–296, 1982.
14. Henn V, Cohen B, Young LR. Visual-vestibular interaction in motion perception and the generation of nystagmus. *Neurosci Res Prog Bull* 1980;**18**:458.
15. Tomlinson RD, Bahra PS. Combined eye-head gaze shifts in the primate. II. interactions between saccades and the vestibulo-ocular reflex. *J Neurophysiol* 1986;**56**:1558.
16. Robinson DA. The use of control systems analysis in the neurophysiology of eye movements. *Ann Rev Neurosci* 1981;**4**:463.
17. Pyykkö I, Schalén L, Wennmo C. Single unit activity in flocculus of alert cat during vestibular, visual and proprioceptive stimulation. *Agressologie* 1983;**24**:215–216.
18. Karlberg M. The neck and human balance. A clinical and experimental approach to 'cervical vertigo'. Thesis. University Hospital of Lund, Sweden, 1995.
19. Richmond FJR, Vidal PP. The motor system: Joints and muscles of the neck. In *Control of Head Movement* (eds. BW Peterson, FJR Richmond), New York: Oxford University Press, pp.1–21, 1988.
20. Dutia MB. The muscles and joints of the neck: their specialisation and role in head movement. *Prog Neurobiol* 1991;**37**:165–178.
21. McLain RF. Mechanoreceptor endings in human cervical facet joints. *Spine* 1994; **19**:495–501.
22. Petersen BW, Goldberg J, Biolotto G, *et al.* Cervicocollic reflex: its dynamic properties and interaction with vestibular reflexes. *J Neurophys* 1985;**54**:90–109.
23. Hikosaka O, Maeda M. Cervical effects on abducens motoneurons and their interaction with vestibulo-ocular reflex. *Exp Brain Res* 1973;**18**:512–530.

24. Pyykkö I, Aalto H, Seidel H, *et al*. Hierarchy of different muscles in postural control *Acta Otolaryngol* 1989;**468**:175–180.

25. Revel M, Minguet M, Gergoy P, *et al*. Changes in cervico-cephalic kinesthesia after a proprioceptive rehabilitation program in patients with neck pain. *Arch Phys Med Rehab* 1994; **75**:895–899.

26. Pompeiano O. The tonic neck reflex: supraspinal control. In *Control of Head Movement*. (eds. BW Peterson, FJR Richmond), New York: Oxford University Press, pp. 108–119, 1988.

27. Botros G. The tonic oculomotor function of the cervical joint and muscle receptors. *Adv Otolarygol* 1979;**25**:214–220.

28. Hirai N, Hongo T, Sasaki S, *et al*. Neck muscle afferent input to spinocerebellar tract cells of the central cervical nucleus in the cat. *Exp Brain Res* 1984;**55**:286–300.

29. Hirai N, Hongo T, Sasaki S, *et al*. The neck and labyrinthine influences on cervical spinocerebellar tract neurones of the central cervical nucleus in the cat. In *Reflex Control of Posture and Movement, Vol 50, Progress in Brain Research*. (eds. R Granit, O Pompeiano), Amsterdam: Elsevier North-Holland: Biomedical Press, pp. 529–536, 1979.

30. Hongo T, Kitama T, Yoshida K. Integration of vestibular and neck afferent signals in the central cervical nucleus. In *Vestibular Control of Posture and Movement, Vol. 76, Progress in Brain Research*, (eds. O Pompeiano, J Allum), Amsterdam, Elsevier North-Holland: Biomedical Press, pp.155–162, 1988.

31. Boyle R, Pompeiano O. Response characteristics of cerebellar interpositus and intermediate cortex neurons to sinusoidal stimulation of neck and labyrinth receptors. *Neuroscience* 1980;**5**:357–372.

32. Wilson VJ, Maeda M, Fuchs JI. Inhibitory interaction between labyrinthine, visual and neck inputs to the cat flocculus. *Brain Res* 1975;**96**:357–360.

33. Popova LB, Ragnarson B, Orlovsky GN, *et al*. Responses of neurons in the central cervical nucleus of the rat to proprioceptive and vestibular inputs. *Arch Ital Biol* 1995;**133**:31–45.

34. Kubin K, Manzoni D, Pompeiano O. Responses of lateral reticular neurons to convergent neck and macular vestibular inputs. *J Neurophysiol* 1981;**46**:48–64.

35. Grüsser O-J, Pause M, Schreiter U. Vestibular neurones in the parieto-insular cortex of monkeys (*Macaca fascicularis*): visual and neck receptor responses. *J Physiol (Lond)* 1990;**430**:559–583.

36. Bronstein AM, Hood JD. The cervico-ocular reflex in normal subjects and patients with absent vestibular function. *Brain Res* 1986;**373**:399–408.

37. Sawyer RN, Thurston SE, Becker KR. The cervico-ocular reflex of normal human subjects in response to transient and sinusoidal trunk rotation. *J Vest Res* 1994;**4**:245–249.

38. van de Calseyde P, Ampe W, Depondt M. ENG: the cervical syndrome neck torsion nystagmus. *Adv Otorhinolaryngol* 1977;**22**:119–124.

39. Barlow D, Freedman W. Cervico-ocular reflex in the normal adult. *Acta Otolaryngol* 1980;**89**:487–496.

40. de Jong JMBV, Bles W, Bovenker G. Nystagmus, gaze shift, and self motion perception during sinusoidal head and neck rotation. In *Vestibular and Oculomotor Physiology* (ed. B Cohen), *Ann NY Acad Sci* 1981;**374**:590–599.

41. Holtmann S, Reiman V, Beimert U. Qantifizierung der Reizparameter beim Halsdrehtest. *Laryngol Rhinol Otol* 1988;**67**:460–464.

42. Jürgens R, Mergner T. Interaction between cervico-ocular and vestibulo-ocular reflexes in normal adults. *Exp Brain Res* 1989;**77**:381–390

43. Doerr M, Schmitt HJ, Thoden U, *et al*. Tonic cervical stimulation: does it influence eye position and eye movements in man? *Acta Otolaryngol* 1991;**111**:2–9.

44. Kobayashi Y, Yagi T, Kamio T. Cervico-vestibular interaction in eye movements. *Auris-Nasus Larynx* 1986;**13**:87–95.

45. Biguer B, Donaldson IM, Hein A, *et al*. Neck muscle vibration modifies the representation of visual motion and direction in man. *Brain* 1988;**111**:1405–1424.

46. Roll R, Velay JL, Roll RP. Eye and neck proprioceptive messages contribute to the spatial coding of retinal input in visually oriented activities. *Exp Brain Res* 1991;**85**:423–431.

47. Taylor JL, McCloskey DI. Illusions of head and visual target displacement induced by vibration of neck muscles. *Brain* 1991;**114**:755–759.

48. Tjell C, Rosenhall U. Smooth pursuit neck torsion test: A specific test for cervical dizziness. *Am J Otol* 1998;**19**:76–81.

49. Tjell C, Tenenbaum A, Sandström S, *et al*. Evaluation of smooth pursuit neck torsion test as a specific test for whiplash associated disorders. In press, 2000.

50. Pompeiano I, Brodal A. The origin of vestibulospinal fibers in the cat. An experimental-anatomical study, with comments on the descending medial longitudinal fasciculus. *Arch Ital Biol* 1957;**95**:166–195.

51. Anderson JH, Soechting JF, Terzuolo CA. Role of vestibular inputs in the organization of motor output to the forelimb extensors. *Progr Brain Res* 1979;**50**:582–596.

52. Nyberg-Hansen R. Origin and termination of fibers from the vestibular nuclei descending in the medial longitudinal fasciculus. An experimental study with silver impregnation methods in the cat. *J Comp Neurol* 1964; **122**:355–367.

53. Wilson VJ, Boyle R, Fukushima K, *et al.* The vestibulocollic reflex. *J Vestib Res* 1995; **5**:147–170.

54. Cawthorne T. The physiological basis for head exercises. *J Chart Soc Physiother* 1944:106–107.

55. Shepard NT, Telian SA, Smith-Wheelock M, *et al.* Vestibular and balance rehabilitation therapy. *Ann Otol Rhinol Laryngol* 1993; **102**:198–205.

56. Gimse R, Tjell C, Björgen IA, *et al.* Disturbed eye movements after whiplash due to injuries to the posture control system. *J Clin Exp Neuropsychol* 1996;**18**:178–186.

57. Gimse R, Björgen IA, Tjell C, *et al.* Reduced cognitive functions in a group of whiplash patients with demonstrated disturbances in the posture control system. *J Clin Exp Neuropsychol* 1997;**9**:838–849.

58. Tjell C. Diagnostic considerations on whiplash associated disorders. Thesis. Karolinska Hospital, Stockholm, Sweden, 1998.

59. Beisinger E. C2 and C3 cervical nerve root syndrome: the influence of cervical spine dysfunction on ENT symptoms. *Man Med* 1997;**35**:12–19.

60. Simon H, Moser M. Der zervikalnystagmus aus manual-medizinischer sicht. *Man Med* 1977;**15**:47–51.

61. Hulse M. Disequilibrium caused by a functional disturbance of the upper cervical spine. Clinical aspects and differential diagnosis. *Man Med* 1983;**1**:18–23.

62. Bjorne A, Berven A, Agerberg G. Cervical signs and symptoms in patients with Meniere's Disease: a controlled study. *J Craniomandib Pract* 1998;**16**:194–202.

63. Wing LW, Hargrove-Wilson W. Cervical vertigo. *Aust NZ J Surg* 1974;**44**:275–277.

64. Mahlstedt K, Westohen M, Konig K. Therapy of functional disorders of the craniovertebral joints in vestibular disease. *Laryngorhinootologie* 1992;**71**:246–250.

65. Stodolny J, Chmielewski H. Manual therapy in the treatment of patients with cervical migraine. *J Man Med* 1989;**4**:49–51.

66. Fitz-Ritson D. The chiropractic management and rehabilitation of cervical trauma. *J Manip Physiol Therap* 1990;**13**:17–26.

67. Uhlemann C, Granowski K-H, Endres U, Callies R. Manual diagnosis and therapy in cervical giddiness. *Man Med* 1993;**31**:77–81.

68. Carlsson J, Rosenhall U. Oculomotor disturbances in patients with tension headaches treated with acupuncture or physiotherapy. *Cephalalgia* 1990;**10**:123–129.

69. Jurk D, Becker R. Traction massage: one possibility for the treatment of giddiness with a cervical spine component. *Man Med* 1989;**27**:87–90.

70. Bracher ES, Almeida CIR, Almeida RR, Duprat AC, *et al.* A combined approach for the treatment of cervical vertigo. *J Manip Physiol Therap* 2000;**23**:96–100.

Chapter 14

Vertebrobasilar incidents and spinal manipulative therapy of the cervical spine

Cameron McDermaid

INTRODUCTION

Vertebrobasilar incidents (VBI) are the most significant adverse events that follow manipulation of the cervical spine. These events usually involve injury to the intimal wall of the vertebral artery with dissection and thrombus formation and sometimes with subsequent embolization. In this chapter, VBI will be used to collectively describe injuries to the cervical vasculature or their sequelae.

At least 165 cases of VBI following cervical manipulation have been reported in the literature from the earliest report to 1993 [1]. The frequency of these events has been estimated to be from 1 in 400 000 [2] to 1 in 1.5 million [3]. These estimates suggest that these events are rare; however, others feel that VBI following cervical manipulation is more common than currently recognized [4]. A better understanding of these events, regardless of their frequency, has implications for patient care and risk management. Better understanding will also help guide future research.

A BRIEF OVERVIEW OF THE CASE LITERATURE

Case reports make up the largest source of information on complications following cervical manipulation. A number of literature reviews have pooled these reports in order to identify factors that may assist in risk management [1,5–7]. While useful, these reviews generally deal only with VBI following cervical manipulation and don't provide a broader context of these types of injuries.

Haldeman *et al.* [8] reviewed the literature up to 1993 that pertained to risk factors for vertebrobasilar artery dissection. They attempted to evaluate the evidence for risk factors for dissection: age, sex, presence of hypertension, migraine, smoking, oral contraceptives, the type of manipulation or minor trauma/neck movement and various co-morbid diseases. The case literature was found to be of little assistance in identifying the type of mechanical trauma, neck movement, manipulation or the patient at risk. The most commonly proposed risk factors for dissection: migraine, hypertension, oral contraceptive use and smoking did not exceed the population prevalence. These findings should be interpreted with caution, however. In general, the case reports lacked many details that would have been useful for their interpretation. These risk factors may have been present, but were not identified in the report. Standardizing the content of case reports would be useful to identify prestroke status, potential risk factors, co-morbid disease and the details of the suspected precipitating event. Standardized and dependable case data would also strengthen comparisons with population-based data.

CERVICAL MANIPULATION AND VBI

What is the relationship between cervical manipulation and VBI? Using a simplistic and monocausal approach, the injuries reported in these cases may be explained in three ways: cervical manipulation is co-incidental to the occurrence of VBI; cervical manipulation is iatrogenic in normal individuals; or cervical manipulation exacerbates a pre-existing and undiagnosed pathology.

VBI following cervical manipulation may be under-reported [1]. However, spurious association is also a risk in case reports [9]. LeBoeuf-Yde *et al* [10] reported a series of cases that failed to burden the statistics of injuries attributed to chiropractors. These six cases included individuals that suffered stroke, bleeding aneurysm, disc herniation, cauda equina and a heart attack in situations where they were unable to or had yet to see their chiropractor. Some of these patients had pre-morbid conditions but at least two had no unusual history. In one case (a case of massive stroke), a CT scan before the stroke had been unremarkable. If the patients reported in the cases had undergone cervical manipulation, it is possible that a post hoc report would have identified manipulation as being iatrogenic. But, while some injuries attributed to cervical manipulation may be coincidental, the close temporal relationship of manipulation to VBI is difficult to discount as being entirely coincidental [8].

If cervical manipulation does have an iatrogenic role in VBI, it must adversely affect normal tissue or tissue that is susceptible to injury. This interaction has been described in two basic models of the mechanism of injury to the vertebral artery following manipulation: trauma to the arterial wall producing vasospasm; and/or trauma to the arterial wall producing tissue damage which is followed by thrombosis and/or embolization [11].

Vasospasm of cerebral and cervical arteries is a major cause of morbidity in severe trauma, subarachnoid haemorrhage or intracranial aneurysm rupture [12,13]. This type of vasospasm may be a reaction to the presence of endothelial factors and may represent a more diffuse phenomenon rather than a specific response to trauma [12]. The role of vasospasm in injuries to the cervical vessels with specific minimal trauma is less clear.

Smith and Estridge [14] have suggested that vasospasm may follow vertebral artery compression. Vasospasm may account for the rapid appearance of symptoms in some cases, relative to the delivery of manipulation, than might be expected with a de-novo intimal injury. Transient spasms causing transient ischaemic attack (TIA)-like symptoms have been detected in the internal carotid artery in the absence of overt vascular injury or pathology [15]. However, the difficulty with imaging transient vasospasm means that the role of vasospasm is poorly understood in the context of VBI.

Intimal injury and subsequent subintimal haematoma, dissection and embolization are better understood and described in the literature. In all types of cervico-cranial dissections, haemorrhage occurs into the medial layer of the vessel [16]. This haemorrhage may be caused by haemorrhage of the vasa vasorum in the medial layer (Figure 14.1a) or by an intimal tear allowing extravasation of blood into the medial layer (Figure 14.1b). Even if the haemorrhage begins in the media, it may still rupture back through the intima proximally, allowing the force of the luminal flow to extend the dissection. Rupture back through the intima can also cause the formation of a false lumen communicating with a true lumen at either end. The injury may dissect subintimally, causing stenosis, or subadventitially, causing an outpouching. This outpouching is distinct from a pseudo-aneurysm, which is caused by arterial rupture and encapsulation of the paravascular haematoma [16]. In the case of subintimal haematoma, luminal stenosis may cause distal ischaemia. In some instances, ischaemia is avoided by the capacity of the collateral circulation to provide adequate perfusion to the brain. This capacity has been demonstrated experimentally [17] and in the presence of complete pathological occlusion [18] of one vertebral artery. Exposure of the basement membrane during intimal disruption can promote platelet aggregation (Figure 14.1c) and may lead to embolization [16] (Figure 14.1d).

Most of the patients in the reported cases have been young and have lacked overt co-morbid disease [1]. However, arterial dissection is one of the most significant causes of stroke in the young [19]. Neck pain and headache, both of which are treated with

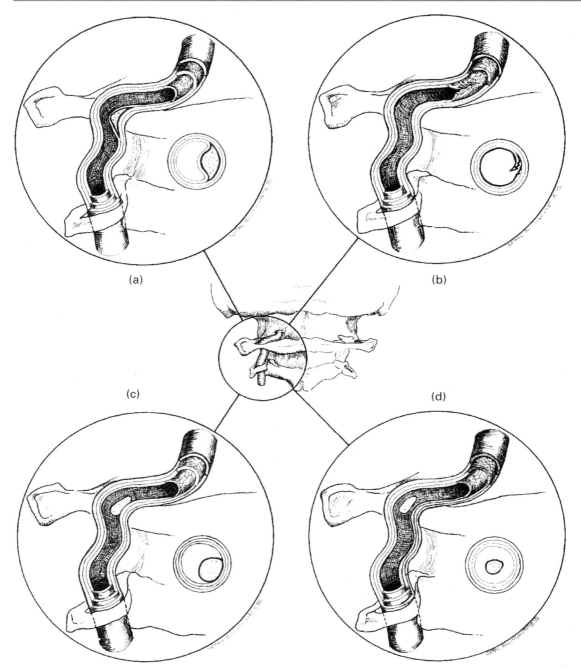

Figure 14.1 *Vascular injury model (see text for explanation).*

manipulation [3], are common presenting complaints of vertebral artery dissection [20]. Is it possible that some of the reported cases had a pre-existing dissection and subsequently presented for care?

Johnson *et al* [21] identified a case in which a 44-year-old man developed acute shoulder and neck pain after a game of cricket. Two to three days later, he underwent a cervical manipulation by a chiropractor with some apparent benefit. Five days later he developed self-limiting vertigo and the subsequent day developed double vision, tinnitus, left orbital headache, vomiting and left arm weakness. The chiropractor referred him to the hospital after he presented with these complaints. He died in hospital approximately 15 days post-manipulation and 18 days after the cricket injury. The vessel demonstrated medial cystic necrosis (a build-up of proteoglycans in the tunica media) and well-established granulation tissue along the entire dissection. It is possible in this case that the cervical manipulation caused a haemorrhage in a pre-existing dissection; however, the sequence of events in this case could not be confirmed. Mas *et al.* [22] identified the case of a 35-year-old woman with a 3-week history of neck pain, who developed basilar-artery territory ischaemia and died following cervical manipulation. Pathological changes were different in the upper and lower part of the dissection. The authors felt that the cervical pain was the first symptom of the dissection and the manipulation precipitated bleeding in an already dissecting vessel.

The initial clinical symptoms of vertebral artery dissection: neck pain and posterior headache, may be attributed to musculo-skeletal pain or tension headache unless focal ischaemic signs appear [20,23]. The pain of dissection may present as sharp in quality, severe in intensity and different from previously experienced pain [23]. None of the 12 patients in one small series of patients with extracranial artery dissection had restriction of cervical spine movements or cervical muscle tenderness [23]. The lack of musculo-skeletal signs in the presence of sudden and unusual neck and occipital pain may be a useful clue to alert the treater to the possibility of arterial dissection. Careful scrutiny for manifestations of bruits, oculosympathetic paralysis or lower cranial nerve palsies may also help detect patients with vertebral artery dissection. Delaying cervical manipulation in cases of unexplained, acute and severe neck pain or occipital headache may prevent injury to an already dissecting vessel and allow for a clearer clinical picture to emerge.

Some patients may be vulnerable to arterial dissection because of a pre-existing arteriopathy or a heritable connective disorder. At least two reported cases have demonstrated frank arteriopathy [21,24]. The former case has been discussed above. The latter case involved a 29-year-old woman who sustained a fatal bilateral internal carotid artery dissection following chiropractic manipulation of the neck. This patient demonstrated pre-existing mediolytic arteriopathy. In the absence of overt arteriopathy, connective tissue changes that are associated with heritable connective tissue disorders may be important. Occult connective tissue disorder may not be uncommon in patients with VBI associated with cervical manipulation [25].

Spontaneous cervical artery dissections are a feature of Ehlers-Danlos syndrome Type IV and may also occur in Marfan's syndrome [26]. However, a heritable vascular defect may play a part in arterial dissection in some individuals, even in the absence of a clinically apparent connective tissue disorder. Patients with cervical artery dissections and unique phenotypes of heritable connective tissue disorders that cannot be identified have been reported [27]. A family history of arterial dissection may be helpful in identifying these cases. Scheivink *et al.* [28] found that intracranial aneurysms and cervical artery dissections occurred in a familial pattern in a small proportion of a series of 175 patients. The possibility of a familial link in subset of patients with spontaneous dissection has also been suggested by others [29,30].

The basic defect in Ehlers-Danlos syndrome Type IV is abnormal Type III collagen. This has led investigators to examine the role of collagen abnormalities in people who experience spontaneous dissection. Van den Berg [31], in a case-control study using 16 subjects with spontaneous cervical artery dissection, used protein analysis to assess the ratios of Type III to Type I collagen. Two of the 16 subjects expressed a low-collagen Type III/I ratio relative to norms set by 41 healthy controls. The authors felt that those subjects with dissection and a relative deficiency of Type III collagen may be expressing the atypical form of Ehlers-Danlos syndrome Type IV, which has no visible phenotypical characteristics. However, the relatively low proportion of patients with dissection in this series who expressed a low Type III to I collagen ratio raises doubt about the extent to which this anomaly contributes to spontaneous dissection or dissection with minimal trauma. This doubt is compounded by the findings of Kuivanieimi *et al.* [32], who found that altered Type III collagen was an unlikely explanation for intracranial aneurysm or cervical artery dissections. Abnormal collagen production has not been demonstrated in other series of patients with cervical artery dissection, even in the suspected presence of a heritable connective tissue disorder [27]. However, collagen may have different role in the aetiology of dissection.

Brandt *et al.* [33] found that the ultrastructural morphology of dermal connective tissue was abnormal in 68% of 25 patients with non-traumatic dissection. Collagen and elastin aberrations were mild in some cases and more marked in others. These aberrations were similar to those seen in Ehlers-Danlos Types I and III, but not in Type IV. No aberrations were noted in a control group of 10 patients without dissection. It is of interest that Type III collagen production was normal in all subjects. It is also of interest that one of the subjects with dissection of the internal carotid artery had mechanical stresses attributed to coughing and chiropractic treatment. This study suggests that abnormal ultrastructural morphology of collagen is more important than abnormal collagen production.

Regardless of the presence or absence of an underlying predisposition, stress that is sufficient to lead to a structural insult must be placed on the vertebral artery. The unique anatomy of the vertebral artery and the biomechanics of the cervical spine as it relates to the vertebral artery may provide the basis for this stress to occur.

The vertebral artery is unique among the cervico-cephalic vessels by virtue of its position and relationship to the adjacent structures. It is usually described as four segments; the pre-transverse segment (V1), the transverse segment (V2), the atlantoaxial segment (V3) and the intracranial segment (V4) [34].

From its usual origin at the subclavian artery, the vertebral artery traverses the subclavian triangle to penetrate the transverse foramen of C6. It may less commonly penetrate at another level, sometimes to the level of C3. The artery fits tightly into the transverse canal as it follows a relatively linear course as it ascends in the V2 segment [34]. The artery has a coating of conjunctive tissue that adheres to the surrounding soft tissue by means of radiated trabeculae. Prominent collagenous fibre bundles are directly or indirectly related to the adventitia and attach to the periosteum of the transverse foramen and the muscular fascia of the inter-transverse musculature throughout the course of the artery [35].

The V3 segment extends from the C3–C2 intertransverse space to the point where it penetrates the dura mater. The vessel has four contours in its course in the V3 segment. The last contour looks like a horizontal crook with the vessel being held in a groove on the posterior slope of the atlanto-occipital joint by a fibrous casing that is reinforced by the transverse and retroglenoid ligaments. The atlanto-occipital dura mater is traversed approximately 10–15 mm from the median line in relation to the atlanto-occipital joint. The intracranial segment (V4) traverses the dura mater and ascends to the occipital foramen to terminate in the basilar artery [36].

The close association of the vertebral artery to its surrounding structures and the hypothesized role of head rotation in VBI [14,37] have directed a great deal of attention on the effects of head movement on the cervical arteries and on the vertebral artery in particular.

Cadaveric specimens have been examined in order to assess the effects of head rotation on the vertebral arteries [38–40]. Vertebral artery patency was reduced or lost in some of these experimental conditions. These studies have utilized prepared cadavers [38,39] or en bloc cervical spine preparations [40]. While interesting, the generalizability of this work to in-vivo events is limited [41].

Case series or individual cases have demonstrated vertebral artery occlusion coincident with symptoms of vertebrobasilar ischaemia [42–49]. Some of these cases have been in the elderly or those with an abnormality in the cervical spine such as instability or spondylitic change. In other cases, structures such as the longus colli muscles have been demonstrated on angiography to be the cause of the occlusion [50]. What is not known is the incidence of vascular occlusion with head rotation, symptomatic or not, in the general population. Studies using Doppler ultrasound have tried to address this question in a variety of studies.

Doppler ultrasound is the most common imaging modality that has been used to assess blood flow at the vertebral artery [51–61] or transcranially [41,62]. Some studies have detected no differences in vertebral artery blood flow [51–53] while others have detected such changes [41,54–62]. The disagreement between these studies may be due to the methods used, the source of subjects, the definitions of blood-flow change, or a low prevalence of vertebral artery-flow changes in the general population. More robust non-invasive gold standards, such as magnetic resonance angiography (MRA), may provide better information about the frequency of vascular occlusion that may accompany clinical vertebrobasilar symptoms. Techniques such as functional MRI may help identify any ischaemic effects of such occlusion.

It is difficult to categorically state that blood-flow alterations with head movement do or do not occur in the general population. Vertebral artery blood flow may change in a subset of individuals and this may explain the diversity of results of the previous studies. Dumas *et al.* [63] have proposed that a combination of an underdeveloped V3 segment and loss of the normal asymmetrical motion of C1 on C2 may predispose to mechanical stresses sufficient to occlude the vertebral artery. In a series of 14 patients, local flow disturbance at the transverse foramen of C2 was detected by MRA in four subjects. These disturbances were not accompanied by a reduction of vertebral artery blood flow downstream from the site of disturbance. The authors also presented the case of one young woman with congenital fusion of C2 and C3 who demonstrated symptomatic vertebral artery occlusion with head rotation. The findings led the authors to conclude that a sufficient extent of underdevelopment of the V3 segment and loss of normal asymmetrical motion was necessary for vertebral artery blood flow alterations to occur.

Even if decreased vertebral artery flow does occur, it may not be symptomatic in all individuals. A lack of symptomatology is probably due to collateral circulation that maintains an adequate blood flow to the posterior cranial circulation. The symptoms that may accompany head movement have been of particular interest to healthcare providers who deliver cervical spine manipulation. Clinically, these symptoms and the presumed role of head rotation in their aetiology have directed risk management procedures for care providers who deliver cervical manipulation.

Provocative positional testing is part of most premanipulative screening protocols [11,64–70]. This testing uses a variety of head positions, usually extension and rotation, to evaluate for symptoms of VBI. If a patient displays symptoms of vertebrobasilar TIA (vbTIA) with testing, cervical manipulation is considered to be contraindicated.

Do these tests predict the risk of injury? A 'critical neck position' has been proposed as an independent and significant risk factor for stroke in the elderly. Weintraub and Khoury [71] examined 64 elderly patients with well documented vbTIA and 30 control subjects using MRA. They found that over 50% of the TIA group had significant vertebral artery compression with head angulation compared with 13% in the control group. Post-study dizziness was seen in 68% of TIA subjects compared to 13% in controls. The vbTIA group in this study had a high prevalence of vascular risk factors such as hypertension, obesity, previous stroke, smoking and diabetes mellitus (87%) compared with the control group (13%). This latter finding is consistent with the findings of Delcker *et al.*[72] who found a higher prevalence of vertebrobasilar TIA in an elderly population with combined vertebral artery and internal carotid disease.

The presence of TIA in an elderly population is a significant risk factor for stroke [73]. Weintraub's study appears to support the use of positional testing as a screening test for ischaemic events in this age group. However, this conclusion is debatable.

Although only percentages of groups were reported, Weinstein's data can be used to estimate the negative predictive value: the probability that a negative test reflects the true absence of the disease of interest. In the context of a screening test for risk of injury, a high negative predictive value is desirable. The negative predictive values for the presence of compression on MRA, the presence of post-test symptoms, and the presence of vascular risk factors are 53%, 61% and 80% respectively. Using symptoms following positional testing, 61% of those tested as 'negative' would truly be negative. Contrast this with a negative predictive value of 80% for a history of vascular disease. Looking at the test another way, the probability of vbTIA being present in this sample is 64% (the prevalence in the sample). If you chose any one person from this sample (vbTIA plus control), there is a 64% chance they would be from the vbTIA group. After applying the likelihood ratio for a negative positional test, the post-test probability only drops to 39%; that is, a person selected from the sample, and who had a negative positional test, still has about a 40% chance of being from the vbTIA group. Using the likelihood ratio for a history of vascular risk factors, the post-test probability drops to approximately 21%. So, it would appear that a history that examines for vascular risk factors is more clinically meaningful than the results of a positional test for risk factors in this age group.

Provocative positional testing has been criticized as useless for detecting those at risk of injury [74] and therefore of having little value in the context of a risk management protocol. There is some case literature that suggests that provocative testing is inadequately sensitive [75–77]. Rivett *et al.* [61] makes the distinction that the test does not predict the likelihood of injury. Rather, it assesses the adequacy of collateral circulation and suggests how significant an injury may be, should it occur.

The ability of provocative testing to identify vertebral artery occlusion as the cause of vertebrobasilar symptoms is debatable. Also, the implications for follow-up for those with a positive test are rarely discussed. Do these patients require further follow-up, investigation and, perhaps, surgical intervention? These issues and the role of provocative positional testing in risk-management protocols have yet to be resolved.

Historical elements are also discussed in the context of risk management and, as has been discussed, may be useful in the elderly or those with a family history of dissection. However, few of the cases that are reported in the literature are of patients for whom a remarkable history was reported [1]. The inadequate documentation in the case literature [8] prevents a clear indication of what historical risks may be important. Moreover, a conventional history may be inadequate for detecting those at risk. Influences that are not engendered in a standard history may be important in the genesis of VBI following cervical manipulation.

If connective tissue abnormalities and/or mechanical factors play such a large part in the aetiology of cervical artery dissection, why do dissections appear to be rare and have a low risk of recurrence [78]. Why do some patients with VBI following manipulation have a history of prior uneventful manipulation [79,80]?

Schievink *et al.* [81] examined a group of 200 consecutive patients from 1970 to 1990 and found that the frequency of spontaneous cervical artery dissection peaked in October; 58% more patients suffered a cervical artery dissection in autumn than during any other season. Weather-related factors or infectious diseases that peak in this season were suggested as possible environmental factors. Grau *et al.* [82] reported three cases of respiratory infection that preceded cervical artery dissection. To examine this relationship further, Grau *et al.* [83] utilized a case-control design using 43 patients with acute cervical artery dissection. They found that recent infection was significantly more common in patients with artery dissection than in those with other causes of cerebral infarction. Like Schievink and colleagues, they noted increased frequency of dissection in the seasons when respiratory infection were most common. In this study, recent infection, rather than mechanical factors such as coughing and sneezing, was independently associated with dissection using multivariate analysis. These infection-related mechanisms may have a role in arterial dissection, as well as other causes of cerebrovascular ischaemia [84] but the nature of these mechanisms is not clearly understood.

CONCLUSION

Very little is known about the mechanisms of VBI following cervical manipulation. Traditional models of injury and risk management have relied heavily on mechanical factors. Despite attempts to provide clinical screening protocols, the evidence suggests that useful risk management strategies have not been satisfactorily developed. The role of pre-existing pathology, heritable connective tissue disorders and low-grade infection requires further study. By looking beyond the traditional models of injury and incorporating new knowledge, a less orthodox, but perhaps more effective, model of risk management may emerge. This work is still in its infancy and, unfortunately, the challenge of how best to ensure the safety of patients who undergo cervical spine manipulation, remains.

REFERENCES

1. Assendelft WJJ, Bouter LM, Knipschild PG. Complications of spinal manipulation. A comprehensive review of the literature. *J Fam Pract* 1996;**42**:475–480.
2. Dvorak J, Orelli FV. How dangerous is manipulation to the cervical spine? Case report and results of a survey. *Man Med* 1985;**2**:1–4.
3. Hurwitz EL, Aker PD, Adams AH, Meeker WC, *et al*. Manipulation and mobilization of the cervical spine. A systematic review of the literature. *Spine* 1996;**21**:1746–1760.
4. Nadereishvilli Z, Norris JW. Stroke from traumatic arterial dissection. *Lancet* 1999;**354**:159–160.
5. Terrett AGJ. Vascular accidents from cervical spine manipulation: Report on 107 cases. *J Aust Chiropractors Assoc* 1987;**17**:15–24.
6. Di Fabio RP. Manipulation of the cervical spine: risks and benefits. *Phys Ther* 1999;**79**:50–65.
7. Vick DA, McKay C, Zengerle CR. The safety of manipulative treatment: Review of the literature from 1925 to 1993. *J Am Osteopath Assoc* 1996;**96**:113–115.
8. Haldeman S, Kohlbeck FJ, McGregor M. Risk factors and precipitating neck movements causing vertebrobasilar artery dissection after cervical trauma and spinal manipulation. *Spine* 1999;**24**:785–794.
9. Terrett AGJ. Misuse of literature by medical authors in discussing spinal manipulative therapy injury. *J Manipulative Physiol Ther* 1995;**18**:203–210.
10. Leboeuf-Yde C, Rasmussen LR, Klougart N. The risk of over-reporting spinal manipulative therapy-induced injuries: A description of some cases that failed to burden the statistics. *J Manipulative Physiol Ther* 1996;**19**:536–538.
11. Terrett AG. Vascular accidents from cervical spine manipulation: The mechanisms. *J Aust Chiropractor's Assoc* 1987;**17**:131–144.
12. Soustiel JF, Bruk B, Shik B, Feinsod M. Transcranial Doppler in vertebrobasilar vasospasm after subarachnoid hemorrhage. *Neurosurgery* 1998;**43**(2):282–291.
13. Marshall LF, Bruce DA, Bruno L, Langfitt TW. Vertebrobasilar spasm: a significant cause of neurological deficit in head injury. *J Neurosurg* 1978;**48**(4):560–564.
14. Smith RA, Estridge MN. Neurologic complications of head and neck manipulations. Report of two cases. *JAMA* 1962;**182**:130–133.
15. Arning C, Schrattenholzer A, Lachenmayer L. Cervical carotid artery vasospasms causing cerebral ischemia. Detection by immediate vascular ultrasonographic investigation. *Stroke* 1998;**29**:1063–1066.
16. Anson J, Crowell RM. Cervicocranial arterial dissection. *Neurosurgery* 1991;**29**(1):89–96.
17. Hoshino Y, Kurokawa T, Nakamura K, Seichi A, *et al*. A report on the safety of unilateral vertebral artery ligation during cervical spine surgery. *Spine* 1996;**21**(12):1454–1457.
18. Macchi C, Catini C. The anatomy and clinical importance of the collateral circles between the vertebral arteries and the cervical, costo-cervical, and occipital branches in 52 living subjects. *Ital J Anat Embryol* 1993;**98**:153–163.
19. Barinagarrementeria F, Amaya LE, Cantu C. Causes and mechanisms of cerebellar infarction in young patients [see comments]. *Stroke* 1997;**28**:2400–2404.
20. Silbert PL, Mokri B, Schievink WI. Headache and neck pain in spontaneous internal carotid and vertebral artery dissections. *Neurology* 1995;**45**:1517–1522.
21. Johnson CP, Lawler W, Burns J. Use of histomorphometry in the assessment of fatal vertebral artery dissection. *J Clin Pathol* 1993;**46**:1000–1003.
22. Mas JL, Henin D, Bousser MG, Chain F, *et al*. Dissecting aneurysm of the vertebral artery and cervical manipulation: A case report with autopsy. *Neurology* 1989;**39**:512–515.
23. Sturznegger M. Headache and neck pain: The warning symptoms of vertebral artery dissection. *Headache* 1994;**34**:187–193.
24. Peters M, Bohl J, Thomke F, *et al*. Dissection of the internal carotid artery after chiropractic manipulation of the neck. *Neurology* 1995;**45**:2284–2286.
25. Schievink WI, Mokri B, Piepgras DG, Parisi J, *et al*. Cervical artery dissections associated with chiropractic manipulation of the neck: the importance of pre-existing arterial disease and injury. *J Neurol* 1996;**243**:96.
26. Schievink WI, Michels VV, Piepgras DG. Neurovascular manifestations of heritable connective tissue disorders. A review. *Stroke* 1994;**25**:889–903.
27. Schievink WI, Wijdicks EF, Michels VV, Vockley J, *et al*. Heritable connective tissue disorders in cervical artery dissections: a prospective study. *Neurology* 1998;**50**:1166–1169.
28. Schievink WI, Mokri B, Michels VV, Piepgras DG. Familial association of intracranial aneurysms and cervical artery dissections. *Stroke* 1991;**22**:1426–1430.
29. Mokri B, Piepgras DG, Wiebers DO, Houser OW. Familial occurrence of spontaneous dissection of the internal carotid artery. *Stroke* 1987;**18**:246–251.

30. Majamaa K, Portimojarvi H, Sotaniemi KA, Myllyla VV. Familial aggregation of cervical artery dissection and cerebral aneurysm. *Stroke* 1994;**25**:1704–1705.

31. van den Berg JS, Limburg M, Kappelle LJ, Pals G, *et al*. The role of type III collagen in spontaneous cervical arterial dissections. *Ann Neurol* 1998;**43**:494–498.

32. Kuivaniemi H, Prockop DJ, Wu Y. Exclusion of mutations in the gene for type III collagen (COL3A1) as a common cause of intracranial aneurysms or cervical artery dissections: Results from sequence analysis of the coding sequence of type III collagen from 55 unrelated patients. *Neurology* 1993;**43**:2652–2658.

33. Brandt T, Hausser I, Orberk E, *et al*. Ultrastructural connective tissue abnormalities in patients with spontaneous cervicocerebral artery dissections. *Ann Neurol* 1998;**44**:281–285.

34. Argenson C, Francke JP, Dintimille H, Papasian S, *et al*. The vertebral arteries (Segments V1 and V2). *Anat Clin* 1980;**2**:29–41.

35. Chopard RP, de Miranda Neto MH, Lucas GA, Chopard MR. The vertebral artery: its relationship with adjoining tissues in its course intra and inter transverse processes in man. *Rev Paul Med* 1992;**110**:245–250.

36. Francke JP, Di Marino V, Pannier M, Argenson C, *et al*. The vertebral arteries (arteria vertebralis). The V3 atlanto-axoidal and V4 Intracranial segments – Collaterals. *Anat Clin* 1981;**2**:229–242.

37. Sherman DG, Hart RG, Easton JD. Abrupt change in head position and cerebral infarction. *Stroke* 1981;**12**:2–5.

38. Toole J, Tucker S. Influence of head position upon cerebral circulation. *Arch Neurol* 1960;**2**:616–623.

39. Brown BSJ, Tatlow WFT. Radiographic studies of the vertebral arteries in cadavers. *JAMA* 1963;**81**:80–88.

40. Selecki B. The effects of rotation of the atlas on the axis: Experimental work. *Med J Aust* 1969;**56**:1012–1015.

41. Petersen B, von Maravic M, Zeller JA, Walker ML, *et al*. Basilar artery blood flow during head rotation in vertebrobasilar ischemia. *Acta Neurol Scand* 1996;**94**:294–301.

42. Matsuyama T, Morimoto T, Sakaki T. Comparison of C1–2 posterior fusion and decompression of the vertebral artery in the treatment of bow hunter's stroke. *J Neurosurg* 1997;**86**:619–623.

43. Morimoto T, Kaido T, Uchiyama Y, Tokunaga H, *et al*. Rotational obstruction of nondominant vertebral artery and ischemia. Case report. *J Neurosurg* 1996;**85**:507–509.

44. Takahashi I, Kaneko S, Asaoka K, Harada T. Rotational occlusion of the vertebral artery at the atlantoaxial joint: is it truly physiological? *Neuroradiology* 1994;**36**:273–275.

45. Kuether TA, Nesbit GM, Clark WM, Barnwell SL. Rotational vertebral artery occlusion: a mechanism of vertebrobasilar insufficiency. *Neurosurgery* 1997;**41**:427–432.

46. Coria F, Rebollo M, Quintana F, Polo JM, *et al*. Occipitoatlantal instability and vertebrobasilar ischemia: case report. *Neurology* 1982;**32**:303–305.

47. Smith DR, Vanderark GD, Kempe LG. Cervical spondylosis causing vertebrobasilar insufficiency: a surgical treatment. *J Neurol Neurosurg Psychiatry* 1971;**34**:388–392.

48. Inui H, Yoneyama K, Kitaoku Y, *et al*. Four cases of vertebrobasilar insufficiency. *Acta Oto-Laryngol* 1998;**533**:S46–S50.

49. Andersson R, Carleson R, Nylen O. Vertebral artery insufficiency and rotational obstruction. *Acta Med Scand* 1970;**188**:475–477.

50. Dadsetan MR, Skerhut HE. Rotational vertebrobasilar insufficiency secondary to vertebral artery occlusion from fibrous band of the longus coli muscle. *Neuroradiology* 1990;**32**:514–515.

51. Theil H, Wallace K, Donat J, Yong-Hing K. Effect of various head and neck positions on vertebral artery blood flow. *Clinical Biomechanics* 1994;**9**:105–110.

52. Weingart JR, Bischoff HP. Doppler sonography of the vertebral artery with regard to head positions appropriate to manual medicine. *Manuelle Medizin* 1992;**30**:62–65.

53. Licht PB, Christensen HW, Hoilund-Carlsen PF. Vertebral artery volume flow in human beings. *J Manipulative Physiol Ther* 1999;**22**:363–367.

54. Licht PB, Christensen HW, Hojgaard P, Hoilund-Carlsen PF. Triplex ultrasound of vertebral artery flow during cervical rotation. *J Manipulative Physiol Ther* 1998;**21**:27–31.

55. Arnetoli G, Amadori A, Stefani P, Nuzzaci G. Sonography of vertebral arteries in De Kleyn's position in subjects and in patients with vertebrobasilar transient ischemic attacks. *Angiology* 1989;**40**:716–720.

56. Haynes MJ. Cervical rotational effects on vertebral artery flow: A case study. *Chiropractic Journal of Australia* 1995;**25**:73–76.

57. Haynes MJ. Doppler studies comparing the effects of cervical rotation and lateral flexion on vertebral artery blood flow. *J Manipulative Physiol Ther* 1996;**19**:378–384.

58. Stevens A. Functional doppler ultrasonography of the vertebral artery and some considerations about manual techniques. *J Man Med* 1991;**6**:102–105.

59. Stevens A. Doppler sonography and neck rotation. *Man Med* 1984;**1**:49–53.

60. Refshauge KM. Rotation: A valid premanipulative dizziness test? Does it predict safe manipulation? *J Manipulative Physiol Ther* 1994;**17**:15–19.

61. Rivett DA, Sharples KJ, Milburn PD. Effect of premanipulative tests on vertebral artery and internal carotid artery blood flow: A pilot study. *J Manipulative Physiol Ther* 1999;**22**:368–375.

62. Sturzenegger M, Newell DW, Douville C, Byrd S, *et al*. Dynamic transcranial Doppler assessment of positional vertebrobasilar ischemia. *Stroke* 1994;**25**:1776–1783.

63. Dumas JL, Salama J, Dreyfus P, Thoreux P, *et al*. Magnetic resonance angiographic analysis of atlanto-axial rotation: anatomic bases of compression of the vertebral arteries. *Surg Radiol Anat* 1996;**18**:303–313.

64. Houle JOE. Assessing hemodynamics of the vertebro-basilar complex through angiothlipsis. *JCCA* 1972;June-July:35–41.

65. George PE, Silverstein HT, Wallace H, Marshall M. Identification of the high risk pre-stroke patient. *ACA J Chiropractic* 1981; **15**:S26–S28.

66. Aspinall W. Clinical testing for cervical mechanical disorders which produce ischemic vertigo. *J Orthop Sports Phys Ther* 1989;**11**:176–182.

67. Rivett DA. Preventing neurovascular complications of cervical spine manipulation. *Phys Ther Rev* 1997;**2**:29–37.

68. Protocol for pre-manipulative testing of the cervical spine. *Aust J Psiother* 1988;**34**:97–100.

69. Rivett DA. The premanipulative vertebral artery testing protocol. A brief review. *NZ J Physiother* 1995;April:9–12.

70. Terrett AG. It is more important to know when not to adjust. *Chiropractic Technique* 1990; **2**:1–9.

71. Weintraub MI, Khoury A. Critical neck position as an independent risk factor for posterior circulation stroke. A magnetic resonance angiographic analysis. *J Neuroimaging* 1995;**5**:16–22.

72. Delcker A, Diener HC, Timmann D, Faustman P. The role of vertebral and internal carotid artery disease in the pathogenesis of vertebrobasilar transient ischemic attacks. *Eur Arch Psychiatry Clin Neurosci* 1993;**242**:179–183.

73. Muuronen A, Kaste M. Outcome of 314 patients with transient ischemic attacks. *Stroke* 1982;**13**:24–31.

74. Cote P, Kreitz B, Cassidy JD, Theil H. The validity of the extension-rotation test as a clinical screening procedure before neck manipulation: A secondary analysis. *J Manipulative Physiol Ther* 1996;**19**:159–164.

75. Bolton PS, Stick PE, Lord RSA. Failure of clinical tests to predict cerebral ischemia before neck manipulation. *J Manipulative Physiol Ther* 1989;**12**:304–307.

76. Lindy DR. Patient collapse following cervical manipulation: a case report. *Br Osteopath J* 1984;**16**:84–85.

77. Rivett HM. Cervical manipulation: Confronting the spectre of the vertebral artery syndrome. *Journal of Orthopaedic Medicine* 1994;**16**:12–16.

78. Schievink WI, Mokri B, Piepgras DG, Kuiper JD. Recurrent spontaneous arterial dissections: risk in familial versus nonfamilial disease. *Stroke* 1996;**27**:622–624.

79. Jentzen JM, Amatuzio J, Peterson GF. Complications of cervical manipulation: A case report of fatal brainstem infarct with review of the mechanisms and predisposing factors. *J Forensic Sci* 1987;**34**:1089–1094.

80. Grayson MF. Horner's syndrome after manipulation of the neck. *BMJ* 1987;**295**:1381–1382.

81. Schievink WI, Wijdicks EF, Kuiper JD. Seasonal pattern of spontaneous cervical artery dissection. *J Neurosurg* 1998;**89**:101–103.

82. Grau AJ, Brandt T, Forsting M, Winter R, *et al*. Infection-associated cervical artery dissection. Three cases. *Stroke* 1997;**28**:453–455.

83. Grau AJ, Brandt T, Buggle F, *et al*. Association of cervical artery dissection with recent infection. *Arch Neurol* 1999;**56**:851–856.

84. Grau AJ, Buggle F, Becher H, *et al*. Recent bacterial and viral infection is a risk factor for cerebrovascular ischemia. Clinical and biochemical studies. *Neurology* 1998;**50**:196–203.

INDEX

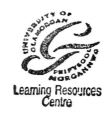